Analgesia, Anaesthesia and Pregnancy

A Practical Guide

Fourth Edition

Analgesia, Anaesthesia and Pregnancy

A Practical Guide

Fourth Edition

Róisín Monteiro
Consultant Anaesthetist at Brighton and Sussex University Hospitals NHS Trust, UK

Marwa Salman
Consultant Anaesthetist at Guy's and St Thomas' NHS Foundation Trust, UK

Surbhi Malhotra
Consultant Anaesthetist at Fiona Stanley Hospital, Perth, Australia

Steve Yentis
Consultant Anaesthetist at Chelsea and Westminster Hospital and Honorary Reader at Imperial College London, UK

CAMBRIDGE
UNIVERSITY PRESS

University Printing House, Cambridge CB2 8BS, United Kingdom

One Liberty Plaza, 20th Floor, New York, NY 10006, USA

477 Williamstown Road, Port Melbourne, VIC 3207, Australia

314–321, 3rd Floor, Plot 3, Splendor Forum, Jasola District Centre, New Delhi – 110025, India

79 Anson Road, #06–04/06, Singapore 079906

Cambridge University Press is part of the University of Cambridge.

It furthers the University's mission by disseminating knowledge in the pursuit of
education, learning, and research at the highest international levels of excellence.

www.cambridge.org
Information on this title: www.cambridge.org/9781108710527
DOI: 10.1017/9781108684729

First edition © W. B. Saunders 2000

Second edition © Cambridge University Press 2007

Third edition © Steve Yentis and Surbhi Malhotra 2013

Fourth edition © Róisín Monteiro, Marwa Salman, Surbhi Malhotra and Steve Yentis 2019

First edition published 2000
Second edition published 2007
Reprinted 2008
Third edition published 2013
Reprinted 2014
Fourth edition published 2019

A catalogue record for this publication is available from the British Library.

Library of Congress Cataloging-in-Publication Data
Names: Yentis, S. M. (Steven M.), author. | Monteiro, Róisín, author. | Salman, Marwa, author. | Malhotra, Surbhi, Dr., author.
Title: Analgesia, anaesthesia and pregnancy : a practical guide / Róisín Monteiro, Marwa Salman, Surbhi Malhotra, Steve Yentis.
Description: Fourth edition. | Cambridge, United Kingdom : Cambridge University Press, 2019. | Steve Yentis' name appears first in
the previous edition. | Includes bibliographical references and index.
Identifiers: LCCN 2018049486 | ISBN 9781108710527 (pbk.)
Subjects: | MESH: Anesthesia, Obstetrical | Analgesia, Obstetrical | Handbooks
Classification: LCC RG732 | NLM WO 39 | DDC 617.9/682–dc23
LC record available at https://lccn.loc.gov/2018049486

ISBN 978-1-108-71052-7 Paperback

....

Contents

III – Operative delivery and the third stage

IV – Anaesthetic problems

V – Problems confined to obstetrics

VI – Problems not confined to obstetrics

Section 3 – Puerperium and after
I – The neonate

Preface

The first edition of this book was written in order to provide useful, practical information and advice to obstetric anaesthetists, in the form of a ready and easily accessible guide to obstetric anaesthesia and analgesia. The book was aimed primarily at trainees, both those starting in the maternity suite and their more experienced colleagues preparing for anaesthetic examinations. We also hoped the book would be of use to more senior anaesthetists and those of all levels involved in teaching obstetric anaesthesia, as well as non-anaesthetists working in the maternity suite. We are pleased that the book has been popular enough to warrant a fourth edition, and welcome two new authors to join the team.

In this fourth edition, we have reviewed and revised each section but kept to the original aims, structure and format, since we are convinced that the need for a short, practically based text still exists. In doing so, we have attempted to bridge the gaps between routine obstetric anaesthesia and analgesia and the care of women with coexisting medical conditions, and between anaesthetic care and advice before pregnancy and that during pregnancy itself.

As before, we have assumed basic anaesthetic knowledge and thus do not include topics such as anaesthetic equipment and drugs, etc., except where there are areas of specific obstetric relevance. We have tried to base the advice given on what we believe would be considered standard UK practice, supported by evidence wherever possible, although we have deliberately not included supporting references for each point made since this would, in our view, detract from the readability and ease of use of this book; readers wishing to obtain such reference lists are directed to the many larger, more comprehensive texts that are currently available.

We hope that the layout of the book is easy to follow. We have tried to provide a brief list of pertinent further reading where possible – though often this has meant that very large topics have been left relatively unreferenced, since there are few journal reviews broad enough in scope.

Finally, we gratefully acknowledge the contributions of Dr D. Bogod, Dr D. Brighouse and Dr C. Elton to the first edition, and Dr A. May to the first and second editions. For this fourth edition, we are also grateful to Dr Aisha Alzouebi for her contributions to the chapters on obstetric topics.

Assisted conception

Infertility affects about one in seven couples, with a small increase in infertility and the number of couples seeking help over the past 10 years. The treatment of infertility has developed rapidly, and the anaesthetist may be involved in many aspects of the patient's treatment, which may be complex. The harvesting of oocytes needs to take place within a defined period of time, or ovulation may have occurred and oocytes will be lost. Couples presenting for infertility treatment are generally anxious, and women are often emotional at the time of oocyte retrieval. It is therefore particularly important for the anaesthetist to understand the couple's anxieties, and to be able to explain the effects of the anaesthetic technique that is to be used.

Problems and special considerations

All of the methods of assisted fertility techniques involve extraction of oocytes from the follicles, either laparoscopically or, with the development of transvaginal ultra-sonography, via the transvaginal route (ultrasound-directed oocyte retrieval, UDOR). The techniques differ in the site of fertilisation and/or replacement of the gamete/zygote:

- **In-vitro fertilisation (IVF).** This term is often (incorrectly) used to encompass all aspects of infertility treatment. IVF involves either UDOR or laparoscopic oocyte retrieval, fertilisation in the laboratory and transfer of the developing embryo into the uterus via the cervix, 48 hours later. UDOR may be painful so may require analgesia, sedation or anaesthesia. Embryo transfer is performed with the patient awake, although there are occasions when the anaesthetist may be requested to provide sedation. The success rate is approximately 15–25%.
- **Gamete intrafallopian transfer (GIFT).** This involves retrieval of oocytes which are placed together with sperm into the fallopian tube It is performed laparoscopically in the majority of cases and has not been shown to have a higher success rate than IVF, so is used less commonly.
- **Zygote intrafallopian tube transfer (ZIFT) or pronuclear stage transfer.** This process involves oocyte retrieval and IVF, with the zygote then being placed in the fallopian tube as for GIFT. It has no significant difference in pregnancy rates to IVF, but has a trend towards increased ectopic pregnancy rates.
- **Intracytoplasmic sperm injection (ICSI).** Fertilisation occurs in the laboratory via injection of sperm into the oocytes, and the developing embryo is transferred into the uterus as for IVF. This technique is used for male infertility. The success rate is approximately 30%.

Management options

Most women who present for assisted conception techniques are healthy and in their thirties or forties. However, it is now recognised that some women may also have a number of comorbidities associated with increasing age. Therefore, a multidisciplinary approach is necessary. It would be logical to minimise drug use and use sedation or regional anaesthesia whenever possible, although this is not suited for laparoscopy (see Chapter 3, *Anaesthesia before confirmation of pregnancy*).

For UDOR, which has become the most common method used for oocyte retrieval, the main anaesthetic techniques are intravenous sedation and regional anaesthesia. It is important to remember that patients requiring UDOR are day cases, and the basic principles of day-case anaesthesia apply. There has been a considerable amount of work to date on the use of propofol with alfentanil, and this combination of drugs would appear to be the technique of choice for intravenous sedation. Propofol may be administered by intermittent boluses or by continuous infusion, with the patient breathing oxygen via a Hudson mask. Many anaesthetists find that they are using levels of sedation close to anaesthesia. There does not seem to be a difference in patient satisfaction or pregnancy rate if sedation or general anaesthesia is used. It is essential that the sedation is administered in a suitable environment with resuscitation facilities and anaesthetic monitoring. Often the assisted conception unit is some distance from the main theatre suite; therefore it may be difficult for the staff working in an isolated environment to maintain their skills in resuscitation.

The desire to minimise the drugs administered to women undergoing ultrasound-guided techniques has led to the use of regional anaesthesia, although there is limited evidence supporting its association with increased pregnancy rates. Careful administration is required to allow same-day discharge; the low-dose spinal that is used for labour analgesia or the short-acting agents used for cervical cerclage can give good operating conditions while satisfying the criteria needed for day-case anaesthesia.

The main considerations for laparoscopy are the type of anaesthesia, the pneumoperitoneum and the effects of the anaesthetic agents on fertilisation and cell cleavage. The length of exposure to the drugs is also important. The effects of nitrous oxide and volatile anaesthetic agents on fertilisation and cleavage rates have been extensively examined. It is generally recognised that all volatile agents and nitrous oxide have a deleterious effect, although opinion is divided as to the extent of the problem. It is also recognised that the carbon dioxide used for the pneumoperitoneum causes a similar effect, and it is difficult to separate the effects of the anaesthetic agents from those of the carbon dioxide.

Of the intravenous agents, the effect of propofol on fertilisation and cleavage appears to be minimal. Propofol accumulates in the follicular fluid, and the amount in the follicular fluid may become significant if there are a large number of oocytes to retrieve. Propofol decreases the fertilisation rates, but there is no significant effect on the cell division rates. This has led to the increased use of propofol as the main agent in total intravenous anaesthesia.

Analgesia following the procedure may be provided with a combination of codeine and paracetamol. Non-steroidal anti-inflammatory drugs such as diclofenac are considered less suitable, as these are thought to interfere with embryo implantation, owing to a disruption in prostaglandin levels. All assisted conception techniques carry the risk of ovarian hyperstimulation (see Chapter 2, *Ovarian hyperstimulation syndrome*), and multiple or ectopic pregnancy.

Key points

- Oocyte retrieval may involve laparoscopy requiring general anaesthesia, although intravenous sedation and regional anaesthesia are suitable for transvaginal ultrasound-directed techniques.
- Couples are usually very anxious and require constant reassurance.

Further reading

Kwan I, Bhattacharya S, Knox F, McNeil A. Pain relief for women undergoing oocyte retrieval for assisted reproduction. *Cochrane Database Syst Rev* 2013; (1): CD004829.

Tsen L. Anesthesia for assisted reproductive technologies. *Int Anesthesiol Clin* 2007; 7: 99–113.

Vlahos NF, Giannakikou I, Vlachos A, Vitoratos N. Analgesia and anesthesia for assisted reproductive technologies. *Int J Gynaecol Obstet* 2009; 105: 201–5.

Ovarian hyperstimulation syndrome

Ovarian hyperstimulation syndrome (OHSS) is a complication of ovarian induction that may be caused by any agent that stimulates the ovaries. Over the last 10 years, the incidence has risen due to the increased use and development of in-vitro fertilisation (IVF) treatments, where the ultimate goal is to produce enough oocytes and embryos. It is thought to be the most common complication of IVF treatment, though the true incidence is unknown, because mild to moderate cases are probably under-reported.

OHSS occurs 3–8 days after treatment with human chorionic gonadotrophin (hCG), and the effects continue throughout the luteal phase. A variety of cytokines and pro-inflammatory mediators such as vascular endothelial growth factor are secreted from the hyperstimulated ovaries, leading to increased vascular permeability and a prothrombotic effect. The condition may become severe enough to warrant intensive care admission.

Problems and special considerations

Clinical manifestations of the syndrome are:

- Enlargement of the ovaries
- Pleural effusion
- Ascites

Additional complications that may occur include:

- Hypovolaemic shock
- Renal failure
- Acute lung injury
- Thromboembolism
- Cerebrovascular disorders

Women undergoing ovarian stimulation who develop OHSS may be classified by the severity of their presenting symptoms and signs (Table 2.1).

Management options

Prophylactic plasma expanders such as human albumin solution may reduce the risk of severe OHSS in women at high risk; these include women with a large number of oocytes retrieved, high oestradiol levels or polycystic ovary syndrome.

Once suspected, the diagnosis of OHSS is made on clinical grounds as there are no specific diagnostic tests. However, the combination of elevated haematocrit with reduced

Table 2.1 Grading of ovarian hyperstimulation syndrome

Grade	Features
Mild	Abdominal distension and discomfort
Moderate	Abdominal pain, nausea, vomiting and diarrhoea Ultrasound evidence of ascites
Severe	Clinical ascites ± hydrothorax, oliguria, haematocrit > 0.45, hypo-osmolality, hyponatraemia, hyperkalaemia, hypoproteinaemia
Critical	Tense ascites/large hydrothorax, haematocrit > 0.55, white cell count > 25×10^9/l, oliguria/anuria, thromboembolism, acute respiratory distress syndrome

Adapted with permission from Royal College of Obstetricians and Gynaecologists. *The Management of Ovarian Hyperstimulation Syndrome.* Green-top Guideline 5. London: RCOG, 2016.

serum osmolality and sodium levels is highly suggestive. Pelvic ultrasound may demonstrate multiple ovarian follicles, enlarged ovaries or free fluid.

Mild to moderate forms of OHSS will be self-limiting and can be managed in the outpatient setting with analgesia, antiemetics and oral hydration, but those women with more severe pathology are likely to require hospitalisation for monitoring and intravenous fluids to correct the hypovolaemia and haemoconcentration.

Ultrasound-guided paracentesis should be considered for women with severe pain, abdominal distension, respiratory compromise or oliguria thought to be secondary to ascites. In women with impaired renal function, dopamine has been given to improve renal perfusion. Ultrafiltration and intravenous reinfusion of ascitic fluid has been used in severe cases. Thromboprophylaxis must be considered.

Monitoring is tailored to the severity of the syndrome, and the following progression is recommended:

- Urea and electrolytes
- Full blood count and packed cell volume
- Plasma/urine osmolality
- Clotting screen
- Chest radiography
- Invasive haemodynamic monitoring may be beneficial for those with a reduced urine output or persistently raised haematocrit despite large volumes of fluid replacement.

Clinicians should be aware that pregnancies complicated by OHSS have an increased risk of pre-eclampsia and preterm delivery.

Key points

- Hyperstimulation comprises ovarian enlargement, pleural effusion and ascites, which may be relentless.
- Severe protein loss may result in shock and renal failure.
- The most severe form occurs in 1–2% of cases treated with human chorionic gonadotrophin.

Further reading

Budev M, Arroliga A, Falcone T. Ovarian hyperstimulation syndrome. *Crit Care Med* 2005; **33**: S301–6.

Royal College of Obstetricians and Gynaecologists. *The Management of Ovarian Hyperstimulation Syndrome*. Green-top Guideline 5. London: RCOG, 2016. www.rcog.org.uk/en/guidelines-researc h-services/guidelines/gtg5 (accessed December 2018).

Sansone P, Aurilio C, Pace MC, *et al.* Intensive care treatment of ovarian hyperstimulation syndrome (OHSS). *Ann N Y Acad Sci* 2011; **1221**: 109–18.

Anaesthesia before confirmation of pregnancy

Many women will require anaesthesia when they are pregnant, and some will be unaware that they are pregnant before attendance for surgery, especially in the first 2–3 months of their pregnancy. Studies have found incidences of up to 2.4% of unrecognised early pregnancy in preoperative testing.

Concerns with anaesthesia and surgery in early pregnancy are related to fetal loss and teratogenicity. A systematic review suggested that miscarriage rates may be slightly increased when surgery occurs in the first trimester; however, whether this is related to anaesthesia, surgery or the underlying pathological process necessitating surgery is difficult to say. A teratogen is a substance that causes structural or functional abnormality in a fetus exposed to that substance. The thalidomide catastrophe initiated the licensing arrangements for new drugs and their use in pregnancy; the current cautious stance of the pharmaceutical industry is reflected in the British National Formulary's statement that no drug is safe beyond all doubt in early pregnancy.

Current evidence suggests that there is no increase in congenital abnormalities in women undergoing surgery and anaesthesia. However, concern has been raised over pre-natal anaesthetic exposure and subtle functional neurocognitive changes. The anaesthetist should have a clear knowledge of the time scale of the developing fetus in order to balance the risks and benefits of any drug given to the mother.

Problems and special considerations

The possible effect of a drug can be considered against the stage of the developing fetus:

- **Pre-embryonic phase (0–14 days post-conception).** The fertilised egg is transported down the fallopian tube and implantation occurs at around 7 days post-conception. The conceptus is a ball of undifferentiated dividing cells during this time and the effect of drugs on it appears to be an all-or-none phenomenon. Cell division may be slowed with no lasting effects or the conceptus will die, depending on the severity of the cell damage.
- **Embryonic phase (3–8 weeks post-conception).** Differentiation of cells into the organs and tissues occurs during this phase, and drugs administered to the mother may cause considerable harm. The type of abnormality that is produced depends on the exact stage of organ and tissue development when the drug is given.
- **Fetal phase (9 weeks to birth).** At this stage, most organs are fully formed, although the cerebral cortex, cerebellum and urogenital tract are still developing. Drugs administered during this time may affect the growth of the fetus or the functional development within specific organs, but structural changes are unlikely.

Management options

The anaesthetist should always consider the possibility of pregnancy in any woman of childbearing age who presents for surgery, whether elective or emergency, and should specifically enquire in such cases. If there is doubt, a pregnancy test should be offered; accepted practice is to delay elective surgery in pregnancy. If pregnancy is confirmed and surgery necessary, it would seem pragmatic to use systemic drugs after weighing up their necessity, benefits and risks while focusing on maintaining normal physiological parameters.

The use of nitrous oxide is now generally considered acceptable, despite its effects on methionine synthase and DNA metabolism, as there is little evidence that it is harmful clinically; however, it may be sensible to avoid as anaesthesia can be delivered safely without its use. Similarly, although the volatile agents have been implicated in impairing embryonic development, clinical evidence is lacking. Some drugs cross the placenta and exert their effect on the fetus – for example warfarin, which may cause bleeding in the fetus.

Key points

- The possibility of pregnancy should be considered in any woman of childbearing age.
- No drug is safe beyond all doubt in pregnancy.

Further reading

Allaert SE, Carlier SP, Weyne LP, *et al.* First trimester anesthesia exposure and fetal outcome: a review. *Acta Anaesthesiol Belg* 2007; **58**: 119–23.

Cohen-Kerem R, Railton C, Oren D, Lishner M, Koren G. Pregnancy outcome following non-obstetric surgical intervention. *Am J Surg* 2005; **190**: 467–73.

Perna RB, Loughan AR, Le JA, Hertza J. Prenatal and perinatal anesthesia and the long-term cognitive sequelae: a review. *Appl Neuropsychol Child* 2015; **4**: 65–71.

Ectopic pregnancy

Ectopic pregnancies occur in approximately 11 per 1000 pregnancies, with nearly 12,000 women diagnosed with an ectopic in the UK each year. There are many risk factors, of which tubal pathology or surgery and the use of an intrauterine device are the most important. Other risk factors are infertility, younger or older maternal age and smoking. The incidence is thought to be increasing as a result of pelvic inflammatory disease.

Ectopic pregnancy accounted for almost 5% of deaths prior to 24 weeks' gestation in the Confidential Enquiries into Maternal Deaths and Morbidity report in 2016 (MBRRACE-UK). Most ectopic pregnancies occur in the fallopian tube, but up to 5% occur elsewhere within the genital tract or abdomen. Typically, the tube initially expands to accommodate the growing zygote, but when it is unable to do so any more, there may be bleeding from the site of implantation or even rupture of the tube.

Problems and special considerations

Diagnosis of ectopic pregnancy may be difficult. Most ectopic pregnancies present 6–8 weeks from the last menstrual period and thus many of the physiological changes of pregnancy are absent or mild – the patient may even be unaware that she is pregnant. Signs and symptoms of an ectopic pregnancy vary. The most commonly reported symptoms are abdominal pain, amenorrhoea and vaginal bleeding. Other symptoms include gastro-intestinal upset and rectal pressure or shoulder-tip pain from intraperitoneal blood. Sudden decompensation may occur due to concealed haemorrhage, leading to haemodynamic collapse.

A common theme in deaths associated with ectopic pregnancy is the failure to consider the diagnosis before collapse; ectopic pregnancy was not considered as a diagnosis in five out of the nine women who died from ectopic pregnancy in the 2016 Confidential Enquiry report. Non-specific abdominal signs including diarrhoea or vomiting may be misinterpreted as other intra-abdominal conditions such as appendicitis or gastroenteritis. Haemodynamic collapse may be misinterpreted as signs of pulmonary embolism, and MBRRACE-UK reported that a third of women who died of ectopic pregnancy received thrombolysis. Ectopic pregnancy must be considered in all women of childbearing age who present with haemodynamic collapse, particularly if anaemic, and it is now recommended that a focused assessment with sonography in trauma (FAST) ultrasound scan should be performed before thrombolysis if pulmonary embolism is considered likely.

A urinary pregnancy test should be performed in all women of reproductive age in whom the diagnosis is unclear or any of the above symptoms or signs are present; the bladder should be catheterised if necessary to facilitate this. Abdominal ultrasound has low specificity, and transvaginal ultrasound is the imaging modality of choice. If ultrasound is not convincing, then diagnosis may be aided by blood tests and laparoscopy. In a less acute situation, serum levels of human chorionic gonadotrophin (hCG) and progesterone are often measured, but these measurements often resemble those levels seen in a normal pregnancy. Previously, the gold standard for diagnosis of an ectopic pregnancy was a laparoscopy; however, its diagnostic accuracy has been questioned when the procedure is performed too early.

The implications for the current and future pregnancies pose a great psychological stress on the patient and her partner. There may be a previous history of ectopic pregnancy, since its occurrence is itself a risk factor for subsequent ectopics.

Management options

Initial management is directed at treating and preventing massive haemorrhage; thus the patient requires at least one large-bore intravenous cannula and careful observation, at least until the diagnosis has been excluded. Similarly, once the decision to operate has been made, surgery needs to occur as soon as possible, since the risk of tubal rupture is always present.

Operative management usually involves laparoscopy unless there is severe haemodynamic instability, in which case laparotomy may be performed. Traditionally, laparoscopy was performed purely for diagnostic purposes, but laparoscopic removal of the zygote with or without tubal resection has become routine in many units.

Anaesthetic management is as for any emergency surgery, given the above considerations. Haematological assistance and admission to the intensive care unit should be available if required. Point-of-care haematological testing may be a useful adjunct. In severe cases, anaesthesia must proceed as for a ruptured aortic aneurysm: full preoperative resuscitation may be impossible, and the patient is prepared and draped before induction of anaesthesia, which may be followed by profound hypotension.

Medical management may be considered in selected cases; thus systemic methotrexate may be offered to suitable women in whom the diagnosis of ectopic pregnancy is absolutely clear and the absence of a viable intrauterine pregnancy has been confirmed. The drug antagonises folic acid and prevents further growth of the trophoblast, which is especially vulnerable at this early stage. Similar outcomes to those following surgical management have been claimed. Local injection of hyperosmolar glucose or potassium chloride, with aspiration of the sac, is an option for clinically stable women with a heterotopic pregnancy. Finally, expectant management has been used in selected patients, although women whose pregnancies are self-limiting cannot yet be identified reliably.

Key points

- Ectopic pregnancy must be considered as a diagnosis in all women of reproductive age presenting with non-specific abdominal symptoms or haemodynamic collapse.
- Severe haemorrhage and/or cardiovascular collapse is always a risk.

Further reading

Elson CJ, Salim R, Potdar N, *et al.*; Royal College of Obstetricians and Gynaecologists. Diagnosis and management of ectopic pregnancy. Green-top Guideline 21. *BJOG* 2016; **123**: e15–55.

Jurkovic D, Wilkinson H. Diagnosis and management of ectopic pregnancy. *BMJ* 2011; **342**: d3397.

Knight M, Nair M, Tuffnell D, *et al.*; MBRRACE-UK. *Saving Lives, Improving Mothers' Care: Surveillance of maternal deaths in the UK 2012–14 and lessons learned to inform maternity care from the UK and Ireland Confidential Enquiries into Maternal Deaths and Morbidity 2009–14.* Oxford: National Perinatal Epidemiology Unit, University of Oxford, 2016.

Evacuation of retained products of conception

Evacuation of retained products of conception (ERPC) may be required at any stage of pregnancy, but it occurs most commonly in early pregnancy following incomplete miscarriage or early fetal demise. It is also required during the puerperium following retention of placental tissue (see Chapter 40, *Removal of retained placenta and perineal suturing*).

Problems and special considerations

ERPC following spontaneous abortion at 8 weeks' gestation may be a minor routine gynaecological emergency for the anaesthetist, but the mother may have lost a much-wanted baby.

The urgency of the procedure varies greatly. The majority of ERPCs are performed as scheduled emergencies in fit young women, and this may lull the inexperienced anaesthetist into a false sense of security. Death may occur from spontaneous abortion; blood loss may be heavy and is frequently underestimated.

The possibility of coexisting uterine or systemic sepsis must always be considered, especially in postpartum ERPC or in a repeat procedure following incomplete evacuation.

Management options

Diagnostic ultrasound scanning is frequently used to confirm a non-viable early pregnancy or the presence of retained placental tissue. Transabdominal and transvaginal ultrasonography are now considered to be complementary to each other, with most women requiring a transvaginal ultrasound. Most units now operate a policy of fully assessing mothers on the day of admission in an early pregnancy advisory unit (EPAU), allowing them home and re-admitting them the following day for planned ERPC. This facilitates planning of medical and nursing staffing levels, reduces prolonged periods of waiting and starvation for the mother, and can be economically advantageous.

Expectant management may be offered as a first-line management strategy, unless there are particular risks of haemorrhage or infection. Medical treatment is increasingly used, and this enables women to be allowed home after treatment with prostaglandin analogues to await events. Analgesia and antiemetics should be offered as required. Non-surgical methods are associated with longer and heavier bleeding, and 15–50% of these women will need surgical management if the products of conception are not fully expelled. If required, surgical management of miscarriage may occur under local, regional or general anaesthetic.

Preoperatively, a full assessment is required. Assessment of blood loss may be difficult; fit young women may lose a significant proportion of their blood volume without becoming hypotensive. Tachycardia should alert the anaesthetist to possible hypovolaemia. Signs of sepsis should be sought, and prophylactic antibiotics may be considered.

General anaesthesia is most commonly used in the UK, although in the absence of uncorrected hypovolaemia or other contraindications, regional anaesthesia is entirely suitable. The puerperal mother in particular may wish to stay awake if offered a choice, and she should be advised to do so if she is at risk of regurgitation.

Rapid-sequence induction of general anaesthesia is indicated for the non-fasting mother requiring urgent surgery (uncommon) and for the mother who is at risk of regurgitation (see Chapter 59, *Aspiration of gastric contents*). Anaesthesia using a laryngeal mask airway or facemask using any standard day-case anaesthetic technique is appropriate for the majority of women needing ERPC. Sedative premedication is rarely needed. Intravenous anaesthesia, for example with propofol, or inhalational anaesthesia, are acceptable, though if the latter is used high concentrations of volatile anaesthetic agents (> 1 minimum alveolar concentration (MAC)) should be avoided because of the uterine relaxation that may ensue.

Oxytocic drugs may be requested by the surgeon, although there is little evidence for their efficacy at gestations of less than 15 weeks. A single intravenous bolus of 5 U oxytocin usually suffices. Ergometrine causes increased intracranial and systemic pressure, and nausea and vomiting, and should not be used routinely.

Spinal anaesthesia produces more rapid and dense anaesthesia than epidural anaesthesia, and an anaesthetic level of at least T8 is recommended. Clinical experience shows that the traditionally taught anaesthetic level of T10 is insufficient to prevent pain occurring when the uterine fundus is manipulated or curetted.

Postoperatively, the aim is rapid recovery and discharge home. Requirement for postoperative analgesia rarely exceeds simple non-opioid drugs. Non-steroidal anti-inflammatory agents may be beneficial in relieving uterine cramps. Routine administration of antiemetics should be considered, since these women are at risk of postoperative nausea and vomiting. Thromboprophylaxis may be indicated depending on risk factors.

Key points
- A sensitive and sympathetic approach to the mother is necessary.
- Prolonged preoperative waiting and starvation reflects poor communication and inefficiency.

Further reading
National Institute for Health and Care Excellence. *Ectopic Pregnancy and Miscarriage: Diagnosis and Initial Management*. Clinical Guideline 154. London: NICE, 2012. www.nice.org.uk/guidance/c g154 (accessed December 2018).

Termination of pregnancy

Termination of pregnancy in the UK is undertaken under the terms of the Abortion Act 1967, with over 200,000 induced abortion procedures occurring each year. For the consideration of anaesthetic procedures and potential problems, patients presenting for a termination of pregnancy broadly fall into two groups:

1. The presence of a maternal problem, the most commonly stated reason being danger to the mental or physical health of the mother. This accounts for up to 98% of terminations and may occur up to 24 weeks' gestation, but usually before 15 weeks.
2. Severe fetal congenital abnormality or early fetal death, two-thirds of which occur before 20 weeks' gestation.

Problems and special considerations

When caring for women who are to undergo a termination of pregnancy, it is important to consider the physiological changes of pregnancy, the psychological state of the woman and the need for routine preoperative assessment of the patient.

Those women in the first group above are usually scheduled to have termination of pregnancy on a gynaecological operating list. Patients in the second group are often looked after in the maternity unit.

Some members of staff may express conscientious objection to performing or being involved in termination of pregnancy, and this must be respected. They cannot be made to participate in such procedures, although they do have a duty to find other staff who will, if that is the patient's wish.

Management options

Termination for maternal indications

Surgical termination of pregnancy is usually a day-case procedure. Assessment should be conducted sympathetically, as these women are often very distressed. Vacuum aspiration may be performed up to 15 weeks' gestation; patients and clinicians are more used to this being performed under general anaesthesia in the UK, although it can be performed with systemic analgesia, local anaesthesia or conscious sedation. After 15 weeks' gestation, dilatation and evacuation (D&E) is necessary, which is also usually performed under general anaesthesia.

As most terminations for maternal indications occur before 15 weeks, these women can usually be regarded as non-pregnant with respect to gastric emptying and acid aspiration unless they have symptoms of reflux.

An anaesthetic technique suitable for day-case anaesthesia should be employed, such as induction with propofol and maintenance with propofol or a volatile anaesthetic agent. There has been concern about concentrations of volatile anaesthetic agents greater than 1 MAC causing uterine relaxation unresponsive to oxytocics. For a termination of pregnancy at less than 15 weeks, standard concentrations of volatile anaesthetic agents do not appear to pose a risk and may be used to maintain anaesthesia. Analgesia may be provided by intravenous fentanyl or alfentanil, with rectal diclofenac (100 mg) at the end of the procedure.

The gynaecologist may request that 5–10 U oxytocin is administered to aid uterine contraction. There is no clear evidence that this is helpful at this stage of pregnancy, and it is not recommended by the Royal College of Obstetricians and Gynaecologists (RCOG).

Termination for fetal abnormality or death

Women who present for termination of pregnancy because of fetal abnormality or intra-uterine death present a difficult clinical problem. A medical termination with vaginal delivery is often aimed for at later gestations, partly because this offers the opportunity for pathological examination of an intact fetus, but also because of limited access to D&E within the NHS. Induction of labour is usually required, and this may be a long and tedious process involving the use of prostaglandin pessaries and oxytocin infusion. The RCOG currently recommends feticide for terminations over 21^{+6} weeks. A discussion regarding analgesic options should be offered, including parenteral opioids and epidural analgesia (see Chapter 76, *Intrauterine death*). It must be remembered that as gestational age increases, the risks associated with termination, including complications such as haemorrhage, uterine perforation and infection, increase.

Termination of a pregnancy at less than 28 weeks is often associated with the retention of products of conception, for which surgical evacuation and anaesthesia are required (see Chapter 5, *Evacuation of retained products of conception*). Either regional or general anaesthesia may be offered to the woman, balancing the risks and benefits of each depending on the clinical condition and whether epidural analgesia is already in place. Rapid-sequence induction and tracheal intubation may be appropriate.

Key points

- Women may present for termination of pregnancy for maternal reasons or because of fetal abnormality or death.
- Such women are distressed and should be dealt with sympathetically.
- Early termination is usually performed as a day-case general anaesthetic procedure.
- Issues surrounding late terminations are as for intrauterine death.

Further reading

Royal College of Obstetricians and Gynaecologists. *Termination of Pregnancy for Fetal Abnormality in England, Scotland and Wales: Report of a Working Party*. London: RCOG, 2010. www.rcog.org.uk/en/guidelines-research-services/guidelines/termination-of-pregnancy-for-fetal-abnormality-in-england-scotland-and-wales (accessed December 2018).

Royal College of Obstetricians and Gynaecologists. *The Care of Women Requesting an Induced Abortion*. Evidence-Based Clinical Guideline 7. London: RCOG, 2011. www.rcog.org.uk/en/guidelines-research-services/guidelines/the-care-of-women-requesting-induced-abortion (accessed December 2018).

Cervical suture (cerclage)

Cervical suture (Shirodkar or McDonald cerclage) is performed to reduce the incidence of spontaneous miscarriage when there is cervical incompetence. Although it can be done before conception or as an emergency during pregnancy, the procedure is usually performed electively in the second trimester. Indications include women with a history of cervical trauma, spontaneous preterm birth, preterm prelabour rupture of membranes (PPROM) or fetal loss between 16 and 34 weeks of pregnancy, and in whom transvaginal ultrasound scans at 16 and 24 weeks indicate a cervical length of less than 25 mm.

It generally takes 15–20 minutes and is performed transvaginally on a day-case basis. A non-absorbable stitch or tape is sutured in a purse-string around the cervical neck at the level of the internal os. This requires anaesthesia, since the procedure is at best uncomfortable, although the suture can often be removed without anaesthesia (usually at 36–37 weeks' gestation unless in preterm labour); spontaneous labour usually soon follows. In patients with a grossly disrupted cervix, for example following surgery, placement of the suture via an abdominal approach may be required. Delivery is usually by elective caesarean section in these cases.

Problems and special considerations

A woman undergoing cervical suturing may be especially anxious if a previous pregnancy has ended in miscarriage. Apart from the possibility of anxiety, anaesthesia is along standard lines, bearing in mind the risks of anaesthesia in the pregnant woman and the possible effects of drugs on the fetus (see Chapter 8, *Incidental surgery in the pregnant patient*). Cerclage may be difficult if the membranes are bulging; the head-down position and/or tocolysis may be required to counteract this.

Management options

Both regional and general anaesthesia are acceptable for the insertion of a cervical suture, with maintenance of normal haemodynamic parameters being paramount. Many authorities advocate spinal anaesthesia as the technique of choice, since only a small amount of drug is administered, although epidural anaesthesia is also acceptable. If spinal or epidural anaesthesia is chosen, standard techniques are used. The procedure itself requires a less extensive block than caesarean section (from T8–10 down to and including the sacral roots) and thus smaller doses are required; however, the reduction is offset by the greater requirements at this early stage of pregnancy compared with the term parturient. Thus the doses required for regional anaesthesia are in the order of 75% of those used for caesarean section. Low-dose techniques have also been used, as for caesarean section; the women have more sensation (though painless) but have less motor block. Short-acting local anaesthetic agents such as prilocaine may be used to facilitate good anaesthesia for a short procedure while allowing faster discharge.

General anaesthesia may also be used; advantages include the relaxing effect of volatile agents on the uterus, and patient comfort if a steep Trendelenburg position is required. This involves administration of several drugs, and the effects on the fetus of many agents in current use are not clear (see Chapter 8, *Incidental surgery in the pregnant patient*). There may also be an increased risk of regurgitation and aspiration of gastric contents, depending on the gestation and severity of symptoms (see Chapter 59, *Aspiration of gastric contents*).

Paracervical and pudendal block and/or intravenous analgesia or sedation may also be used, but most authorities would recommend avoiding paracervical block because of potential adverse effects on uteroplacental perfusion.

Key points
- Cervical suture is usually performed in the second trimester.
- Patients may be especially anxious because of previous miscarriage.
- Standard techniques for the parturient are used; spinal anaesthesia may be preferable.

Further reading
National Institute for Health and Care Excellence. *Preterm Labour and Birth*. NICE Guideline NG 25. London: NICE, 2015. www.nice.org.uk/guidance/ng25 (accessed December 2018).

Incidental surgery in the pregnant patient

Non-obstetric surgery may occur in 0.5–2% of pregnancies; pregnant women may present with the same surgical conditions as the non-pregnant population, or with problems related to their pregnancy. Most pregnant women are relatively young and fit, although there is an increasing number of women with systemic disease who are becoming pregnant because of advances in medical or surgical management of their condition. Points of particular relevance to anaesthetists are therefore any underlying condition in addition to the reason for surgery, the effects of pregnancy on its management and the effect upon the fetus.

Problems and special considerations

Surgical diagnosis of the acute abdomen may be difficult because of the physical presence of the gravid uterus. Non-specific signs such as white cell count may be unreliable (up to 15 × 10^9/l in normal pregnancy). The differential diagnosis may also include obstetric conditions such as placental abruption and HELLP (haemolysis, elevated liver enzymes and low platelet count) syndrome.

The risks of aortocaval compression, difficulties with airway management and aspiration of gastric contents are present as for any pregnant woman, and depend to a certain extent on the stage of pregnancy and the reason for surgery; most will treat such risks as clinically relevant during the second trimester (see Chapter 59, *Aspiration of gastric contents*).

Surgical technique may be hindered by the pregnancy, and the operation itself may be more difficult than in the non-pregnant patient. For example, laparoscopic procedures may be impossible. Surgery that normally requires the non-supine position, such as back surgery, may pose particular problems.

Since surgery is generally withheld during pregnancy unless absolutely necessary, patients who do present for surgery tend to be more severely affected; thus careful pre-operative assessment and management are especially important. Problems of emergency surgery include inadequate preparation and investigation and an increased incidence of vomiting and dehydration.

The fetus is at risk from the primary effects of the mother's illness (e.g. dehydration, sepsis), the possible teratogenic effects of any drugs that are given to the mother, especially during the first trimester (see Chapter 3, *Anaesthesia before confirmation of pregnancy*), alterations in uteroplacental blood flow or oxygenation during anaesthesia and surgery, and possible premature onset of labour provoked by the illness, drugs or surgery itself.

Management options

In general, surgery is delayed until the second trimester if possible, because by then the major fetal organs will have already developed; in addition, the risk of premature labour is lower and the surgery easier than in the third trimester. Elective surgery should be postponed until after pregnancy. Once 24 weeks' gestation is reached, surgery should be undertaken at a location where emergency caesarean section is possible.

Perioperative management requires attendance by senior surgical and obstetric staff, with investigations and scans as required. The neonatal team should be informed once the fetus reaches 24 weeks' gestation. Anaesthetic management includes thorough preoperative assessment, taking into account the altered physiology of pregnancy (see Chapter 11, *Physiology of pregnancy*) when interpreting history, examination and investigations, and planning management. Particular attention should be paid to general assessment, as for emergency surgery in any patient. A sensitive discussion regarding risk to the pregnancy should be included in the preoperative assessment (see Chapter 3, *Anaesthesia before confirmation of pregnancy*). Current evidence suggests that miscarriage rates and premature delivery may be slightly increased, particularly when surgery occurs in the first and third trimester respectively. However, whether this is due to the anaesthetic, the surgery or the underlying pathological process is difficult to establish.

Depending on the stage of pregnancy, the airway may be more difficult, antacid administration should be considered, and the supine position should be avoided, although the efficacy of lateral tilt when the uterus is still small is uncertain. The disadvantages of regional anaesthesia (e.g. hypotension, increased peristalsis, problems with managing the block during difficult or prolonged surgery) must be weighed against those of general anaesthesia (airway problems, risk of awareness, less familiarity with general anaesthesia in the pregnant population etc.).

Although general anaesthesia involves the administration of more drugs with possible effects on the fetus, it also allows the use of volatile agents that relax the uterus. In general, drugs with good safety records during pregnancy should be used; most anaesthetic drugs do not have licences for use in pregnancy (mainly because of the costs involved in extending their licences), but newer drugs should probably be avoided until more is known about their actions. The only standard anaesthetic drug that has excited controversy in recent years is nitrous oxide, because of its effects on methionine synthase and DNA metabolism. Although there is a theoretical risk of its affecting the fetus, there is no evidence to support this clinically and many authorities, if not most, would now consider its use acceptable if needed.

General anaesthetic management would thus usually consist of rapid-sequence induction with standard agents, tracheal intubation and maintenance of anaesthesia with a volatile agent, as for any emergency general anaesthetic. Other drugs would be used as standard, but those that might increase uterine tone (e.g. ketamine, β-blockers) or vasoconstriction should be avoided if possible. Certain drugs given near to delivery may cross the placenta and affect the fetus (e.g. non-steroidal anti-inflammatory drugs, which can prevent the ductus arteriosus from closing). Prophylactic administration of tocolytic drugs has not been shown to be of any benefit, but uterine tone should be monitored perioperatively to allow administration of tocolytics if indicated. Traditional fears about the detrimental effects of high levels of maternal oxygen causing uteroplacental vasoconstriction are now known to be unfounded, and fetal arterial partial pressure of oxygen increases (up to a maximum of about 8 kPa (60 mmHg)) as maternal arterial oxygen content increases, so long as maternal hypotension is avoided. Phenylephrine is considered the vasopressor of choice as it has the most evidence supporting its use; however, other α-agonists (e.g. metaraminol) may also be used. Maternal arterial partial pressure of carbon dioxide should be kept in the normal (pregnant) range during controlled ventilation, to avoid fetal acidosis with associated myocardial depression, and uterine artery vasoconstriction.

With regard to fetal monitoring, between 18 and 24 weeks' gestation, the fetal heart rate should be recorded pre- and post-procedure. From 24 weeks, cardiotocography monitoring with simultaneous electronic fetal heart rate and contraction monitoring should be performed before and after the procedure as a minimum. Intraoperative monitoring necessitates the presence of staff suitably trained to interpret preterm monitoring in the presence of anaesthesia and surgery, and abdominal surgery makes it more difficult to place the monitor. It may be difficult to arrange midwifery and surgical nursing care both before and after surgery, and the most appropriate area for the mother's postoperative care needs careful consideration.

Key points

- Surgical diagnosis and management may be difficult.
- Maternal risks are those of anaesthesia in the pregnant state.
- Fetal risks are related to the mother's condition and maternal drugs, and include the premature onset of labour.
- Anaesthetic management should focus on maintaining normal uteroplacental blood flow.

Further reading

American College of Obstetricians and Gynecologists. ACOG Committee Opinion No. 474: nonobstetric surgery during pregnancy. *Obstet Gynecol* 2011; **117**: 420–1.

Cheek TG, Baird E. Anesthesia for nonobstetric surgery: maternal and fetal considerations. *Clin Obstet Gynecol* 2009; **52**: 535–45.

Melnick DM, Wahl WL, Dalton VK. Management of general surgical problems in the pregnant patient. *Am J Surg* 2004; **187**: 170–80.

Reitman E, Flood P. Anaesthetic considerations for non-obstetric surgery during pregnancy. *Br J Anaesth* 2011; **107** (Suppl 1): i72–8.

Chapter

9

Intrauterine surgery

Fetal surgery is an attractive option in cases where an isolated abnormality would be otherwise fatal to the fetus or neonate, and is clearly amenable to correction, such as neck tumours with airway obstruction, sacrococcygeal teratomas, obstructive uropathy and diaphragmatic hernia. However, results of intrauterine surgery are variable depending on the type of surgery, and there is no clear consensus on its place. There are three main types of intrauterine surgery:

- Ex-utero intrapartum treatment (EXIT). This occurs immediately before delivery, and the fetus remains attached to the placenta, allowing brief procedures such as tracheal intubation or tracheostomy for airway obstruction to occur. Corrective surgery may then occur post-delivery.
- Open procedures such as correction of a meningomyelocoele. A vertical uterine incision may be required for access, necessitating caesarean delivery if the pregnancy proceeds.
- Minimally invasive procedures such as intrauterine blood transfusion in haemolytic disease or laser ablation of communicating vessels in twin-to-twin transfusion syndrome.

Problems and special considerations

Each procedure must be assessed on a risk–benefit basis, since there is a risk of up to 50% fetal loss associated with premature labour, haemorrhage, abruption and infection. Surgery is technically difficult because of the small size of the fetus and its mobility when small, but leaving the surgery until later may result in increased end-organ damage caused by the malformation. The optimal timing for most procedures is uncertain, although most open ones have been performed at around 18–24 weeks. Percutaneous procedures (e.g. transfusions) may be performed later or at intervals.

Maternal risks include haemorrhage, uterine scarring and amniotic fluid embolism. Postoperatively, the mother may be confined to bed and receive β_2-agonists, with the risks of deep-vein thrombosis and pulmonary oedema, respectively.

Each lesion must be carefully defined and a chromosomal abnormality or other malformation excluded. For example, intrauterine placement of intraventricular shunts is no longer considered suitable for treatment of hydrocephalus, since the risk–benefit ratio cannot be calculated for individual fetuses because of the difficulty in predicting outcome antenatally. Since most conditions that might be amenable to intrauterine surgery are rare or uncommon and already associated with poor outcome, it is difficult to demonstrate that outcome after fetal surgery is better than that after conventional postpartum therapy, because any expected improvement will be small.

Management options

Anaesthetic management is along the lines of that for incidental surgery during pregnancy, with maintenance of uteroplacental perfusion the main concern (see Chapter 8, *Incidental surgery in the pregnant patient*). Local anaesthetic infiltration of the abdominal wall, with or without conscious sedation, may be adequate for percutaneous procedures, although there may be a need for emergency caesarean section if fetal bradycardia occurs, and so adequate preparation and facilities are required for this. Regional anaesthesia is a suitable alternative if extensive percutaneous procedures are required.

Fetal and maternal general anaesthesia for corrective surgery is administered by using standard techniques, though placental transfer of anaesthetic agents may be desirable in this scenario, unlike during caesarean section. Total uterine relaxation may be required, and this may be achieved with 2–3 MAC of an inhalational agent; this may result in maternal haemorrhage or hypotension, both of which must be anticipated and treated aggressively. Alternatively, magnesium sulfate or glyceryl trinitrate may be used. Fetal injection of a neuromuscular blocking drug may be required to stop fetal movement. Analgesics may also be injected into the fetus, since there is increasing evidence that the fetus can experience pain. Fetal monitoring may be difficult, but pulse oximetry, ultrasonography and cardiotocography have been used. Bleeding may be excessive in prolonged open procedures.

Key points

- The place of intrauterine surgery is uncertain.
- To be suitable for intrauterine surgery, malformations must be clearly defined, fatal if untreated and amenable to corrective surgery.
- General principles of anaesthesia are as for incidental surgery during pregnancy.

Further reading

De Buck F, Deprest J, Van de Velde M. Anesthesia for fetal surgery. *Curr Opin Anaesthesiol* 2008; **21**: 293–7.

Garcia PJ, Olutoye OO, Ivey RT, Olutoye OA. Case scenario: anesthesia for maternal–fetal surgery: the ex utero intrapartum therapy (EXIT) procedure. *Anesthesiology* 2011; **114**: 1446–52.

Tran KM. Anesthesia for fetal surgery. *Semin Fetal Neonatal Med* 2010; **15**: 40–5.

Chapter

10
Anatomy of the spine and peripheral nerves

Although not exclusive to obstetric anaesthesia, a sound knowledge of the anatomy pertinent to epidural and spinal anaesthesia is fundamental to obstetric anaesthetists. In addition, knowledge of the relevant peripheral nerves is important in order to differentiate central from peripheral causes of neurological impairment.

The structures involved in obstetric neuraxial anaesthesia comprise the vertebrae and sacral canal, vertebral ligaments, epidural space, meninges and spinal cord. The important peripheral aspects are the lumbar and sacral plexuses and the muscular and cutaneous supply of the lower part of the body.

Vertebrae (Figure 10.1)

The vertebral column has two curves, with the cervical and lumbar regions convex anteriorly and the thoracic and sacral regions concave. Traditionally, T4 is described as the most posterior part (most dependent in the supine position), although T8 has been suggested by recent imaging studies. L3–4 is the most anterior part (uppermost in the supine position), although this curve may be flattened by flexing the hips. In the lateral position, the greater width of women's hips compared with their shoulders imparts a downward slope from the caudal end of the vertebral column to the cranial end.

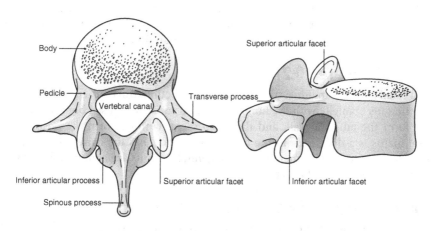

Figure 10.1 A lumbar vertebra, seen from superior and lateral aspects. Reproduced with permission from Yentis SM, Hirsch NP, Smith GB. *Anaesthesia and Intensive Care A–Z*, 4th edn. Churchill Livingstone. © Elsevier 2009.

There are seven cervical vertebrae, twelve thoracic, five lumbar, five fused sacral and three to five fused coccygeal. A number of ligaments connect them (see below). Vertebrae have the following components:

- **Body.** This lies anteriorly, with the vertebral arch behind. It is kidney-shaped in the lumbar region. Fibrocartilaginous vertebral discs, accounting for about 25% of the spine's total length, separate the bodies of C2 to L5. Each disc has an outer fibrous annulus fibrosus and a more fluid inner nucleus pulposus (the latter may prolapse through the former: a 'slipped disc'). The bodies of the thoracic vertebrae are heart-shaped and articulate with the ribs via superior and inferior costal facets at their rear. The bodies of the sacral vertebrae are fused to form the sacrum, which encloses the sacral canal; the coccygeal vertebral bodies are fused to form the triangular coccyx, the base of which articulates with the sacrum.
- **Pedicles.** These are round in cross-section. They project posteriorly from the body and join the laminae. Each intervertebral foramen is formed by the pedicles of the vertebra above and below.
- **Laminae.** These are flattened in cross-section. They complete the vertebral arch by meeting in the midline at the spinous process. The superior and inferior articular processes bear facets for articulation with adjacent vertebrae; those of the thoracic vertebrae are flatter and aligned in the coronal plane, whereas those of the lumbar vertebrae are nearer the sagittal plane.
- **Transverse processes.** In the lumbar region these are thick and pass laterally. The transverse processes of L5 are particularly massive but short. The transverse processes of thoracic vertebrae are large and pass backwards and laterally; they bear facets that articulate with the tubercles of the ribs (except T11 and T12).
- **Spinous process.** These project horizontally backwards in the lumbar region; in the thoracic region they are longer and inclined at about 60 degrees to the horizontal. The spinous process of T12 has a notched lower edge.

The cervical vertebrae have a number of features that distinguish them from the others, including the foramen transverarium in the transverse processes, bifid spinous processes and the particular characteristics of C1 and C2.

A line drawn between the iliac crests (Tuffier's line) usually crosses the L3–4 interspace (slightly higher than in the non-pregnant state because of rotation of the pelvis), although this is unreliable, and it has been shown that even experienced anaesthetists can be one or more interspaces lower (or more commonly, higher) than that intended.

Sacral canal (Figure 10.2)

The sacral canal is 10–15 cm long, triangular in cross-section, runs the length of the sacrum and is continuous cranially with the lumbar vertebral canal. The fused bodies of the sacral vertebrae form the anterior wall, and the fused sacral laminae form the posterior wall. The sacral hiatus is a deficiency in the fifth laminar arch, has the cornua laterally and is covered by the sacrococcygeal membrane. Congenital variants are common, possibly contributing to unreliable caudal analgesia.

Vertebral ligaments (Figure 10.3)

- **Anterior longitudinal ligament.** This is attached to the anterior aspects of the vertebral bodies, and runs from C2 to the sacrum.

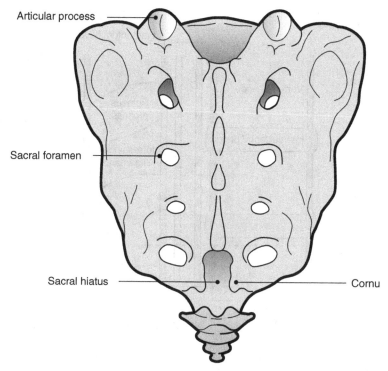

Articular process

Sacral foramen

Sacral hiatus

Cornu

Figure 10.2 Sacrum, posterior aspect. Reproduced with permission from Yentis SM, Hirsch NP, Smith GB. *Anaesthesia and Intensive Care A–Z*, 4th edn. Churchill Livingstone. © Elsevier 2009.

- **Posterior longitudinal ligament.** This is attached to the posterior aspects of the vertebral bodies, and runs from C2 to the sacrum.
- **Ligamentum flavum (yellow ligament).** This is attached to the laminae of adjacent vertebrae, forming a V-shaped structure with the point posteriorly. It is more developed in the lumbar than in the thoracic region.
- **Interspinous ligament.** This passes between the spinous processes of adjacent vertebrae.
- **Supraspinous ligament.** This is attached to the tips of the spinous processes from C7 to the sacrum.

In addition, there are posterior, anterior and lateral sacrococcygeal ligaments. Other ligaments are involved in the attachments of C1 and C2 to the skull. The ligaments may become softer during pregnancy because of the hormonal changes that occur.

Epidural space

- **Boundaries.** The space extends from the foramen magnum to the sacrococcygeal membrane. It is triangular in cross-section in the lumbar region, its base anterior; it is very thin anteriorly and up to 5 mm wide posteriorly. It lies external to the dura mater of the spinal cord and internal to the ligamenta flava and vertebral laminae posteriorly, the posterior longitudinal ligament anteriorly and the intervertebral foramina and vertebral pedicles laterally. Magnetic resonance imaging suggests the space is divided into

(a)

(b)

Figure 10.3 Vertebral ligaments: (a) longitudinal section and (b) transverse section through A–B. Reproduced with permission from Yentis SM, Hirsch NP, Smith GB. *Anaesthesia and Intensive Care A–Z*, 4th edn. Churchill Livingstone. © Elsevier 2009.

segments by the laminae. The space may extend through the intervertebral foramina into the paravertebral spaces.

- **Contents.** These include epidural fat, epidural veins (Batson's plexus), lymphatics and spinal nerve roots. The veins become engorged in pregnancy as a result of the hormonal changes and any aortocaval compression. Connective tissue layers have been demonstrated by radiology and endoscopy within the epidural space, in some cases dividing it into right and left portions.

- **Pressure.** A negative pressure is usually found in the epidural space upon entering it; the reason is unclear but may involve anterior dimpling of the dura by the epidural needle, sudden posterior recoil of the ligamentum flavum when it is punctured, stretching of the dural sac during extreme flexion of the back, transmitted negative intrapleural pressure via thoracic paravertebral spaces and/or relative overgrowth of the vertebral canal compared with the dural sac. Occasionally a positive pressure is found.

Meninges

- **Pia mater.** This delicate and vascular layer adheres closely to the brain and spinal cord. Between it and the arachnoid mater is the cerebrospinal fluid (CSF) within the subarachnoid space containing blood vessels, the denticulate ligament laterally along its length and the subarachnoid septum posteriorly. The pia terminates as the filum terminale, which passes through the caudal end of the dural sac and attaches to the coccyx.
- **Arachnoid mater.** This membrane is also delicate and lies between the dura externally and the CSF internally. The potential subdural space lies between the dura and arachnoid mater, which fuses with the dura at S2.
- **Dura mater.** This fibrous layer has an outer component that is adherent to the inner periosteum of the vertebrae, and an inner one that lies against the outer surface of the arachnoid. The dura projects into the epidural space, especially in the midline. It ends at about S2.

Spinal cord

The spinal cord ends inferiorly level with L3 at birth, rising to the adult level of L1–2 (sometimes T12 or L3) by 20 years. Below this level (the conus medullaris), the lumbar and sacral nerve roots (comprising the cauda equina) and filum terminale occupy the vertebral canal. The main ascending and descending tracts are shown in Figure 10.4.

The blood supply of the spinal cord is of relevance to obstetric anaesthetists, since cord ischaemia may result in neurological damage:

- **Anterior spinal artery.** This descends in the anterior median fissure and supplies the anterior two-thirds of the cord. The anterior spinal artery syndrome (e.g. arising from profound hypotension) thus results in lower motor neurone paralysis at the level of the lesion, and spastic paraplegia, reduced pain and temperature sensation below the level, with normal joint position sense and vibration sensation.
- **Posterior spinal arteries.** These descend along each side of the cord, one anterior and one posterior to the dorsal nerve roots.
- **Radicular branches.** These arise from local arteries (from the aorta) and feed the spinal arteries. Those at T1 and the lower thoracic/upper lumbar level (artery of Adamkiewicz – usually unilateral) are the most important. The cord at T3–5 and T12–L1 is thought to be most at risk from ischaemia. The conus medullaris and cauda equina are supplied by a vascular plexus arising from the artery of Adamkiewicz above and pelvic vessels below. In 15% of the population, the artery of Adamkiewicz is the

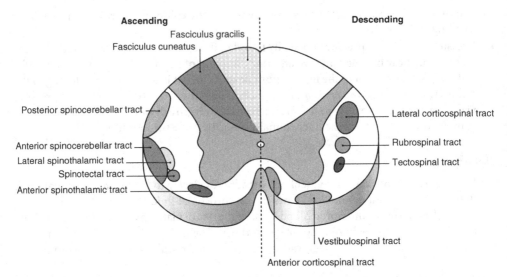

Figure 10.4 Ascending and descending tracts of the spinal cord. Reproduced with permission from Yentis SM, Hirsch NP, Smith GB. *Anaesthesia and Intensive Care A–Z*, 4th edn. Churchill Livingstone. © Elsevier 2009.

main source of arterial blood to the conus medullaris and cauda equina; compression during delivery may result in permanent paraplegia.

Venous drainage is via the internal iliac, intercostal, azygos and vertebral veins.

Peripheral nerves of the lower body

The lumbar and sacral plexuses are shown schematically in Figure 10.5. They form at the posterior of the pelvis, and their branches pass round the interior of the pelvis, where they may be exposed to pressure during labour and delivery (Figure 10.6; see also Chapter 53, *Peripheral nerve lesions following regional anaesthesia*).

Peripheral cutaneous innervation may be characterised according to the dermatomal distribution or peripheral nerves (Figures 10.5 and 10.7, Table 53.1). Both representations may vary considerably between individuals. Peripheral motor innervation may also be considered according to myotomal innervation or peripheral nerves (Table 10.1).

Dermatomal innervation of the upper body is also important when determining the upper extent of regional blockade.

Key points

- A clear understanding of the anatomy of the spine and peripheral nerves is essential when delivering neuraxial anaesthesia and analgesia, and when assessing neurological complications related to delivery.

Further reading

Richardson J, Groen G. Applied epidural anatomy. *Contin Educ Anaesth Crit Care Pain* 2005; **5**: 98–100.

Westbrook JL. Anatomy of the epidural space. *Anaesth Intensive Care Med* 2012; **13**: 551–4.

(a)

T12
L1 — Iliohypogastric nerve
— Ilioinguinal nerve
— Genitofemoral nerve
L2 — Lateral cutaneous nerve of thigh
L3
L4

Femoral nerve   Obturator nerve

(b)

L4
L5
S1
S2 — Superior gluteal nerve
— Inferior gluteal nerve
S3
S4

Posterior cutaneous nerve of thigh   Sciatic nerve

Perforating cutaneous nerve

Pudendal nerve

Figure 10.5 Plan of (a) lumbar plexus and (b) sacral plexus. Reproduced with permission from Yentis SM, Hirsch NP, Smith GB. *Anaesthesia and Intensive Care A–Z*, 4th edn. Churchill Livingstone. © Elsevier 2009.

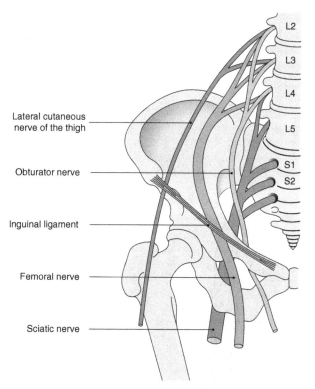

L2
L3
L4
L5
S1
S2

Lateral cutaneous nerve of the thigh

Obturator nerve

Inguinal ligament

Femoral nerve

Sciatic nerve

Figure 10.6 Relationship of peripheral nerves with the pelvis. Adapted with permission from Holdcroft A, Thomas TA. *Principles and Practice of Obstetric Anaesthesia*. Blackwell Science Ltd. © John Wiley & Sons Ltd 1999.

Table 10.1 Motor innervation of lower limbs by myotomes and peripheral nerves

Joint	Movement	Myotomes	Nerve supply
Hip	Flexion	L1–3	Lumbar plexus
		L2–4	Femoral nerve
	Extension	L5–S2	Sacral plexus
		L5–S2	Sciatic nerve
	Abduction	L5–S2	Sacral plexus
	Adduction	L2–4	Obturator nerve
Knee	Extension	L2–4	Femoral nerve
	Flexion	L5–S2	Sciatic nerve
		S1–2	Tibial nerve[a]
Ankle/foot	Dorsiflexion	L4–5	Deep peroneal nerve[b]
	Eversion	L5–S1	Superficial peroneal nerve[b]
	Plantar flexion	S1–2	Tibial nerve[a]
	Inversion	L4–5	Tibial nerve[a]

[a] Branch of sciatic nerve.
[b] Branch of common peroneal nerve, itself a branch of the sciatic nerve.

Figure 10.7 Dermatomes of upper and lower body. Reproduced with permission from Yentis SM, Hirsch NP, Smith GB. *Anaesthesia and Intensive Care A–Z*, 4th edn. Churchill Livingstone. © Elsevier 2009.

Physiology of pregnancy

Pregnancy is associated with major physiological changes throughout the body. These are caused both by hormonal factors (influential from conception onwards) and by the mechanical changes due to the enlarging uterus (of increasing significance as pregnancy progresses). It is important to understand the normal physiological changes occurring during pregnancy, in order to predict the risks and effects of analgesic and anaesthetic intervention, and also to anticipate the impact of pregnancy on any coexisting medical condition.

Hormonal changes

Following fertilisation, the corpus luteum in the ovary secretes progesterone, oestrogens and relaxin. The placenta takes over the hormone-producing function of the corpus luteum from 6–8 weeks' gestation onwards and secretes in addition human chorionic somatomammotrophin (hCS; previously known as human placental lactogen and chorionic growth hormone-prolactin).

Human chorionic gonadotrophin (hCG) can be measured by radioimmunoassay and detected in the blood 6 days after conception, and in the urine 2–3 weeks after conception. It is therefore a useful early diagnostic test of pregnancy. It is produced by the syncytiotrophoblast, and levels rise rapidly during the first 8 weeks of pregnancy, falling to a plateau thereafter.

Progesterone is responsible for most of the hormonally mediated changes occurring during pregnancy. It causes:

- Smooth muscle relaxation
- Generalised vasodilatation
- Bronchodilatation
- Dilatation within the renal tract
- Sluggish gastrointestinal tract motility and constipation

It is thermogenic, causing an increase in basal temperature during pregnancy. It may be responsible for the nausea and vomiting that are common in early pregnancy. Progesterone is a neurotransmitter and, together with increased endogenous endorphins, is implicated in the elevated pain threshold experienced by pregnant women. It also decreases the minimum alveolar concentration (MAC) of inhalational anaesthetic agents. Progesterone has also been demonstrated to enhance conduction blockade in isolated nerve preparations, and it is therefore thought likely to play a role in the decreased requirement for local anaesthetic agents for neuraxial anaesthesia.

Mechanical changes

The uterine fundus progressively enlarges and becomes palpable abdominally by the beginning of the second trimester, at the level of the umbilicus by 20 weeks' gestation and the xiphisternum by 36 weeks.

Fetal head engagement in the maternal pelvis at the end of pregnancy reduces the fundal height and may alleviate some symptoms attributable to mechanical factors. In multiple pregnancies, the uterus expands to a greater extent and more rapidly, and therefore the mechanical effects are usually greater.

Following delivery the uterus involutes rapidly, and should not be palpable above the maternal umbilicus. It has usually returned to within the pelvis by 72 hours after delivery.

Cardiovascular and haemodynamic changes

Pregnancy

- Blood volume increases throughout pregnancy secondary to hormone-mediated fluid retention, and reaches approximately 45–50% more than pre-pregnant values by term.
- Cardiac output, heart rate and stroke volume all increase as pregnancy progresses. Cardiac output increases by approximately 40–50% by term, with most of the increase occurring by 20 weeks' gestation. The increased blood flow is distributed primarily to the uterus, where blood flow increases from approximately 50 ml/minute at 10 weeks' gestation to 850 ml/minute at term. Approximately 1 litre of blood is contained within the uterus and the maternal side of the placenta.
- There is a propensity for arrhythmias that is caused by hormonal effects, increased sympathetic discharge and the stimulation of stretch-activated cardiac ion channels secondary to increased blood volume and cardiac chamber size. The resulting membrane depolarisation may lead to a shortened refractory period, slowed conduction and a mismatch of depolarisation and refractoriness.
- The electrocardiogram in pregnancy may show sinus tachycardia, ectopic beats, shortening of the PR and uncorrected QT intervals, a Q wave and T wave inversion in the lateral leads or lead III, or left axis deviation.
- Renal blood flow increases by 80% over non-pregnant levels by the middle of the second trimester. Glomerular filtration rate and creatinine clearance increase by 50% during pregnancy.
- Systemic vascular resistance falls (peripheral vasodilatation mediated by progesterone, prostacyclin and oestrogens), and there is a decrease in both systolic and diastolic blood pressures, which reach a nadir during the second trimester and then increase gradually towards term, although remaining lower than pre-pregnancy values.
- Aortocaval compression can occur from the middle of pregnancy onward if the supine position is adopted. This is due to mechanical compression of the aorta and inferior vena cava. Venous return is dependent on the competence of collateral circulation via the azygos and ovarian veins. Studies have demonstrated that uterine blood flow decreases primarily as a result of aortic rather than venous compression (see Chapter 13, *Aortocaval compression*).
- Central venous and pulmonary arterial pressures are unchanged during normal pregnancy.

Labour and delivery

- Cardiac output increases by 25–50% in labour, with an additional 15–30% increase during contractions. This increase in cardiac output is mediated through increased sympathetic nervous system activity, and is therefore significantly attenuated by epidural analgesia.
- Central venous pressure increases during contractions, partly due to sympathetic activity and partly from the transfer of up to 500 ml of blood from the intervillous space. The latter is unaffected by epidural analgesia, as is the increase in central venous pressure which occurs when the Valsalva manoeuvre is performed during pushing.
- Autotransfusion of around 500 ml of blood (from the placenta) occurs during the third stage. There is a sustained increase in cardiac output and central venous pressure for several hours after delivery secondary to intravascular fluid shifts. These haemodynamic changes may be significant in women with cardiac disease or those with pre-eclampsia.

Respiratory changes

Pregnancy

- Progesterone increases the sensitivity of the respiratory centre to carbon dioxide and also acts as a primary respiratory stimulant. These effects are enhanced by oestrogens, and the combined hormonal effect causes an increase in minute ventilation of 45–50%. A sensation of breathlessness is common and is experienced by up to 70% of pregnant women. Physicians should, however, maintain a high index of suspicion when evaluating breathlessness in pregnancy, especially if it is associated with other clinical features. Persistent breathlessness on lying down is an abnormal sign and must be investigated.
- The partial pressure of carbon dioxide in arterial blood ($PaCO_2$) is re-set to approximately 4 kPa during the first trimester and remains at that level throughout pregnancy. A partially corrected respiratory alkalosis is found in normal pregnant women.
- Oxygen consumption increases progressively during pregnancy to 35% above pre-pregnancy levels.
- Functional residual capacity (FRC) decreases to 80% of pre-pregnancy values as pregnancy progresses, caused by increased intra-abdominal pressure and upward displacement of the diaphragm by the enlarging uterus. Total lung capacity remains unchanged. FRC remains greater than closing capacity throughout pregnancy while the woman remains in an upright position, but falls when a recumbent position is adopted. It has been estimated that airway closure within normal tidal ventilation may occur in as many as 50% of all supine pregnant women during the second half of pregnancy. Consideration should therefore be given to continuous administration of oxygen to women particularly at risk (e.g. those who are obese, and those with respiratory disease).

Labour and delivery

- Massive hyperventilation occurs during labour (unless there is effective analgesia), with minute ventilation increasing to 3–4 times prelabour values.

- $PaCO_2$ falls to below 2 kPa in some women. This respiratory alkalosis is associated with a metabolic acidosis, since maternal aerobic requirement for oxygen (increased by hyperventilation, hyperdynamic circulation and uterine activity) cannot be met, resulting in a progressive lactic acidosis.
- Effective epidural analgesia abolishes these effects during the first stage of labour but not during the second, when the additional uterine activity and work of pushing produce a further oxygen demand that cannot be met.
- The increased oxygen consumption and reduced oxygen reserves put pregnant women at a significant risk of hypoxia during periods of apnoea, e.g. at the induction of general anaesthesia.

Gastrointestinal changes

Pregnancy

- Lower oesophageal sphincter pressure is reduced because of the smooth muscle relaxant effect of progesterone.
- Intragastric pressure rises as a mechanical consequence of the enlarging uterus.
- The overall effect of these changes is a decrease in gastro-oesophageal barrier pressure, with a concomitant increase in risk of regurgitation and aspiration of gastric contents.
- 75–85% of pregnant women complain of heartburn during the third trimester, and a significant number will have a demonstrable hiatus hernia.
- Gastric emptying is not delayed during pregnancy.
- There is some evidence that gastric volume is increased, and the pH of the intragastric volume may be lower than in the non-pregnant individual.
- Plasma albumin concentration falls due to physiological haemodilution, thus increasing the unbound fraction of highly protein-bound drugs. This may have implications for dose calculation and serum-level monitoring of drugs such as phenytoin, which should be based on measurement of the free drug concentration.

Labour and delivery

- Gastric emptying is now thought to be normal in labour in most cases. However, opioid administration by any route will delay gastric emptying.
- The risk of pulmonary aspiration of gastric contents means that rapid-sequence induction of general anaesthesia, preceded by measures to reduce the acidity of the gastric contents, is required (see Chapter 59, *Aspiration of gastric contents*).
- Studies suggest that gastric volume (but not acidity) may remain elevated for 48 hours after delivery.

Haematological changes

Total blood volume increases by approximately 1.5 litres during pregnancy, with plasma volume increasing by 30–50% and red cell mass increasing by 20–30% (thus causing the so-called 'physiological anaemia' of pregnancy). The magnitude of the increase is greater in women with multiple pregnancy and greatly reduced in women with pre-eclampsia. Plasma volume changes are maximum by mid-pregnancy, returning to normal by approximately 6 weeks postpartum.

The haemoglobin concentration falls by 10–20 g/l by mid-pregnancy; the red cell indices remain approximately constant apart from a small increase in the mean cell volume, unless women become iron/folate-deficient. Postpartum, the haemoglobin concentration usually takes up to 4–6 weeks to reach pre-pregnancy levels.

The white blood cell count increases, peaking at $10–15 \times 10^9/l$ around mid-pregnancy and increasing further in labour (to up to $30 \times 10^9/l$), returning to normal non-pregnant levels by 6–7 days postpartum. Most of the increase is in neutrophils. (Note that the use of steroids in preterm labour can also increase white cell count.)

The platelet count usually remains within the normal range in pregnancy, although population mean counts are slightly lower, with the lower normal limit usually given as approximately $100–120 \times 10^9/l$.

Pregnancy represents a state of hypercoagulability; there is increased hepatic production of coagulation factors, especially fibrinogen (increases by approximately 50%) and factor VIII (approximately doubles), but others also increase (II, X and von Willebrand factor). Resistance to activated protein C also increases. Fibrinolytic inhibitors decrease, as do factor XI and protein S activity.

Musculoskeletal changes

The pregnant woman has increased ligamentous laxity, secondary to increased relaxin release, which may lead to increased joint mobility and instability. This may put the woman at risk of musculoskeletal trauma if she has received epidural analgesia, and this risk is considerably higher if she has received either regional or general anaesthesia, when she is unable to safeguard her position. Care is therefore required when positioning, with special attention being paid to the hips and back. The wedged supine position and the use of lateral tilt are compromises and do not reliably relieve aortocaval compression. Women should be encouraged to remain sitting upright or in the full lateral position whenever possible. Walking and standing in labour should also be encouraged.

Key points

- An understanding of the normal physiological changes of pregnancy is essential when caring for the parturient, both in normal pregnancy and delivery and when pathology occurs.

Further reading

Feghali M, Venkataramanan R, Caritis S. Pharmacokinetics of drugs in pregnancy. *Semin Perinatol* 2015; **39**: 512–19.

Jarvis S, Nelson-Piercy C. Common symptoms and signs during pregnancy. *Obstet Gynaecol Reprod Med* 2014; **24**: 245–9.

Antenatal care

Antenatal care includes a wide range of functions, including:

- Provision of information to mothers about the importance of diet and lifestyle, and about choices available to them during their pregnancy.
- Screening for pre-existing maternal conditions and risk factors, including those that may influence the anaesthetic care of the woman, and the construction of an individualised peripartum management plan.
- Assessment of maternal wellbeing during pregnancy and screening for development of pregnancy-specific and non-specific conditions.

Maternal assessment

Specific maternal conditions and their assessment and management are addressed in subsequent chapters. For routine antenatal care in the UK, ten antenatal appointments are currently recommended for nullipara with uncomplicated pregnancies, and seven for multipara, with regular urine and blood pressure checks and further checks (e.g. for anaemia) at specified intervals. This may be midwifery- or obstetrician-led, depending on the progress of the pregnancy, previous complications or the presence of comorbidities. Anaesthetic involvement may be ad hoc or via formal clinics, in which anaesthetists can assess women referred to them and arrange further referral or investigations and discuss management options. A checklist for midwives and obstetricians, listing those conditions that warrant anaesthetic referral, is useful (Table 12.1).

Fetal assessment

It is possible to make detailed assessments of fetal wellbeing in the antenatal period that allow monitoring of fetal growth and development, and enable the detection of fetal hypoxia. A decision to deliver the baby early may be made on the outcome of these assessments, and the obstetric anaesthetist may be involved in this decision making. The most commonly used methods of antenatal assessment are symphysis–fundal height measurement, serial ultrasonography, serial Doppler flow studies and cardiotocography.

- **Symphysis–fundal height measurement** should be performed from 24 weeks of pregnancy and may enable the prediction of a small-for-gestational-age (SGA) fetus. Measurements obtained are plotted on customised growth charts, and a single value below the 10th centile or multiple ones suggesting a slow rate of growth may trigger further assessment by ultrasound.

Table 12.1 Checklist for antenatal anaesthetic referral

Obstetric	Placenta accreta/percreta
	Three or more fetuses
Cardiovascular/respiratory/neurological	All except mild, without functional limitation, and without history of previous surgery
Haematological	Coagulopathy, including anticoagulant therapy
	Sickle cell variants
	Thrombocytopenia
Musculoskeletal	Severe back or neck problems or previous surgery
	Spina bifida
	Scoliosis
Anaesthetic	Previous difficulties, e.g. intubation or failed or poor regional analgesia or anaesthesia
	Family history of malignant hyperthermia or suxamethonium apnoea
Other	Severe obesity
	Severe allergy to drugs or latex
	Severe anxiety/needle phobia
	Severe connective tissue disease
	Poor venous access, e.g. intravenous drug use
	Refusal of blood products
	Inability to give consent
	Language/communication barrier

- **Serial ultrasonography.** Routine scanning is offered at 10–13 weeks and 18–20 weeks. The head circumference is measured in association with the abdominal circumference. If the fetus is starving, glycogen stores in the liver will be depleted and there will be an increase in the ratio of head circumference to abdominal wall circumference (asymmetrical growth restriction). There may also be a generalised growth restriction (symmetrical growth restriction). The liquor volume is also used as an indicator of fetal wellbeing and placental function, poor placental function being reflected in a reduced liquor volume. As a measure of this volume, the anterior–posterior distance across the liquor (the liquor column) is measured using a transducer. A column of less than 3 cm is indicative of oligohydramnios and one less than 2 cm represents very severe oligohydramnios. The amniotic fluid index may also be used to measure the liquor volume; this is the sum of the liquor column in each of the four liquor quadrants and is normally 8–20 cm.
- **Serial Doppler flow studies.** Both maternal uterine blood flow and fetal umbilical artery blood flow may be measured using Doppler techniques. The pattern of flow is influenced by resistance of the placental vasculature and reflects placental function as follows:
  1. Normal flow continues through systole and diastole, as there is little resistance to flow through the placenta. The systolic/diastolic flow velocity ratio (SD ratio) is widely used to indicate resistance to arterial flow; several other derived indices (e.g.

pulsatility index) have also been used to indicate fetal perfusion and oxygenation. The use of these techniques for screening for high-risk fetuses is controversial, and they may be reserved for monitoring known high-risk cases.

2. Just absent end-diastolic flow may indicate the need for delivery of the baby. Wide absence of end-diastolic flow suggests the need to deliver the baby urgently.

3. Reversal of end-diastolic flow suggests the need for immediate delivery of the baby. Plans for timing and mode of delivery may be based on the evidence of the Doppler studies. The anaesthetist should understand that the anaesthetic management should optimise the placental flow, and that meticulous care should be taken to avoid sudden cardiovascular changes and in particular supine hypotension.

In specialised fetal medicine units, blood flow may also be measured by using Doppler techniques in the fetal abdominal aorta, renal or middle cerebral arteries.

- **Cardiotocography.** This will only record the fetal heart during the time of the trace and cannot provide historical or predictive information. The pattern of the trace may be indicative of fetal compromise and may be used to plan the mode of delivery, e.g. either induction of labour or caesarean section (see Chapter 20, *Intrapartum fetal monitoring*). It is important that the anaesthetist communicates with the obstetrician and understands how compromised the fetus is when asked to give analgesia or anaesthesia to these mothers. The degree of urgency for the delivery will depend on the condition of the fetus. It should be remembered that women in these circumstances may be very anxious and upset and will need extra support during delivery.

Key points

- Antenatal assessments may identify mothers and fetuses at special risk.
- High-risk mothers should be referred for antenatal anaesthetic assessment.
- Meticulous care should be taken to maintain optimal placental perfusion if investigations indicate fetal hypoxaemia.
- Communication between medical and midwifery staff is crucial.

Further reading

Everett TR, Peebles DM. Antenatal tests of fetal wellbeing. *Semin Fetal Neonatal Med* 2015; **20**: 138–43.

Grivell RM, Alfirevic Z, Gyte GM, Devane D. Antenatal cardiotocography for fetal assessment. *Cochrane Database Syst Rev* 2015; (9): CD007863.

National Institute for Health and Care Excellence. *Antenatal Care for Uncomplicated Pregnancies.* Clinical Guideline **62**. London: NICE, 2008 (updated 2017). www.nice.org.uk/guidance/CG62 (accessed December 2018).

Aortocaval compression

Aortocaval compression (supine hypotensive syndrome) was first reported in 1931. The inferior vena cava and aorta become compressed by the pregnant uterus (the vena cava may be totally occluded), causing reduction in venous return and cardiac output, thus compromising the mother, the fetus or both. Vasovagal syncope may follow aortocaval compression. Maternal symptoms and signs vary from asymptomatic mild hypotension to total cardiovascular collapse, partly dependent on the efficacy of the collateral circulation bypassing the inferior vena cava. Onset of symptoms and signs is associated with lying in the supine or semi-supine position, and in most cases is relieved by turning to the full lateral position.

Problems and special considerations

Aortocaval compression is not confined to the woman at term. The condition has been reported in the fifth month of pregnancy. Women with multiple pregnancy or polyhydramnios are at increased risk because of the increased size of the gravid uterus.

It is important to appreciate that a normal blood pressure and lack of maternal symptoms do not exclude a significant fall in cardiac output and placental perfusion.

Onset of symptoms may occur within 30 seconds, but may be delayed by 30 minutes. Severity of symptoms is not a reliable guide to the severity of hypotension.

Slight changes in maternal position may cause significant change in symptoms. A 15-degree lateral tilt does not always relieve aortocaval compression, and even a 45-degree tilt does not guarantee abolition of hypotension.

Catastrophic hypotension, and even cardiac arrest, may occur if general anaesthesia is induced in a woman who is experiencing severe aortocaval compression (e.g. in the supine position). Even mild degrees of aortocaval compression may lead to severe hypotension after spinal or epidural anaesthesia.

It is impossible to perform effective cardiopulmonary resuscitation on a pregnant woman in the supine position, and the uterus must be displaced off the vena cava and aorta by tilting the pelvis or using manual displacement.

Management options

Women in late pregnancy will not voluntarily adopt positions in which aortocaval compression occurs, and therefore the condition is largely iatrogenic, occurring after a woman has been placed in the supine position by her midwifery or medical attendants. A history suggestive of aortocaval compression in late pregnancy may indicate an increased risk of developing the condition during labour and delivery. All healthcare staff must be aware of aortocaval compression and of the need to avoid the supine position. This is particularly important if the woman is unable to change her own position because of administration of analgesia or anaesthesia.

Uterine displacement (usually to the left, although occasionally improved symptomatic relief will be obtained by displacement to the right) must be used during all vaginal examinations, for fetal blood sampling, and for both vaginal and operative delivery, and is especially important if regional analgesia or anaesthesia is used. This can be achieved manually or by use of table tilt or a wedge under the hip. Use of uterine displacement rather than the full lateral position is a compromise between maternal safety and obstetricians' convenience. Use of the full lateral position for caesarean section has been reported.

Extreme vigilance is necessary during general anaesthesia, as the mother will not be able to report symptoms. During regional anaesthesia for operative delivery, complaints of faintness, dizziness, restlessness and nausea should alert the anaesthetist to the onset of hypotension. Pallor, particularly of the lips, yawning and non-specific feelings of anxiety are also warning signs of aortocaval compression. Continuous fetal monitoring may indicate signs of fetal distress when the mother adopts the supine or semi-supine position, and occasionally this may be the only indicator of the condition. Turning the mother into the full left lateral position should be the first step in the treatment of hypotension or cardiotocographic abnormalities.

Key points

- No pregnant woman should lie supine beyond 16–18 weeks.
- The uterus must be displaced off the aorta and vena cava during vaginal examinations and during caesarean section. This can be done manually, with a wedge under the hip, or by using lateral tilt of the operating table.
- Manual displacement of the uterus is essential for effective cardiopulmonary resuscitation in advanced pregnancy.

Further reading

Cluver C, Novikova N, Hofmeyr GJ, Hall DR. Maternal position during caesarean section for preventing maternal and neonatal complications. *Cochrane Database Syst Rev* 2013; (3): CD007623.

Lee A, Landau R. Aortocaval compression syndrome: time to revisit certain dogmas. *Anesth Analg* 2017; **125**: 1975–85.

Gastric function and feeding in labour

Physiological changes in pregnancy affect the volume, acidity and emptying of gastric secretions as well as sphincter mechanisms in the lower oesophagus. Interventions in labour such as analgesia may also affect these changes adversely. General anaesthesia is occasionally necessary in emergency situations, and the presence of a full stomach (and thus the risk of aspiration of gastric contents) should always be assumed in such patients (see Chapter 59, *Aspiration of gastric contents*). The increasing incidence of obesity in the pregnant population has raised concerns that these patients may be at more risk of aspiration should they need a general anaesthetic for operative delivery.

Problems and special considerations

Increased circulating progesterone associated with pregnancy relaxes smooth muscle and causes relaxation of the lower oesophageal sphincter, whereas placental gastrin increases the volume and decreases the pH of gastric contents. The enlarging uterus increases intragastric pressure and there is an increase in small and large bowel transit time. However, evidence suggests that gastric emptying per se is not affected by pregnancy, although it may be decreased in labour if opioids are given.

Epidural analgesia with local anaesthetic solutions in labour is associated with normal gastric emptying, whereas subarachnoid or epidural opioids (fentanyl or diamorphine) in large doses cause a modest decrease in gastric emptying. Systemic opioid analgesia causes a much greater and prolonged decrease in gastric emptying. There are some randomised trials that have demonstrated large gastric volumes and a high incidence of vomiting in women allowed to eat solid food, even when pain was adequately controlled with a low-dose fentanyl/bupivacaine epidural. Previous studies suggested that oral intake of food during labour may be associated with a longer duration of labour and also possibly an increase in caesarean section rate, but recent evidence suggests that this is not the case.

The risk of gastroesophageal reflux is considerably reduced within 48 hours of delivery, owing to the decreasing progesterone level and the relief of raised intra-abdominal pressure. Nevertheless, the period of risk of aspiration extends to a poorly defined time after delivery, and appropriate general anaesthetic management in the early postpartum period remains somewhat controversial.

Routine withholding of food and fluids in labour has been challenged by a number of authors, particularly those who are not anaesthetists. They point out that absolute starvation is not popular with mothers, that aspiration associated with emergency general anaesthesia nowadays is uncommon owing to the increase in use of regional anaesthesia, and that there may be risks associated with prolonged starvation. On the other hand, there is little evidence that a period of starvation during labour is harmful, although it may be unpleasant. Starvation is associated with ketosis, but this has not been found to affect the duration or outcome of labour.

Management options

There are three approaches to the treatment of feeding in labour. The traditional approach is to assume that all women in labour are at risk of an event that will require emergency general anaesthesia, and that they are therefore at risk of aspiration of large volumes of acid gastric contents. As a consequence of this assumption, all women in labour are starved, allowed only sips of water to drink and given regular H_2-antagonists and antacids (see Chapter 59, *Aspiration of gastric contents*). This regimen has become less common in recent years for the reasons discussed above. In addition, women who know that a unit's policy is not to allow any oral intake are more likely to 'binge' before admission in labour, potentially negating any benefit from the policy.

Another approach is to assume that women in labour require food and fluid and to give these liberally. Often no H_2-blockers are given. A more rational approach is to stratify management on the basis of risk factors such as morbid obesity, upper gastrointestinal tract abnormalities or an increased likelihood of operative intervention. Current guidance from the National Institute for Health and Care Excellence (NICE) recommends that parturients should be advised that they may consume a light diet during labour unless they have received opioids or they become at a higher risk of receiving general anaesthesia. H_2-receptor antagonists should be considered for the higher-risk group. For those who do eat and drink during labour, substances that are associated with slower gastric emptying (those with high fat or sugar content) should be discouraged in favour of low-residue foods and isotonic drinks.

If intravenous water is required in labour, the most sensible fluid to provide might be 5% or 10% dextrose. Unfortunately, this has been associated with fluid overload in the mother and hyponatraemia in the neonate. However, modest volumes (< 1 litre) do not significantly affect neonatal plasma sodium concentrations. Many units give relatively low volumes of intravenous saline, dextrose–saline or Hartmann's solution when intravenous fluid is considered necessary.

Key points

- Solid food ingested during labour is not predictably absorbed.
- Women treated with epidural analgesia may have normal gastric emptying unless large boluses of opioid are given.
- Opioids given parenterally markedly decrease gastric emptying.
- Acid aspiration prophylaxis should be given to all women at risk of intervention in labour.

Further reading

National Institute for Health and Care Excellence. *Intrapartum Care for Healthy Women and Babies.* Clinical Guideline 190. London: NICE, 2014 (updated 2017). www.nice.org.uk/guidance/cg190 (accessed December 2018).

O'Sullivan G, Liu B, Hart D, Seed P, Shennan A. Effect of food intake during labour on obstetric outcome: randomised controlled trial. *BMJ* 2009; **338**: b784.

Singata M, Tranmer J, Gyte GM. Restricting oral fluid and food intake during labour. *Cochrane Database Syst Rev* 2013; (8): CD003930.

Sperling JD, Dahlke JD, Sibai BM. Restriction of oral intake during labour: whither are we bound? *Am J Obstet Gynecol* 2016; **214**: 592–6.

Drugs and pregnancy

Pregnancy may interact with drugs in a number of different ways. Firstly, the pregnant state confers alterations in both pharmacokinetics and pharmacodynamics; secondly, the fetus may be affected by drugs administered to the mother, and in many cases this may restrict the use of certain drugs; and thirdly, there may be further passage of certain drugs to the neonate in breast milk (see Chapter 162, *Drugs and breastfeeding*). Because of these considerations, special licensing requirements exist for drugs to be used in pregnancy, which have not been met by many drugs in current use.

Pharmacokinetics

Each of the traditional components of pharmacokinetics may be altered in the pregnant, as opposed to the non-pregnant, state.

- **Absorption of drug.** This depends on the route of administration and, in general, is little affected by pregnancy. However, absorption of enterally administered drugs may be affected by pregnancy-associated gastrointestinal upsets including vomiting and delayed gastrointestinal motility. However, a higher cardiac output increases intestinal blood flow, which may counter these effects, and there is little evidence to suggest altered bioavailability of drugs sufficient to alter dosage. Enterally administered drug absorption may be delayed in labour, particularly after administration of opioids. Drugs administered intramuscularly are often absorbed more rapidly due to increased tissue perfusion. Owing to the increased minute ventilation and cardiac output, absorption of inhalational agents is more rapid.
- **Distribution of drug.** This is affected by the increased blood volume and body fluids, and altered plasma protein profile, which vary as gestation progresses. The first two result in a greater volume of distribution. Decreased plasma protein binding can lead to increased availability of free drug, resulting in an increased risk of toxicity, particularly of highly protein-bound drugs such as phenytoin and local anaesthetics. In addition, the fetus represents an additional compartment to which drugs will distribute, depending on their lipid solubility, pKa and protein binding. The increased cardiac output will tend to redistribute drugs more quickly unless they are extensively bound to the tissues. During labour, acute changes in plasma pH (e.g. acidosis associated with maternal exhaustion or alkalosis associated with pain-induced hyperventilation) may affect both protein binding and degree of dissociation of drug.
- **Metabolism of drugs.** Drugs broken down by the major organs (usually the liver) may be handled in the same way as in the non-pregnant state, unless there is hepatic impairment, e.g. in HELLP (haemolysis, elevated liver enzymes and low platelet count)

syndrome. Changes in the activity of enzymes involved in phase I and phase II metabolism, such as the cytochrome P450 family and uridine 5'-diphosphate glucuronosyltransferases (UGTs), may affect drug metabolism, and have been shown to alter concentrations of drugs such as nifedipine and lamotrigine. For drugs with a narrow therapeutic window, dosage alterations may be required in pregnancy to maintain disease control or avoid toxicity. Some drugs are metabolised by plasma cholinesterases, which are reduced in pregnancy and may lead to a longer duration of drug action; the clinical duration of suxamethonium may be prolonged.

- **Elimination.** Since glomerular filtration rate (GFR) is increased in pregnancy, clearance of many drugs is increased unless renal function is impaired, e.g. in pre-eclampsia. Variation in renally eliminated drugs in pregnancy does not merely reflect changes in GFR, suggesting changes in renal tubular transport also. Another route of elimination is in breast milk, although this represents a relatively small amount of total drug elimination. Inhalational agents are excreted via the lungs more rapidly in the pregnant than the non-pregnant state.

Pharmacodynamics

The effects of most drugs are unchanged in pregnancy. However, notable and important exceptions are anaesthetic agents. Thus the minimum alveolar concentration (MAC) of inhalational agents is reduced, as is the minimal blocking concentration of local anaesthetics. While the volume of distribution of thiopental is increased during pregnancy, it is clinically more effective, resulting in a similar dose requirement in the pregnant state. The cause of this decrease in anaesthetic requirement is thought to be progesterone and/or a metabolite thereof. In addition, a given amount of epidural local anaesthetic solution produces a more extensive block than in non-pregnant subjects, possibly related to the reduction in epidural space caused by epidural venous engorgement, although progesterone has also been suggested as a cause.

Fetal effects of drugs

Drugs may affect the fetus at any stage of pregnancy. During the first trimester, the developing organ systems and overall body structure are especially at risk, particularly between the third and tenth weeks; administration of certain drugs during this period may result in congenital malformations. During the second and third trimesters, the growth and development of fetal tissues may be affected. Finally, drugs given before delivery may affect fetal oxygenation indirectly (e.g. by causing maternal hypotension or respiratory depression), may affect labour (e.g. β-agonists), or may have neonatal effects after birth (e.g. opioids and non-steroidal anti-inflammatory drugs).

Many drugs are known to be harmful when given during pregnancy, but for many others, precise information is not always available. Thus, in general, drugs are not prescribed unless the benefits are felt to outweigh any possible risk, especially during the first trimester. Where possible, older drugs of which clinicians have greater experience are preferred over newer ones, and this is also true of anaesthetic agents.

Licensing of drugs in pregnancy

Many drugs, including anaesthetic agents, are not licensed for use in pregnancy, mainly because of the prohibitive costs to the manufacturer of performing the appropriate studies required and the relatively limited addition such licensing would make to the market. For example, the data sheets of many drugs, including fentanyl, contain the sentence 'safety in human pregnancy has not been established' or words to that effect, while that of propofol specifically warns against its use in obstetrics. Even in the case of thiopental, the data sheet merely states that there is 'epidemiological and clinical evidence' of its safety in pregnancy, whereas those of atracurium, vecuronium and suxamethonium state that they should only be used in pregnancy 'if the potential benefits outweigh any potential risks'. In 2015 the US Food and Drug Administration (FDA) created a pregnancy exposure registry, which may result in more data surrounding drug use in pregnancy.

Key points
- Pharmacokinetics and pharmacodynamics in pregnancy may be altered from those in the non-pregnant state.
- Most drugs administered to the mother will pass to the fetus to a degree.
- Many drugs pass into breast milk.
- Most anaesthetic drugs are not licensed for use in pregnancy.

Further reading

Henderson E, Mackillop L. Prescribing in pregnancy and during breast feeding: using principles in clinical practice. *Postgrad Med J* 2011; **87**: 349–54.

Howell PR, Madej T. Administration of drugs outside of product licence: awareness and current practice. *Int J Obstet Anesth* 1999; **8**: 30–6.

World Health Organization. *Breastfeeding and Maternal Medication: Recommendations for Drugs in the Eleventh WHO Model List of Essential Drugs*. Geneva: WHO, 2002. http://whqlibdoc.who.int/hq/2002/55732.pdf (accessed December 2018).

Placental transfer of drugs

The placenta is a complex structure composed of both maternal and fetal tissues. In order for a substance to reach the fetal circulation, it must cross the endometrial arteries, intervillous spaces, syncytiotrophoblast, fetal connective tissue, and the endothelium of fetal capillaries. Nevertheless, it is basically a semi-permeable biological membrane and as such obeys the laws that govern transport across such membranes.

Most transfer of drugs across the placenta occurs by simple diffusion. In addition, some drugs will reach the fetal circulation through facilitated diffusion, whereby a carrier molecule aids transfer down the concentration gradient (e.g. glucocorticoids), or through active transport (e.g., noradrenaline). All drugs administered to the mother will reach the fetus, albeit to a variable extent depending on the factors discussed below.

Factors determining placental transfer

Molecular weight and lipid solubility

The molecular weight of the drug, its degree of ionisation, its lipid solubility and the degree to which it is protein-bound will all affect the readiness with which it crosses the placenta. The majority of anaesthetic drugs are small (molecular weights < 500 Da) and lipid-soluble; thus they cross the placenta readily. The main exceptions are the neuromuscular blocking drugs, which are less lipid-soluble, more highly ionised quaternary ammonium compounds, and in the doses used in normal clinical anaesthesia do not cross the placenta to any significant extent. However, if used in large doses or over a prolonged period of time (e.g. to facilitate artificial ventilation in the intensive care unit) they do reach the fetal circulation in doses that may have a clinical effect necessitating ventilatory support. Opioids also cross the placenta, fentanyl being highly lipid-soluble, and morphine being only 35% protein-bound.

Changes in maternal or fetal pH may alter the degree of ionisation and protein binding of a drug, and thus alter its availability for transfer. This is most likely to occur if the pKa of a drug is close to physiological pH, and becomes clinically relevant in the acidotic fetus. Once drug transfer to the fetus has occurred, acidosis results in increased ionisation of the drug, which is then unable to equilibrate with the maternal circulation by diffusion back across the placenta. This results in drug accumulation in the fetus ('ion trapping'), and is particularly relevant for local anaesthetics, which all have a pKa greater than 7.4.

Maternal drug concentration

Drug transfer occurs down a concentration gradient (which is usually from mother to fetus but can also occur from fetus to mother). The drug concentration on the maternal side depends on the route of administration, total maternal dose, volume of distribution and drug clearance and metabolism. The highest maternal blood concentration of a drug will be achieved following intravenous administration; epidural and intramuscular administration result in similar maternal blood concentrations. Systemic drug absorption will be greater from more vascular tissues, such as the paracervical region. The increase in blood volume and cardiac output that accompanies normal pregnancy has an effect on maternal drug concentration; the volume of distribution and plasma clearance of drugs such as thiopental is increased.

Placental factors

The area of placenta available for transfer is important. Physiological shunting occurs in the placenta, and in maternal disease such as pre-eclampsia the placenta itself may present an increased barrier to transfer. Although there is evidence that some drug metabolism occurs within the placenta itself, this is not clinically significant.

Fetal drug concentration

Once a drug has reached the fetus it is subject to redistribution, metabolism and excretion. The fetus has less plasma protein-binding capacity and less mature enzyme systems than the mother, and will therefore eliminate drugs less effectively. Some transfer of drugs occurs back across the placenta to the mother if the maternal concentration falls below that in the fetus (unless ion trapping occurs – see above).

Uteroplacental blood flow

This is the other major factor influencing placental transfer. Any reduction in blood flow to the placenta will inevitably reduce transfer of drugs (and nutrients) to the fetus. Reduction in uteroplacental flow may occur as a result of generally reduced maternal blood flow (hypotension, reduced cardiac output states, aortocaval compression, generalised vasoconstriction) or direct obstruction of flow (aortocaval compression, uterine contraction, umbilical cord compression).

Problems and special considerations

All general anaesthetic agents cross the placenta readily, and in normal clinical practice their effects on the fetus are only of significance immediately after delivery. The compromised fetus, or one in whom the interval between uterine incision and delivery has been prolonged, may be depressed at birth, but rarely requires more than simple resuscitative measures.

Pethidine (and all other opioids) crosses the placenta readily. It has maximal effect in the fetus 3–4 hours after maternal administration and minimal effect if given to the mother within an hour of delivery. (This is contrary to traditional midwifery teaching, which recommends that pethidine is not given if delivery is expected within 2–3 hours.) Both pethidine and its active metabolite norpethidine have prolonged half-lives in the fetus and cause respiratory depression and reduced sucking ability. While remifentanil rapidly crosses the placenta, it is also rapidly metabolised by the neonate, reducing the likelihood of side effects. Opioid side effects are reversed by naloxone.

Local anaesthetics cross the placenta by simple diffusion, but the extent of placental transfer is also dependent on maternal plasma protein binding (bupivacaine and ropivacaine are highly protein-bound, and therefore cross less readily than lidocaine, which is less protein-bound).

Key points

- The major determinants of transfer by simple diffusion are the maternal–fetal drug concentration gradient, molecular weight of the drug, lipid solubility, degree of drug ionisation and extent of protein binding.
- Uteroplacental blood flow is also important.
- Opioids given to the mother for labour analgesia cross the placenta freely and may cause fetal respiratory and neurobehavioural depression, which are reversible with naloxone.

Further reading

Griffiths SK, Campbell JP. Placental structure, function and drug transfer. *Contin Educ Anaesth Crit Care Pain* 2015; **15**: 84–89.

Littleford J. Effects on the fetus and newborn of maternal analgesia and anesthesia: a review. *Can J Anesth* 2004; **51**: 586–609.

Prescription and administration of drugs by midwives

In the UK, regulations for the prescription and administration of drugs by midwives fall under the responsibility of the Nursing and Midwifery Council (NMC), which issues codes and standards relating to the practical application of Acts such as the Medicines Act 1968 (now broadly repealed by the Human Medicines Regulation 2012), the Misuse of Drugs Act 1971, and the Medicinal Products: Prescription by Nurses Act 1992, and their subsequent amendments. From 2019, the Royal Pharmaceutical Society's Competency Framework for all Prescribers will be adopted as the NMC's standards of competency for prescribing practice.

Many of the NMC's publications on the matter are not legally binding but would be taken into account if there were to be medicolegal or regulatory action concerning administration of drugs. Against this background of central control, the setting up of, and adherence to, local policies is strongly encouraged, in recognition of the differing requirements from unit to unit.

A compromise must exist between: (1) supporting the midwife's role as an independent practitioner, (2) reducing the workload on medical staff by not requiring them to treat common and relatively minor conditions, (3) permitting the rapid administration of drugs that may have real benefits to mothers and reduce morbidity or mortality, and (4) restricting the use of potentially harmful drugs or reducing the incidence of adverse effects. Whether a particular drug should be allowed to be given thus depends on the incidence, importance and potential severity of the condition for which it is indicated and the efficacy, method of administration and safety profile of the drug concerned. In recent years, many NHS trusts have developed strategies for improving safety in administering drugs, along with improved methods of assessing competency for nursing and midwifery staff.

Drugs that midwives can administer without medical prescription

Registered midwives may prescribe and administer any of the drugs that are specified under midwives' exemptions; this includes drugs such as lidocaine, oxytocin and pethidine (Table 17.1). As of 2011, midwifery students may also administer drugs on the midwives' exemption list (apart from controlled drugs), under the direct supervision of a midwife. Exemptions are distinct from prescribing, which requires the involvement of a pharmacist and the completion of an accredited prescribing course. The NMC attributes professional accountability for any prescribing decisions to the prescribing midwife.

There is regional variation according to local policies, and individual trusts bear ultimate responsibility for approving drug policies within their maternity services. Local regulations are usually decided by a panel including representatives of midwives, pharmacists and

Table 17.1 Sample standing orders for drugs that may be prescribed and administered by midwives without medical prescription

Analgesics	Opioids (usually pethidine, up to two intramuscular doses)
	Paracetamol; codydramol; cocodamol
	Entonox
	Diclofenac
Local anaesthetics	Lidocaine for infiltration/local application
Gastrointestinal	Liquid antacids
	Laxatives
	Cyclizine; prochlorperazine
Oxytocics	Oxytocin; ergometrine; carboprost
Haematological	Iron/folate oral preparations
	Anti-D immunoglobulin
	Hepatitis B vaccine/immunoglobulin
	Vitamin K (neonatal)
Other	Adrenaline 1:1000 intramuscular (for anaphylaxis)
	Gelofusine; Hartmann's solution; 0.9% saline
	Naloxone (adult and neonatal)
	Topical clotrimazole/nystatin; hydrocortisone
	Transcutaneous electrical nerve stimulation (TENS)

obstetricians; anaesthetic staff may also be involved, for example in helping with analgesic or local anaesthetic drug policies.

Midwives in different units may interpret the NMC's guidelines differently, especially with regard to epidural top-ups; for example, midwives in certain units may be prepared to administer epidural drugs prescribed by a doctor (i.e. an anaesthetist) whereas those in others may not. This is rarely a problem with local anaesthetic drugs alone but may be problematic with mixtures of local anaesthetics and opioids, e.g. fentanyl, which are both controlled drugs and unlicensed for epidural use. In all cases, midwives' willingness to give epidural drugs is only on the understanding that ultimate responsibility for administering the drug is with the anaesthetist.

The regulations are regularly reviewed, with recent attention being paid to administration of intravenous fluids to reflect (1) the widespread competence of midwives in venous cannulation and (2) the number of women choosing to deliver at home and therefore the potential for severe haemorrhage away from hospitals.

Key points

- The Nursing and Midwifery Council (NMC) issues professional guidelines and codes for administration of drugs by midwives.

- Midwives are able to administer several drugs without a doctor's prescription, according to the NMC's recommendations and local policies.
- Midwives may administer certain drugs unlicensed for use in labour, e.g. epidural fentanyl, if covered by local policies and on the written prescription of a doctor.

Further reading

Nursing and Midwifery Council. *Standards for Medicines Management*. London: NMC, 2007 (updated 2015). www.nmc.org.uk/standards/standards-for-post-registration/standards-for-medicines-man agement (accessed December 2018).

Royal Pharmaceutical Society. *Safe and Secure Handling of Medicines: a Team Approach*. London: RPS, 2005 (updated 2018). www.rpharms.com/resources/professional-standards/safe -and-secure-handling-of-medicines (accessed December 2018).

Local anaesthetics

Bupivacaine, lidocaine, ropivacaine and levobupivacaine (the S-enantiomer of bupivacaine) are all licensed for obstetric epidural use in the UK, and heavy (hyperbaric) 0.5% bupivacaine and heavy 2% prilocaine are the only local anaesthetics licensed for obstetric spinal use (levobupivacaine is licensed for non-obstetric spinal anaesthesia). These local anaesthetics are all amides. There are no local anaesthetics in the ester group in use in British obstetric anaesthesia, although chloroprocaine is used in the USA owing to its speedy onset and offset, and possible reduced incidence of fetal ion trapping because of its rapid breakdown by plasma esterases in the maternal circulation (see Chapter 16, *Placental transfer of drugs*).

Pharmacology

Local anaesthetics act by reducing permeability of the nerve cell membrane to sodium, preventing development of a propagated action potential. The local anaesthetic binds to receptor sites within the sodium channels of the nerve membrane. Increasing lipid solubility allows the local anaesthetic drug to penetrate the nerve membrane more readily, and is associated with increased potency (bupivacaine and levobupivacaine have greater lipid solubility than lidocaine and ropivacaine).

Increased capacity for protein binding increases the duration of action of the local anaesthetic. Bupivacaine and levobupivacaine are 95% protein-bound and ropivacaine is 94% protein-bound, and these drugs therefore have a longer duration of action than lidocaine, which is only 64% protein-bound.

The speed of onset of local anaesthetic activity is related to the degree of ionisation of the drug. The non-ionised form of the drug diffuses across the nerve sheath to reach the nerve membrane. The degree of ionisation is dependent on the pKa of the drug. Bupivacaine, ropivacaine and levobupivacaine all have a pKa of 8.2 and are therefore more ionised (and thus have a slower onset of anaesthetic action) at body pH than lidocaine, which has a pKa of 7.7. Addition of bicarbonate to local anaesthetic solutions speeds onset time and may improve the quality of the block.

The development of the minimum local analgesic concentration/dose (MLAC/D) technique, using an up–down sequential allocation model, has enabled relative analgesic potency ratios to be determined for epidural analgesia (and to a lesser extent, spinal analgesia/anaesthesia). In this technique, the first patient in a study group is given a set volume of a certain concentration (MLAC) or a set volume containing a certain dose (MLAD). If the target response is achieved (e.g. pain scores < 1 cm on a scale of 0–10 cm), the next patient receives a 20% decrease in concentration/dose; if the target response is not achieved the next patient receives a 20% increase. The process is repeated and the median effective dose (ED_{50}) may be derived from the resultant graph of responses. This technique has allowed the potencies of different local anaesthetics and the effect of additives (e.g. opioids) to be compared. Studies have suggested the relative potencies of epidural ropivacaine : levobupivacaine : bupivacaine to be 0.7:0.9:1.0. They have also shown that the MLAC of bupivacaine increases as labour progresses, suggesting increased analgesic requirements as further pain fibres are recruited.

The amide local anaesthetics are metabolised by the liver and excreted via the kidney.

Toxicity

Systemic toxicity of local anaesthetics is manifest as central nervous system (CNS) excitability (caused by inhibition of inhibitory fibres) that may lead to convulsions and, later, to CNS depression. Local anaesthetics also affect the cardiovascular system. Toxic doses cause depolarisation of cardiac cell membranes and systemic vasodilatation; this may lead to cardiovascular collapse. The parturient appears to be particularly sensitive to local anaesthetic toxicity; suggested reasons for this include greater uptake due to increased vascularity and cardiac output, increased free fraction of the drug due to altered protein binding, and altered cardiomyocyte electrophysiology and neuronal susceptibility due to hormonal changes.

Resuscitation of the pregnant patient is notoriously difficult. In recent years, lipid rescue has become established as the treatment of choice in local anaesthetic toxicity; experience in pregnancy is limited, but its use is advocated in parturients as for non-pregnant patients.

The margin between the systemic concentration of local anaesthetic causing CNS symptoms and signs and that causing cardiovascular signs is smaller for bupivacaine than for the other local anaesthetic agents in clinical use, and it is this problem that has stimulated the development of newer local anaesthetics. Bupivacaine appears to be particularly cardiotoxic in pregnancy, causing ventricular arrhythmias and asystolic cardiac arrest. Both ropivacaine and levobupivacaine appear to have a wider safety margin than bupivacaine.

The addition of adrenaline to lidocaine reduces its systemic absorption and therefore permits administration of larger doses (up to 7 mg/kg body weight, compared with 3 mg/kg if adrenaline is not used), while prolonging its action. This is not the case with bupivacaine, the maximum dose of which is 2 mg/kg.

Amide local anaesthetics have a minimal chance of causing allergic reactions, unlike the ester group.

Differential block

The ideal local anaesthetic for obstetric analgesia would provide complete sensory analgesia of rapid onset and long duration without any motor blockade. Although bupivacaine provides long-lasting sensory block, this is accompanied (especially at increasing dosage) by motor blockade. Ropivacaine has similar action at higher concentrations, but at lower concentrations is claimed to produce differential sensory block by preferential action on C fibres. The extent to which this is clinically significant is still unproven, and the increasing use of very low concentrations of local anaesthetic combined with opioids for labour analgesia may make any difference clinically irrelevant.

Key points

- All the local anaesthetics used in British obstetric anaesthetic practice are amides.
- Anaesthetic potency is proportional to lipid solubility.
- Duration of action is proportional to extent of protein binding.
- Speed of onset of action is proportional to the amount of non-ionised drug present.
- Systemic toxicity is manifest by CNS excitability followed by cardiovascular depression. The margin of safety between CNS and cardiovascular toxicity is lowest for bupivacaine. Lipid rescue is recommended for local anaesthetic toxicity.

Further reading

Association of Anaesthetists of Great Britain and Ireland. *Management of Severe Local Anaesthetic Toxicity*. London: AAGBI, 2010. www.aagbi.org/sites/default/files/la_toxicity_2010_0.pdf (accessed December 2018).

Bern S, Weinberg G. Local anesthetic toxicity and lipid resuscitation in pregnancy. *Curr Opin Anaesthesiol* 2011; **24**: 262–7.

Normal labour

A large number of pregnant women are assessed as being 'low-risk' and are predicted to have a normal labour, but the diagnosis of normal labour is retrospective.

The parameters for normal labour are:

- Contractions once in every 3 minutes, lasting 45 seconds
- Progressive dilatation of the cervix
- Progressive descent of the presenting part
- Vertex presentation with the head flexed and the occiput anterior
- Labour not lasting less than 4 hours (precipitous) or longer than 18 hours (prolonged)
- Delivery of a live healthy baby
- Delivery of a complete placenta and membranes
- No complications

A low-risk mother would traditionally have midwife-led care. Low-risk multiparous women may choose to give birth at home or in a midwifery-led unit, where the rate of intervention is lower and neonatal outcome the same. There is a small increase (of about 4 per 1000 births) in adverse neonatal outcomes for low-risk nulliparous women who choose a home birth.

A labour record is kept to measure and record the vital signs of the mother and fetus, together with the progress of labour. It also serves as a record of events should an adverse outcome occur, especially if there is subsequent medicolegal involvement (see Chapter 170, *Medicolegal aspects*; Chapter 171, *Record keeping*). A list of items recorded would normally include:

- Fetal heart rate every 15 minutes
- Cervical dilatation at least every 4 hours
- Descent of the presenting part
- Colour of the liquor
- Fetal pH if relevant
- Amount of oxytocics given
- Strength and frequency of uterine contractions
- All drugs administered, including those for an epidural
- Maternal blood pressure, pulse rate and temperature
- Urine volume and analysis for ketones, protein or glucose
- Fluid input

The most commonly used means of charting the progress of labour is the partogram, which presents the data in a graphical form. 'Normal' curves may be printed on the partogram, obtained from large numbers of healthy primigravidae and multigravidae, against which it is easier to assess the progress of labour. An example of a partogram is shown in Figure 19.1.

First stage of labour

During the latent phase, the cervix effaces and then cervical dilatation begins. This may be associated with painful contractions. A woman is said to be in established labour once regular contractions occur and there is progressive cervical dilatation from 4 cm. The rate of cervical dilatation should be around 0.5 cm per hour for a primiparous woman and 1 cm per hour for a multigravid woman.

It is standard practice to perform a vaginal examination every 4 hours to assess the dilatation of the cervix, or more frequently if there is cause for concern. The fetal heart may be monitored intermittently by auscultation using Pinard's stethoscope or by cardiotocographic monitoring (see Chapter 20, *Intrapartum fetal monitoring*). The cardiotocogram (CTG) is recorded either intermittently or continuously depending on the condition of the fetus. Continuous recording of fetal heart rate may be done using either an abdominal transducer or a clip applied to the fetal head. Radiotelemetry is available in some units, and this allows the woman to be mobile while her baby is monitored. Uterine contractions may be monitored externally by an abdominal transducer or internally by an intrauterine catheter. The fetal heart rate and the uterine contractions are recorded together.

Second stage of labour

The second stage of labour commences at full dilatation of the cervix and terminates at the delivery of the baby.

At full dilatation of the cervix, the character of the contractions changes and they are usually, but not invariably, accompanied by a strong urge to push. In normal labour, there is an increase in circulating oxytocin secondary to Ferguson's reflex, with consequent increased strength of uterine contractions at full dilatation. Higher-dose epidural analgesia is thought to diminish the effect of this reflex.

The second stage of labour can be divided into passive and active stages, and this is particularly relevant when epidural analgesia is used. With epidural analgesia, especially using older, higher-dose techniques, the labouring woman may not have the normal sensation at the start of the second stage of labour. Therefore, the active stage of pushing should only commence when the vertex is visible or the woman has a strong urge to push. In normal labour, the active stage usually commences at full dilatation. Traditionally, the second stage is limited to 2 hours because of the risk of fetal acidosis; up to 3 hours is often allowed in the presence of epidural analgesia, in recognition of the slower descent of the fetal head. It is difficult for a woman to push efficiently for more than 1 hour, and after this time fetal acidosis is felt to be more likely. If there is not good progress, the advice of the obstetrician should be sought. Intramuscular oxytocics are given to hasten the delivery of the placenta and to stimulate uterine contraction: 10 U oxytocin (Syntocinon) intramuscularly after delivery of the anterior shoulder (so as not to exacerbate shoulder dystocia if present) is now considered the drug of choice, as it is associated with fewer side effects than oxytocin/ergometrine (Syntometrine).

Figure 19.1 Example of a partogram for assessing and recording the progress of labour. Reproduced with permission from Perinatal Institute, Birth Notes Version 17.1 (May 2017). © Perinatal Institute.

Third stage of labour

The third stage of labour is the complete delivery of the placenta and membranes and the contraction of the uterus. It is usually managed actively by administering an oxytocic as above, but it may also be managed physiologically without oxytocics. This may prolong the third stage and increase the risk of postpartum haemorrhage.

During the third stage of labour there is a major redistribution of (and increase in) maternal circulating blood volume. This is potentially dangerous to those women who have cardiac disease, who may be precipitated into heart failure immediately postpartum.

Figure 19.1 (cont.)

Departure from a normal labour

Certain signs may trigger departure from a normal labour and/or necessitate transfer to obstetric-led care:

- Maternal tachycardia (> 120 beats/minute on two occasions 30 minutes apart)
- Maternal hypertension (diastolic blood pressure (DBP) ≥ 110 mmHg or systolic blood pressure (SBP) ≥ 160 mmHg, or two consecutive readings of DBP ≥ 90 mmHg or SBP ≥ 140 mmHg)
- Proteinuria (2+ on urinalysis) and a single reading of raised blood pressure of 140/ 90 mmHg
- Pyrexia of 38 °C on a single reading, or 37.5 °C on two consecutive readings 1 hour apart
- Vaginal blood loss other than a show

- Rupture of membranes more than 24 hours before the onset of established labour
- Significant meconium
- Abnormal presentation or lie
- A high (> 4/5 palpable) or free-floating head in a primiparous woman
- Anhydramnios or polyhydramnios
- Fetal heart rate < 110 or > 160 beats/minute
- A fetal heart rate deceleration
- Reduced fetal movements reported in the last 24 hours
- A delay in the first or second stage of labour
- A retained placenta or a third/fourth-degree tear
- A request for regional analgesia; this does not in itself confer 'abnormality' to an otherwise uncomplicated labour, but may require transfer to obstetric-led care depending on local policy.

Key points

- Normal labour can be anticipated but can only be diagnosed after delivery.
- Routine recording of labour is a standard of care in maternity units.
- The partogram is used to chart labour, and for reference should a bad outcome or legal proceedings occur.
- The first stage comprises cervical effacement and dilatation.
- During the second stage, the baby passes through the birth canal.
- The placenta and membranes are delivered during the third stage.

Further reading

Ferguson E, Owen P. The second stage of labour. *Hosp Med* 2003; **64**: 210–13.

National Institute for Health and Care Excellence. *Intrapartum Care for Healthy Women and Babies.* Clinical Guideline 190. London: NICE, 2014 (updated 2017). www.nice.org.uk/guidance/cg190 (accessed December 2018).

Steer P, Flint C. Physiology and management of normal labour. *BMJ* 1999; **318**: 793–6.

Chapter

20

Intrapartum fetal monitoring

Fetal monitoring is an important part of intrapartum care since labour is a stressful event for the fetus, and the ability of the fetus to maintain oxygenation is tested with each uterine contraction. Fetal wellbeing can be monitored routinely using the following methods:

- Assessment of liquor colour
- Fetal heart auscultation
- Fetal heart cardiotocography (CTG)
- Fetal electrocardiography (ECG) waveform analysis
- Fetal blood sampling (FBS) and oximetry

Special considerations

A low-risk pregnancy uncomplicated by any obstetric or medical problems will need a low level of fetal monitoring during labour, whereas a high-risk pregnancy (e.g. one complicated by hypertensive disease of pregnancy or poor intrauterine growth) will need increased intrapartum monitoring (see Chapter 19, *Normal labour*). The labour itself can also be assessed as either low- or high-risk; it is generally recognised that a spontaneous labour is usually low-risk whereas an augmented labour or an induced labour is usually high-risk.

Liquor colour

When the membranes are ruptured, the liquor may be observed for the presence of meconium; this may indicate fetal hypoxia, which can cause the anal sphincter to relax allowing the fetus to pass meconium. Meconium may range from 'light' or grade-1 staining (in which a small amount of meconium diluted in a large volume of amniotic fluid gives the latter a greenish or yellowish discolouration), through 'moderate' or grade-2 staining (definite green/brown-coloured waters) to 'heavy' or grade-3 staining (thick, dark green/black-coloured fluid). Although such grading is commonly used, it has poor consistency between observers and poor predictive value for identifying degrees of fetal compromise. However, the appearance of thick new meconium is an indication for urgent delivery. If meconium is aspirated into the lungs of the neonate, severe lung damage may ensue; therefore, it should be aspirated from the neonate's mouth before intermittent positive-pressure ventilation is started. A paediatrician should be present at the delivery if meconium is observed. Meconium is more commonly seen in post-term labour.

Fetal heart rate and CTG

Fetal heart monitoring is recommended as follows:

1. **Low-risk** (low-risk pregnancy and normal labour). Intermittent monitoring with a Pinard's stethoscope is said to be as effective as CTG monitoring. Structured intermittent monitoring involves listening immediately after a contraction for a minimum of 60 seconds and repeating this every 15 minutes in the first stage of labour (every 5 minutes in the second stage). The maternal heart rate must also be recorded hourly to differentiate between maternal and fetal heart rates. It has been suggested that CTG monitoring in the low-risk group may lead to unnecessary intervention and increased anxiety.

2. **High-risk** (high-risk pregnancy and induced or augmented labour). Continuous CTG monitoring of the fetal heart rate is recommended. This records both the fetal heart rate and the uterine contractions (and thus the effect of the latter on heart rate can be observed). The monitor uses either an external transducer or a 'clip' applied to the fetal head. It is generally recommended that women with epidural analgesia have continuous fetal monitoring, although there is some evidence to suggest that women who have a mobile (low-dose) epidural may not need this. The need for continuous fetal monitoring during epidural analgesia is related to: (1) the cardiovascular instability that may follow administration of local anaesthetic solutions into the epidural space, (2) the transient fetal bradycardia that may follow administration of epidural or spinal opioids, and (3) any pre-existing maternal or fetal risk factors that contributed to the decision to have an epidural (e.g. previous caesarean section).

There are four features of the fetal heart rate that are especially important:

- **Baseline rate:** normally 110–160 beats/minute.
- **Variability:** normally 5–25 beats/minute. Opioids or other sedative drugs may cause a flat trace with a loss of beat-to-beat variability, which makes interpretation difficult.
- **Accelerations from baseline** (> 15 beats/minute for 15 seconds): two in 20 minutes are normally present. The significance of absent accelerations on an otherwise normal CTG is uncertain and so does not form part of the National Institute for Health and Care Excellence (NICE) description of CTGs (Table 20.1).
- **Decelerations from baseline:** normally absent. Decelerations are classified as early, variable and late. Early decelerations are synchronous with the contraction; they are benign and may be associated with compression of the fetal head in the pelvis. They mirror the uterine contractions and should be associated with good beat-to-beat variability. Variable decelerations vary in their shape, size and occurrence. They may or may not indicate fetal hypoxia. Late decelerations continue after the contraction has finished and are more ominous, especially if associated with other abnormalities, such as reduced variability.

The NICE guidelines give three descriptions of the CTG trace (reassuring, non-reassuring and abnormal; Table 20.1) and, based on this, give four management categories:

- **Normal:** all features are reassuring.
- **Suspicious:** one of the features is non-reassuring. This should prompt correction of any potential precipitating causes (such as hypotension or uterine hyperstimulation) and a plan for further review.
- **Pathological:** two non-reassuring features or one 'abnormal' feature is present. In addition to a review by a senior midwife and obstetrician and correction of any potential causes, fetal scalp stimulation, blood sampling and/or expedition of birth should be considered.

Table 20.1 Description of the CTG trace features

	Reassuring	Non-reassuring	Abnormal
Baseline (beats/minute)	110–160	100–109 or 161–180	< 100 or > 180
Variability (beats/minute)	5–25	< 5 for 30–50 minutes or	< 5 for > 50 minutes or
		> 25 for 15–25 minutes	> 25 for > 25 minutes or
			sinusoidal
Decelerations	None or Early or Variable with no concerning characteristics[a] for < 90 minutes	Variable with no concerning characteristics for > 90 minutes	Variable with concerning characteristics in > 50% contractions for > 30 minutes (or less if any maternal or fetal risk factors)
		Variable with concerning characteristics in < 50% contractions for > 30 minutes	Late decelerations for > 30 minutes
		Variable with concerning characteristics in > 50% contractions for < 30 minutes	Acute bradycardia or a single deceleration lasting > 3 minutes
		Late decelerations in > 50% contractions for < 30 minutes with maternal/fetal clinical risk factors	

[a] Concerning characteristics in variable decelerations include duration > 60 seconds; reduced variability within the deceleration; failure to return to baseline; biphasic shape; no shouldering.

Adapted from National Institute for Health and Care Excellence. *Intrapartum Care for Healthy Women and Babies*. Clinical Guideline 190. London: NICE, 2014 (updated 2017). www.nice.org.uk/guidance/cg190.

- **Need for urgent intervention:** acute bradycardia, or a single prolonged deceleration for 3 minutes or more. Delivery should occur if a bradycardia lasts 9 minutes.

Fetal heart rate monitoring has low specificity and sensitivity. Any trace that causes concern, especially in a high-risk pregnancy, is an indication for a fetal blood sample to be taken, unless there is evidence of acute fetal compromise, in which case urgent delivery is indicated. The CTG trace should be kept for at least 25 years in case of a later medicolegal claim.

Use of the CTG may be combined with fetal ECG waveform analysis (see below).

Fetal ECG waveform analysis

This requires application of an electrode to the scalp of the fetus following rupture of the membranes. It is thought that ST changes in the fetal ECG are associated with hypoxaemia.

Although this technique has not reduced the caesarean section rate, it is associated with a decrease in interventions during labour. Problems associated with its use include poor signal quality, difficulties in interpretation, poor compliance with guidelines and deterioration in the clinical status of the fetus without any ECG alert. Recently, European guidelines have been agreed with regard to ST waveform analysis, but it is not currently included in the NICE guidance.

Fetal blood sampling

When the fetus becomes hypoxic, there is a build-up of lactic acid and a reduction in the fetal pH. Fetal blood sampling allows a more accurate assessment of fetal wellbeing than the CTG and is likely to be performed whenever there is anxiety about the CTG or when there is meconium in the liquor. It is thought that the use of FBS may help reduce intraoperative interventions. The sample should be taken with the mother in the left lateral position and should not be taken immediately after a prolonged deceleration. Recommended actions for values of fetal pH and lactate are as follows:

- pH ≥ 7.25; lactate ≤ 4.1 mmol/l – should be repeated if the fetal heart rate abnormality continues.
- pH 7.21–7.24; lactate 4.2–4.8 mmol/l – borderline; should be repeated within 30 minutes, or delivery considered if there has been a rapid fall since the last sample.
- pH ≤ 7.20; lactate ≥ 4.9 mmol/l – indicative of significant acidosis and a need for urgent delivery of the baby.

Fetal gas tension measurement and oximetry

Non-invasive continuous transcutaneous measurement of oxygen and carbon dioxide tensions has been developed. This method requires the application of a suction ring to the baby's head; therefore the cervix needs to be dilated. Fetal oxygen saturation may also be measured by using special pulse oximeters; however, the technique is not yet reliable enough for routine use. Preliminary results suggest that fetuses normally have saturations of 30–60%.

These techniques may be influenced by skin contact, uterine contractions, caput on the baby's head and fetal hair.

Key points

- Good communication between anaesthetist, midwife and obstetrician is important.
- Fetal monitoring includes assessment of liquor colour, auscultation, cardiotocography and fetal scalp blood pH measurement.
- Fetal heart rate monitoring has poor specificity and sensitivity but this may be improved by ST analysis.

Further reading

Hinshaw K, Ullal A. Peripartum and intrapartum assessment of the fetus. *Anaesth Intensive Care Med* 2010; **11**: 324–32.

National Institute for Health and Care Excellence. *Intrapartum Care for Healthy Women and Babies.* Clinical Guideline 190. London: NICE, 2014 (updated 2017). www.nice.org.uk/guidance/cg190 (accessed December 2018).

Viswanatha RK, Talaulikar VS, Arulkumaran S. Intrapartum fetal surveillance. *Obstet Gynaecol Reprod Med* 2017; **27**: 363–72.

Pain of labour

The pain of primiparous labour is said to be one of the most severe pains experienced, reported to be exceeded only by the pains of traumatic amputation and causalgia. Approximately 50% of women report severe or very severe pain during labour. Painless childbirth is a reality for only a small minority of women, although labour pain can be modified by a number of non-pharmacological manoeuvres.

The pain pathways involved in labour and delivery are extensive, involving afferent fibres from T10 down to S4.

Pain pathways

The uterus, lower uterine segment and cervix are all supplied by afferent Aδ and C fibres, which accompany the thoracolumbar and sacral sympathetic outflows. The pain of the first stage of labour is therefore referred to the dermatomes supplied by the same spinal cord segments that receive input from the uterus and cervix: T10–L1 during the first half of the first stage and then the lower lumbar and sacral dermatomes as labour progresses.

The second stage of labour may also involve somatic pain caused by distension and tearing of pelvic structures and by abnormal pressure on perineal skeletal musculature.

Modification of labour pain

Psychological factors

There is considerable evidence that preparation for childbirth can significantly modify the degree of pain experienced. This was the basis of the 'childbirth without fear' movement, which was popular in the 1960s. Although there can be little doubt that fear, fatigue and anxiety enhance pain perception, it is misleading for the majority of mothers to suggest that good antenatal education will lead to painless childbirth. Such expectations may in fact have the reverse effect, since the mother may develop complete loss of self-confidence when she begins to experience significant labour pain.

Women whose pregnancy is unplanned or unwanted are likely to experience more pain, as are those who have no birth partner to support them during labour. Conversely, the continuous presence of a midwife or female birth partner (doula) has been shown to reduce the amount of pain reported.

Cultural factors and ethnic group also have an influence on pain behaviour during labour, although it is likely that women from different cultures and of different racial groups actually experience similar levels of pain.

Promise of a finite duration of labour (as with active management of labour) may improve the ability to tolerate labour pain, although not necessarily reduce the level of pain experienced.

Physical factors

First labours are acknowledged to be more painful than subsequent labours, and older primiparae experience more painful labours than do younger women. Malpresentations, especially occipito-posterior positions, increase the pain of labour. Augmentation of labour by oxytocic drugs is reported to increase labour pain, and obstructed labour is more painful than normal labour. Tiredness is well known to reduce pain tolerance and is likely to occur if either the latent or the active phase of labour is prolonged.

There is a positive correlation between menstrual pain and labour pain, which has been postulated to be caused by excessive prostaglandin production.

Physiological factors

Progesterone may increase pain thresholds, and there is some evidence that in rats there is activation of endogenous opioid systems during late pregnancy. Experimental work in humans appears to confirm this.

Untreated pain causes an increase in circulating maternal catecholamines and other stress hormones. This may be detrimental to the mother with coexisting medical disease, and is also detrimental to the fetus. Maternal pain and acidosis are associated with reduced uteroplacental blood flow and fetal acidosis.

Key points

- The pain of childbirth is one of the most severe pains experienced.
- Pain from afferent Aδ and C fibres is referred to the dermatomes of T10 to S4 and is augmented during the second stage of labour by somatic pain from stretching and tearing of pelvic structures.
- Labour pain may be modified by antenatal education, and by the presence of a supportive partner.

Non-pharmacological analgesia

Many women wish to avoid intervention in labour, including the use of pharmacolo-gical methods of analgesia. The use of psychoprophylaxis ('childbirth without fear') dates from the 1950s, and since then a variety of relaxation techniques have been introduced. Relaxation techniques, self-hypnosis, acupuncture, aromatherapy, reflexol-ogy, water labour/birth and transcutaneous electrical nerve stimulation (TENS) are now widespread.

Problems and special considerations

Fear of the unknown is a major factor in the experience of pain. Provision of antenatal education about the process of labour and the common complications that occur is an essential first step in the provision of analgesia for labour. Translations of information leaflets and availability of interpreters must be considered, especially in units delivering a significant number of women for whom English is not their first language. It is desirable to have an independent interpreter rather than a family member whenever possible. Videos about pain relief in labour are readily available and provide information in a format that is familiar and accessible to the majority of the population. Attendance at parentcraft classes should be encouraged.

Relaxation techniques

These range from simple breathing exercises to formal yoga techniques. There is a vast range of literature in the lay press about such techniques. The association between tension, anxiety and pain is well recognised, and the use of relaxation techniques should be encouraged for all pregnant women.

Self-hypnosis

Practitioners of hypnosis differentiate between a hypnotic state and deep relaxation. Hypnosis has been successfully used not only for pain relief in labour but also to provide anaesthesia for caesarean section. Hypnosis is time-consuming, requires con-siderable antenatal preparation, and is not freely available to the majority of women. Not all women are susceptible to its effects. While current evidence suggests that women taught self-hypnosis have reduced requirements for pharmacological analgesia overall, there is no decrease in the use of epidurals nor an increase in the rate of normal vaginal delivery.

Acupuncture, aromatherapy and reflexology

Acupuncture has much evidence to support its use in certain areas of medicine, but properly conducted studies in obstetric practice are few. What evidence there is from the few studies published mostly concerns manual acupuncture and suggests there may be a beneficial effect on pain and analgesic requirements in labour, including a reduced need for epidural analgesia.

Practitioners of aromatherapy and reflexology are becoming more numerous, and include an increasing number of midwives. The use of such analgesic techniques is dependent on the availability of a practitioner. The available evidence does not suggest a reduction in pain or analgesic requirements with aromatherapy. The National Institute for Health and Care Excellence (NICE) recommends that these techniques should not be provided in labour, but their use should be supported if women wish to use them.

Water

For decades, mothers have been advised to have warm baths to help them relax in early labour, and use of the pool for labour analgesia is an extension of this advice. Women who have had a lot of back pain during pregnancy often find the birthing pool particularly helpful. Benefit is thought to derive from inhibition of pain transmission and support of the gravid uterus by the warm water. Enthusiasts for the pool claim reduced rates of virtually all forms of medical intervention in labour, whereas some obstetricians view the pool as an unnecessary additional hazard for the labouring mother. The evidence regarding the first stage of labour suggests a reduction in labour pain and analgesic requirements with no effect on outcome of labour or neonatal status, and NICE recommends that water immersion should be an available option for women in labour.

Continuous fetal monitoring using telemetry that is suitable for use in water is available in some units, but if not, the mother with an at-risk fetus should be advised against using the pool. Similarly, the use of the pool is inadvisable in mothers needing intravenous infusions or any form of continuous maternal monitoring. Mothers requesting pharmacological analgesia should be asked to leave the birthing pool, though Entonox is usually allowed. In an emergency situation the mother should be helped out of the pool; an evacuation net may be required, and staff should be trained in its use.

TENS

The mechanism of action of TENS is through interference with transmission of efferent pain signals by electrical stimulation, according to the gate theory of pain. Particular benefit for TENS is claimed for women in early labour, those with backache associated with a posterior position, and women with a prolonged latent phase of labour.

The advantages of TENS are the absence of any effect on the fetus and the lack of any significant side effects for the mother. Meta-analysis of randomised controlled trials of TENS in labour suggests only limited evidence of its efficacy, and TENS is not supported by NICE for women in established labour, but it remains popular with mothers and midwives.

Water blocks

This technique involves the injection of small volumes of sterile water (0.1 ml) subcutaneously, or more commonly intracutaneously, over four spots lateral to the lumbosacral spine. It is thought that the mechanism of action is similar to that of TENS. Although it can be intensely painful for up to 30 seconds after injection, meta-analysis suggests a reduction in pain scores lasting up to 2 hours. Water blocks are common in certain countries but rarely used in the UK, and are not recommended by NICE.

Doulas

It is recognised that the constant presence of a supportive and encouraging second person reduces the pain scores of women in labour and may result in a reduced intervention. Some cultures ban the father from the labour room and provide a female partner for the labouring woman. There has been a resurgence of interest in use of birth partners, or doulas, in both the USA and the UK. The constant presence of the midwife during labour is also thought to reduce demand for analgesia and other interventions.

Management options

Anaesthetists should be aware of the benefits and limitations of non-pharmacological analgesia and be able to advise mothers when use of these methods of pain relief is or is not appropriate. It is important that anaesthetists realise that maternal satisfaction with pain relief in labour is not necessarily related to the degree of analgesia obtained. Many women benefit from the sense of control they gain from employing non-pharmacological methods of analgesia.

Non-pharmacological methods of pain relief have the major advantage of minimal or absent fetal and maternal adverse effects, and as such their use by mothers in normal, uncomplicated labour should be encouraged. However, prolonged use of these methods of pain relief by mothers with pregnancy or labour complications may increase the risk of ultimate recourse to general anaesthesia for delivery. For this group of women a change from non-pharmacological to regional analgesia is advisable.

Key points

- There is evidence for efficacy of several non-pharmacological methods of analgesia, and many women request them.
- Those techniques for which evidence of efficacy is limited or lacking still have minimal, if any, adverse effects, and women should not be denied them if that is their wish.
- Antenatal education should include all methods of analgesia available in a particular unit.

Further reading

Bohren MA, Hofmeyr GJ, Sakala C, Fukuzawa RK, Cuthbert A. Continuous support for women during childbirth. *Cochrane Database Syst Rev* 2017; (7): CD003766.

Cluett ER, Burns E, Cuthbert A. Immersion in water during labour and birth. *Cochrane Database Syst Rev* 2018; (5): CD000111.

Dowswell T, Bedwell C, Lavender T, Neilson JP. Transcutaneous electrical nerve stimulation (TENS) for pain relief in labour. *Cochrane Database Syst Rev* 2009; (2): CD007214.

Madden K, Middleton P, Cyna AM, Matthewson M, Jones L. Hypnosis for pain management during labour and childbirth. *Cochrane Database Syst Rev* 2016; (5): CD009356.

National Institute for Health and Care Excellence. *Intrapartum Care for Healthy Women and Babies.* Clinical Guideline 190. London: NICE, 2014 (updated 2017). www.nice.org.uk/guidance/cg190 (accessed December 2018).

Chapter

23

Inhalational analgesic drugs

The only agent licensed for inhaled analgesia in the UK is Entonox, which is a mixture of 50% nitrous oxide and 50% oxygen. Its advantages are that it is inexpensive, is almost universally available (including for use in the community), has a long record of safety, and is acceptable to many mothers and midwives; it is used in almost two-thirds of deliveries in the UK. Its low blood solubility means that blood levels rapidly reach a maximum after inhalation and fall once a contraction has passed and inhalation has ceased. It does not appear to have any detrimental effect on the fetus. The main disadvantage of Entonox is that it provides only limited pain relief.

Volatile anaesthetic agents such as methoxyflurane and trichloroethylene have been used for analgesia in labour, but these drugs have been withdrawn for non-obstetric reasons. They were administered using a draw-over vaporiser and breathing system and provided analgesia of slow onset because of their high blood solubility, with residual effects between contractions. Other volatile agents, including sevoflurane and desflurane, have also been studied, but none is widely used. A premixed preparation of isoflurane and Entonox (Isoxane) has been described, but this too is not widely available.

Problems and special considerations

Entonox is presented as a premixed agent, available in cylinders for community use and piped from central tanks in hospital maternity units. The mixture is stable under most conditions, but at very low temperatures the constituent gases separate out. This is relevant for community midwives practising in parts of the UK in winter, who must be aware that they need to invert Entonox cylinders several times before use to ensure adequate mixing.

Nitrous oxide is a relatively weak analgesic that exerts its effect through N-methyl-D-aspartate (NMDA) antagonism, thus benefiting 30–50% of mothers who use it, but with little effect on actual pain scores. Some women report benefit through distraction and concentration on breathing technique. Use of more than 50% nitrous oxide improves analgesic efficacy, but at the cost of increased maternal sedation and decreased inspired concentration of maternal oxygen. The use of the 50:50 mixture of nitrous oxide and oxygen represents a compromise between analgesic efficacy and maternal and fetal safety.

The efficacy of Entonox can be improved with good technique. About 45 seconds of use is required to achieve maximal effect, so the mother should be instructed to start inhaling as soon as she becomes aware of a contraction, and to continue inhalation until the contraction subsides. It is also important to ensure that if a facemask is used it is applied firmly to the face to avoid entraining air.

The mother administers the gas to herself from a demand valve via either facemask or mouthpiece. Maternal sedation may occur even with 50% nitrous oxide, especially if systemic opioids such as pethidine have been given, and it is therefore important that Entonox is self-administered, not administered by the midwife or by the woman's partner. The mother should also take a break from Entonox when not having a contraction. Overzealous use can lead to hyperventilation, hypocapnia, alkalosis and vasoconstriction.

Some mothers find inhalation of dry gases unpleasant, and in asthmatics this may provoke bronchospasm. Entonox also causes unacceptable nausea in a small number of women, and dizziness is common.

Although Entonox crosses the placenta readily, it is excreted by the neonatal lungs after delivery. Entonox does not have adverse effects on the fetus, but the maternal hyperventilation associated with its use may cause placental vasoconstriction and impair fetal oxygenation. Similarly, the combination of pethidine and Entonox has been associated with a high incidence of maternal arterial oxygen desaturation and should be avoided if there is evidence of fetal compromise.

There has been recent concern about the pollutant effects of Entonox. Many labour wards do not have any means of scavenging exhaled Entonox, and this is increasingly considered unacceptable. Scavenging equipment is available but obviously has resource implications.

Volatile anaesthetic agents cause dose-dependent uterine relaxation, although this can be overcome at low concentrations (< 0.5 MAC) by oxytocic drugs. They also have cardiorespiratory side effects, although these are usually minimal at low concentrations.

Key points

- Entonox provides acceptable (but incomplete) analgesia to up to half of the mothers who use it. It is appropriate for low-risk mothers in uncomplicated labour and for mothers awaiting regional analgesia.
- Entonox should not be recommended for high-risk mothers or as a supplement to inadequate systemic analgesia.

Further reading

Likis FE, Andrews JC, Collins MR, *et al.* Nitrous oxide for the management of labor pain: a systematic review. *Anesth Analg* 2014; **118**: 153–67.

Richardson MG, Lopez BM, Baysinger CL. Should nitrous oxide be used for labouring patients? *Anesthesiol Clin* 2017; **35**: 125–43.

Sutton CD, Butwick AJ, Riley E, Carvalho B. Nitrous oxide for labor analgesia: utilization and predictors of conversion to neuraxial analgesia. *J Clin Anaesth* 2017; **40**: 40–5.

Chapter 24

Systemic analgesic drugs

A variety of opioid analgesics has been used in the UK to reduce the pain of labour, and none has been found adequate for the majority of mothers. Pethidine is the most commonly used systemic analgesic in England and Wales, whereas in Scotland diamorphine is also common. Shorter-acting opioids such as fentanyl, alfentanil and remifentanil have also been used (see Chapter 25, *Intravenous patient-controlled analgesia for labour*). All opioid agents, given in equianalgesic doses, have similar advantages and disadvantages, and the widespread use of pethidine is largely due to historical reasons.

The major advantages of systemic opioid analgesia for labour are ease of administration, low cost, midwife autonomy of use and acceptability by many mothers. The major disadvantages are failure to provide adequate analgesia for many women (a third of women using pethidine will request epidural analgesia), general opioid side effects for the mother and rapid placental transfer to the fetus.

Drugs and administration

Midwives in the UK are authorised to give a total of 200 mg pethidine to a labouring mother, provided that the dose is divided, without a doctor's prescription. It is common practice to give 100 mg intramuscularly as the first dose. Blood levels of pethidine following intramuscular injection are unpredictable, and it is not possible to achieve therapeutic levels reliably with this standardised approach to administration. There is also little correlation between the weight of the mother, the amount of pethidine given and subsequent plasma concentration of pethidine. Pethidine has a long-acting metabolite, norpethidine, which accumulates in both the mother and fetus and has significant opioid activity. Its half-life is 21 hours in the mother and 63 hours in the fetus, compared with 3–7 hours and 13–23 hours respectively for pethidine. Norpethidine also has proconvulsant activity, and therefore on theoretical grounds pethidine is not an ideal analgesic for women with epilepsy or pre-eclampsia.

Intravenous administration of pethidine, either by medical staff or as patient-controlled analgesia (PCA; see Chapter 25), is more likely to achieve therapeutic plasma concentrations of the drug, but the intramuscular route remains the most commonly used.

Diamorphine is also used in some units, in doses of 5.0–7.5 mg intramuscularly. A recent UK-based randomised controlled trial found that diamorphine provided a modest improvement in analgesia over pethidine at the expense of a significantly longer labour.

Morphine has also been used but produces similar effects to pethidine and diamorphine; it is therefore rarely used in labour other than for miscarriage or terminations around 18–22 weeks.

Fentanyl has been used intravenously to provide labour analgesia, usually as PCA (see Chapter 25). The advantages are a rapid onset and short duration of action due to its high lipid solubility and volume of distribution. The general risks and benefits of opioid analgesics in labour apply, although severe neonatal depression is uncommon.

Remifentanil is a very short-acting opioid with characteristics that make it ideal for PCA in labour. It has been used to provide analgesia for women unable to have epidural analgesia, or in certain units as a less effective alternative to epidural analgesia for women not wishing to have an epidural but wanting something more effective than other methods of pain relief. It is only administered by PCA (see Chapter 25).

Side effects

These are common to all opioid drugs. Maternal side effects include:

- Altered respiratory pattern – hypoventilation occurs between contractions, but inadequate analgesia is accompanied by hyperventilation during contractions
- Reduced gastric motility
- Nausea and vomiting
- Sedation, dysphoria and euphoria

Mothers should be warned of the implications for other modes of analgesia if opioids are administered because of these side effects; for example, a period of 4 hours has traditionally been advocated after pethidine administration before an epidural solution containing fentanyl can be given, although this restriction is no longer widespread. Labouring women should also not go into a birthing pool if drowsy, or for at least 2 hours after opioids.

Drugs such as promethazine and promazine are still occasionally administered with pethidine in an attempt to reduce the incidence of nausea and vomiting, and these drugs considerably enhance the sedative effects of pethidine, sometimes to the extent that the mother has no clear recall of the events surrounding delivery.

All opioids cross the placenta freely because of their low molecular weight and high lipid solubility, and the fetus is particularly susceptible due to its reduced metabolism and elimination in comparison to the mother and its immature blood–brain barrier. Fetal effects include:

- Loss of heart-rate variability – the typical 'flat' cardiotocographic trace that results may make interpretation of any other changes difficult, but alone is not usually associated with worsening fetal acid–base balance.
- Neonatal respiratory depression, especially if given within 2–4 hours of delivery for pethidine or diamorphine (reversible with naloxone, although it is important to remember that naloxone is a short-acting drug and may need to be given either as an infusion or in repeated boluses). Studies have shown an increased need for neonatal resuscitation with maternal parenteral opioids in comparison with epidural analgesia.
- Depression of neonatal neurobehavioural scores for up to 3 days – the significance of this is not clear.
- Smaller likelihood of successful breastfeeding in babies whose mothers have received pethidine in labour, although there may be other psychosocial factors relevant to these findings.

Management options

The advantages of intramuscular opioid analgesia (simplicity of administration, low cost and acceptability to many midwives and mothers) have to be balanced against the disadvantages for both mother and baby, and the fact that the quality of analgesia is generally poor, although it may be useful in very early labour or prelabour. For mothers with significant medical disease and those at increased risk of operative delivery, regional analgesia is usually preferable. However, women unable to have regional analgesia (e.g. those with coagulation disorders) may benefit from PCA as an alternative.

Women receiving systemic opioid analgesia should be considered at risk of gastric stasis and advised accordingly regarding oral intake. Concurrent administration of H_2-antagonists should also be considered. In some units, metoclopramide is given concurrently to women receiving opioids as a non-sedating antiemetic.

Key points

- Pethidine is the most commonly used opioid analgesic for labour in the UK.
- Other opioids have similar risks and benefits.
- Patient-controlled analgesia (PCA) may improve efficacy and reduce side effects.
- Systemic opioid analgesia is not advisable for women at increased risk of operative delivery.
- Neonatal respiratory depression and impaired neurobehavioural scores may follow maternal administration of opioids.

Further reading

Littleford J. Effects on the fetus and newborn of maternal analgesia and anesthesia: a review. *Can J Anaesth* 2004; **51**: 586–609.

Phillips SN, Fernando R, Girard T. Parenteral opioid analgesia: does it still have a role? *Best Pract Res Clin Anaesthesiol* 2017; **31**: 3–14.

Smith LA, Burns E, Cuthbert A. Parenteral opioids for maternal pain management in labour. *Cochrane Database Syst Rev* 2018; (6): CD007396.

Intravenous patient-controlled analgesia for labour

The risk of side effects (particularly sedation and respiratory depression) associated with systemic opioids, traditionally given intramuscularly, led in the 1980s/1990s to the investigation of small, repeated doses of opioid that were self-administered by the patient herself (patient-controlled analgesia, PCA). Originally developed for postoperative analgesia (see Chapter 41, *Postoperative analgesia*), PCA was extended to administration of opioids in labour. Experience with older opioids (morphine, diamorphine, pethidine) was limited by their slow onset, long duration of action and persistence of side effects, but newer drugs (especially fentanyl and more recently remifentanil) are more suited to the PCA technique and are now in widespread use.

Choice of drug

The ideal drug for PCA in labour would have a very rapid onset, produce intense effective analgesia, and have a rapid offset with no or minimal side effects. Over the years, a succession of drugs and regimens has been used as drugs closer to meeting this ideal have become available:

- **Pethidine** was the first drug studied for PCA during labour (e.g. 10–20 mg with a lockout of 10 minutes), but is slow in onset and offset, with a risk of cumulation over time (including of its metabolite norpethidine).
- **Morphine** or diamorphine PCA has received less attention, but is sometimes used in early miscarriage or termination (e.g. 18–22 weeks), when effects on the fetus are no longer a concern.
- **Fentanyl** became a useful alternative to epidural analgesia in women unable to have the latter for medical reasons (e.g. 20–50 µg bolus with a lockout of 5–6 minutes). Use of fentanyl bolus doses has been reported to cause less neonatal depression than intravenous boluses of pethidine. However, its use has largely been superseded by that of remifentanil.
- **Alfentanil**, with its rapid onset and offset due to its small volume of distribution and low pKa, may seem well suited for labour analgesia, but there has been no evidence of benefit over the more familiar fentanyl PCA.
- **Remifentanil** is a very short-acting mu-opioid receptor agonist that is rapidly hydrolysed by red blood cell and tissue esterases and thus is thought to have the characteristics that are ideal for PCA in labour, despite not being licensed for this indication. Furthermore, studies suggest that fetal and neonatal effects are less than with other opioids, since the drug is rapidly metabolised after crossing the placenta. While uterine vein to maternal artery concentration ratio is 0.88, uterine artery to uterine vein

concentration ratio is 0.29, illustrating its high placental transfer followed by rapid fetal metabolism and redistribution. Although analgesia is incomplete, there exist two groups of women who might particularly benefit from remifentanil PCA: first, those unable to have an epidural sited for medical reasons; and second, those who do not necessarily want to have an epidural, but who just want analgesia that is more effective than the other methods.

Remifentanil's analgesic efficacy seems to lie between that of pethidine and neuraxial techniques. Current evidence suggests that remifentanil PCA is associated with improved patient satisfaction and pain scores and decreased conversion to epidural analgesia, in comparison with pethidine. While pain scores are better with epidural analgesia, patient satisfaction appears to be similar.

Regimens used usually include a 20–50 µg bolus with a lockout of 1–3 minutes. Background infusions are not recommended because of safety concerns (see below).

Side effects

All opioids share the same range of side effects, but common side effects of remifentanil PCA in practice include maternal drowsiness, nausea, pruritus and dizziness. However, the biggest concern is respiratory depression; this may be noted in nearly a third of women using remifentanil PCA. There have been several case reports of cardiac or respiratory arrest and even perimortem caesarean section associated with its use. Problems have been hypothesised to be patient-related (e.g. increased sensitivity), equipment-/administration-related (e.g. a bent arm resulting in a larger bolus dose when unbent), or due to the use of additional parenteral opioids in opioid-naive women. An increased prevalence of respiratory arrest has been noted in women using remifentanil PCA after an intrauterine death; this may be due to altered pharmaco-kinetics or a tendency to reduced monitoring/observation/presence of staff in these circumstances. It is vital, therefore, that midwifery staff are instructed not to leave a woman alone for a moment if she is receiving remifentanil PCA.

Remifentanil appears to result in fewer problems for the neonate than pethidine. Loss of beat-to-beat variability may be seen with remifentanil use, although this tends to be less marked than with pethidine. The need for neonatal resuscitation appears to be lower with remifentanil.

There may be some benefits of remifentanil PCA over epidural analgesia; the RemiPCA SAFE Network (which has collected data from over 20 hospitals worldwide, although only three from the UK) has noted an association between the use of remifentanil PCA and a lower incidence of pyrexia, a reduced need for oxytocin infusion and a shorter duration of labour than with epidural analgesia.

Management options

For its successful use, there must be locally developed guidelines, appropriate to the obstetric unit, which are strictly adhered to. In addition to careful monitoring of mother and baby, a member of staff who has been trained to observe for possible side effects (e.g. respiratory depression, bradycardia) must be present at all times. Suggested minimum standards for remifentanil PCA include oxygen saturation monitoring with regular doc-umentation of respiratory rate, sedation level and pain scores. A dedicated cannula with an anti-syphon valve should be used. Supplemental oxygen must be administered, and resuscitation drugs and equipment including naloxone and a bag-valve mask must be available.

If a unit plans to use remifentanil PCA, the staff need to be regularly trained and exposed to its use in order to gain familiarity and facilitate safe use.

Key points

- Intravenous PCA is thought to be a more logical and safer method of administering opioids during labour than intramuscular injection.
- Remifentanil PCA provides analgesia that is superior to other opioids, but inferior to neuraxial techniques.
- Remifentanil should only be used if a local protocol is adhered to and appropriate safety precautions are in place.

Further reading

Hinova A, Fernando R. Systemic remifentanil for labor analgesia. *Anesth Analg* 2009; **109**: 1925–9.
Muchatuta NA, Kinsella SM. Remifentanil for labour analgesia: time to draw breath? *Anaesthesia* 2013; **68**: 231–5.
Schnabel A, Hahn N, Broscheit J, *et al.* Remifentanil for labour analgesia: a meta-analysis of randomised controlled trials. *Eur J Anaesthesiol* 2012; **29**: 177–85.
Van de Velde M, Carvalho B. Remifentanil for labor analgesia: an evidence-based narrative review. *Int J Obstet Anesth* 2016; **25**: 66–74.

Chapter 26

Epidural analgesia for labour

The caudal route was the first approach used for epidural analgesia and anaesthesia in childbirth and was described in 1901. It has now been superseded by the lumbar route, with continuous lumbar epidural analgesia for labour described in the 1940s.

The use of epidural analgesia varies widely between different units in the UK, some small units having no provision and others having an epidural rate of over 50%.

It is generally accepted that epidural analgesia provides the most consistently effective form of pain relief during labour, and there are other benefits such as the ability to top up for instrumental delivery or caesarean section, and an improved fetal acid–base status if the mother is exhausted. Conversely, side effects and complications do exist, and the provision of a 24-hour epidural service is expensive. There are therefore differing (and often strong) views on the place of epidural analgesia in labour, held by mothers, midwives, obstetricians and obstetric anaesthetists.

Contraindications

The contraindications of epidural analgesia are the same as those in the non-pregnant population, but in the context of the above benefits, especially avoidance of general anaesthesia if an epidural catheter is in situ. The most common reasons for being unable to recommend epidural analgesia are coagulation disorders (whether iatrogenic or pathological), sepsis (local or systemic), and spinal neurological abnormality or the presence of metal or other implants around the lumbar region.

Consent

The modern emphasis on informed consent and the placement of mothers at the centre of their care have highlighted the difficulties that can exist when providing epidural analgesia for labour. There are many factors that may impair the usual consenting process, both antenatally and during labour itself; these are discussed further in Chapter 169, *Consent*.

Equipment

Provision of epidural analgesia for labour virtually always involves the insertion of an epidural catheter, usually with one of a variety of disposable epidural packs that are available. In the UK, these usually include a 16 G or 18 G Tuohy epidural needle, a multi-orifice catheter and a filter. Single, end-hole epidural catheters are popular in North America but are rarely used in the UK. Most epidural packs include a loss-of-resistance (LOR) syringe (strictly, called an LOR 'device' as they do not meet the standard for 'syringes') for identifying the epidural space.

If analgesia is to be provided by continuous infusion or patient-controlled epidural analgesia (PCEA), a suitable infusion syringe or pump will be required. Dilute solutions of local anaesthetic and opioid for either intermittent top-up or infusion may be prepared 'in-house' by the hospital pharmacy or may be purchased from an external manufacturer.

Technique

Epidural analgesia is traditionally commenced at or near the onset of established labour. However, it may be initiated earlier, for example before induction of labour or in those with significant risk factors such as morbid obesity or an unfavourable airway. Women who request epidural analgesia in advanced labour may have difficulty in adopting or maintaining the desired position for epidural placement, which may be challenging for the anaesthetist. These patients should be advised that delivery may precede the onset of effective labour analgesia.

Either a midline or a paramedian technique may be used to approach the epidural space. Both techniques are equally possible and acceptable in the lumbar spine, and the final choice of approach is usually determined by personal preference.

The epidural space is usually identified by LOR to the injection of saline, using a continuous injection technique. Although previously popular, because the presence of clear fluid must indicate dural puncture, the use of LOR to air is no longer advocated, as this is associated with a number of disadvantages including patchy block, subcutaneous emphysema, pneumocephalus and air embolism.

The continuous technique involves the operator's hand exerting a continuous pressure on the syringe plunger as the needle is advanced. Because saline is non-compressible, when the needle tip lies in the ligament or the ligamentum flavum there will be resistance to injection, which is lost as the epidural space is entered. With the intermittent technique, usually with air, the plunger is tested after each incremental advance of the needle. However, this technique is used less now as air is not routinely used for LOR; it is also thought that the intermittent technique may be associated with a higher incidence of dural puncture.

Once the epidural space has been identified, the epidural catheter is inserted through the needle, leaving 3–5 cm within the epidural space, and is secured to the mother's back. With shorter lengths inserted, the spread of the block is usually better, but there is a greater chance of the catheter falling out; longer lengths are associated with lower replacement rates but more one-sided blocks.

Ultrasound has been used to assist in locating the epidural space, for example by identifying the midline and/or depth of space before needle insertion. A number of studies have established that there is a considerable degree of error when manual palpation is used to identify the desired intervertebral level for neuraxial blockade. Insertion of a spinal needle at a higher space than intended carries the potential risk of injury to the conus. In addition, patients with impalpable bony landmarks or structural deformity of the spine may be exposed to additional risks associated with repeated punctures or failure to establish regional anaesthesia. Pre-procedural ultrasonography enables the operator to determine the optimal site for puncture and the needle trajectory, and allows a reliable estimation of the depth of the epidural space, which may reduce the number of attempts required for successful placement of a central neuraxial block.

Although the ultrasound-guided technique has established advantages, it is not without its limitations. Image acquisition may be challenging in obese patients, and there remains a margin of error in the identification of intervertebral levels, albeit smaller than that with clinical assessment. Learning the technique requires consistent practice, ideally in routine cases. It has been suggested that competency in neuraxial scanning may be achieved after the performance of a minimum of 30–40 scans.

Epidural drugs

In the 1970s and 1980s, the only drug used widely in the UK to provide epidural analgesia was bupivacaine, used in concentrations of 0.25–0.5%. During the past 30–40 years a variety of drug mixtures has been assessed. The most commonly used combination in the UK is now bupivacaine and fentanyl (0.1–0.125% bupivacaine with 2–2.5 µg/ml fentanyl). The reason for adding opioids to local anaesthetic is to enhance the quality of analgesia and to reduce the total dose of local anaesthetic given, with the intention of reducing both motor block and rates of instrumental vaginal delivery.

In North America, combinations of up to four drugs (bupivacaine, sufentanil, adrenaline and clonidine) have been recommended, but the benefit of using such mixtures, given the potential for drug errors, has been questioned. More recently, levobupivacaine (0.1–0.125%) or ropivacaine (0.2%) has been used alone or in combination with opioids.

These 'low-dose' mixtures are given as intermittent top-ups of 10–15 ml, infusions of 10–12 ml/hour, or PCEA. For the latter, several different methods have been described, but typical regimens consist of boluses of 8–15 ml with no background infusion, or boluses of 4–6 ml with a background infusion of 4–8 ml/hour. Suitable lockout periods are 5–20 minutes.

Infusions and PCEA have been shown to have similar efficacy to intermittent boluses, although the two former techniques have been associated with better maternal satisfaction and a lower workload for staff. The main advantages of PCEA techniques are the reduced consumption of local anaesthetic, and therefore reduced motor blockade, and improved patient satisfaction as mothers are also in control of their pain relief.

Recently, more sophisticated methods of drug delivery have been explored. These include programmed intermittent bolus administration (in which mandatory boluses are given, e.g. 10 ml low-dose solution every 30 minutes, instead of boluses on demand) and computer-integrated PCEA (in which basal infusion rates are adjusted according to the woman's demands/usage during the previous hour). A 'programmed intermittent mandatory bolus' technique has also been described, in which mandatory boluses are given unless the woman has received a self-administered bolus within a set time frame. Such techniques have been developed with the aim of reducing drug requirements and/or improving the quality of analgesia. They currently require sophisticated equipment and are not widely used.

Side effects and complications of epidural analgesia

Epidural analgesia is highly effective but is an invasive technique that has associated side effects and the potential for life-threatening complications (Table 26.1). It must not, therefore, be used unless there is adequate care from a suitably trained birth attendant and the ability to access advanced resuscitation facilities rapidly if required.

Epidural local anaesthetics cause sympathetic blockade and hypotension. Administration of intravenous fluids, vasopressor agents, or a combination of both, can prevent and/or treat this. Currently used low-dose combinations of local anaesthetic and opioid cause minimal

Table 26.1 Risk of side effects and complications of epidural analgesia

Side effect/complication	Risk
Backache	Thought to be unchanged
Caesarean section	Thought to be unchanged
Length of the first stage of labour	Thought to be unchanged
Second stage of labour	Average increase ~15–20 minutes
Need for instrumental delivery	~1:4
Itching	1:10
Need for adjustment of epidural catheter and/or other analgesia	1:10
Heavy leg(s)	1:20
Difficulty passing urine	1:20
Significant fall in blood pressure	1:50
Failure of epidural	1:50
Headache	1:200
Temporary nerve palsy	1:2000
Permanent nerve palsy	1:13,000
Total spinal	1:15,000
Paraplegia	1:100,000
Infection complications	1:50,000–100,000

haemodynamic disturbance, but it is mandatory to establish venous access before initiating epidural analgesia, although routine preloading with intravenous fluids has been abandoned in many units unless there are other indications such as dehydration.

Local anaesthetics also cause motor blockade, commonly graded by using various versions of the Bromage score (Table 26.2). The scoring system has been modified several times from the original one, described in 1965, to account for the less intense motor block that occurs with modern, low-dose techniques. Because such variety of scores exists, it is important that staff are familiar with the system in use in their unit. Motor blockade can be minimised by using the lowest concentration of local anaesthetic compatible with adequate analgesia. Addition of opioid facilitates reduction of local anaesthetic dose, but motor blockade may still occur.

Epidural opioids may cause nausea, vomiting, urinary retention, itching and respiratory depression. Each of these side effects occurs less commonly with fentanyl than with other opioids.

The effect of epidural opioids on gastric emptying is uncertain. Boluses of fentanyl (50–100 µg) have been shown to delay gastric emptying by up to 45 minutes, but low-dose continuous infusions do not appear to have this effect.

There has been considerable debate about the effect of epidural analgesia on the outcome of labour. Meta-analysis suggests that epidural analgesia may prolong the second stage of

Table 26.2 Bromage score for assessing motor power following epidural analgesia

Score	Original Bromage scoring system	Examples of modified Bromage scoring system	
1	Unable to move feet or knees	Unable to flex ankles	Unable to move legs at all
2	Able to move feet only	Able to flex ankles but not knees	Able to move legs but unable to raise against gravity
3	Just able to move knees	Able to flex ankles and knees but unable to straight leg raise	Able to raise legs against gravity but not against resistance
4	Able to flex knees and feet fully	Able to sustain straight leg raise	Able to raise legs against gravity and resistance

labour, with a resultant increase in the need for instrumental delivery, but not caesarean section.

Key points

- Most units in the UK offer a 24-hour epidural service for labour.
- Modern techniques consist of low-dose local anaesthetic (usually bupivacaine) with opioid (usually fentanyl in the UK and fentanyl or sufentanil elsewhere).
- PCEA techniques are associated with reduced usage of local anaesthetic.
- Use of epidural analgesia may prolong the second stage of labour and increase the likelihood of instrumental delivery.

Further reading

Anim-Somuah M, Smyth RM, Cyna AM, Cuthbert A. Epidural versus non-epidural or no analgesia for pain management in labour. *Cochrane Database Syst Rev* 2018; (5): CD000331.

Loubert C, Hinova A, Fernando R. Update on modern neuraxial analgesia in labour: a review of the literature of the last 5 years. *Anaesthesia* 2011; **66**: 191–212.

Sng BL, Sia ATH. Maintenance of epidural labour analgesia: the old, the new and the future. *Best Pract Res Clin Anaesthesiol* 2017; **31**: 15–22.

Epidural test doses

The purpose of the epidural test dose is to detect intravenous or subarachnoid placement of the catheter. As such, it must be formulated to produce an easily detected result when in one of these two situations, without compromising the safety of the mother or the fetus.

Problems and special considerations

As with all screening procedures, the sensitivity and specificity of the test dose are all-important when assessing its ability to protect the mother from the unwanted effects of intravenous or subarachnoid administration. Sensitivity is the ability of the test dose to detect accurately a misplaced catheter; failure to do so represents a false-negative result. Specificity is the ability of the test dose not to produce a false-positive result, i.e. incorrectly alerting the anaesthetist when the catheter is actually in the right place.

Accidental catheterisation of the epidural veins is common in obstetric practice, since these vessels act as collateral conduits of venous blood from the lower limbs to the heart and are therefore dilated when the inferior vena cava is compressed by the gravid uterus. Venous cannulation occurs about 1 in 20 times and is usually detected before the test dose is given, by the ability to aspirate blood.

Subarachnoid puncture occurs about 1 in 100 times, with the incidence decreasing as the practitioner becomes more experienced. Again, the vast majority of dural punctures are detected by the free flow of cerebrospinal fluid through the needle or catheter.

It follows that it is very rare for a test dose to be used in a situation where the catheter is actually intravenous or subarachnoid. This means that, in addition to the sensitivity and specificity of the test, it is also important to know what proportion of positive test results will actually indicate misplacement of the catheter; this is known as the positive predictive value of the test, and it is often lower than might be expected from the sensitivity and specificity.

A test dose, designed to improve safety, should not in itself compromise the safety of the mother or fetus. This is a particular problem when trying to detect intravenous placement, as many tests rely on the use of adrenaline to produce tachycardia in these circumstances. Intravenous adrenaline may stress the maternal cardiovascular system and temporarily reduce placental perfusion, so doses must be carefully chosen.

Although initial confirmation of the correct placement of the epidural catheter is particularly important, the possibility of later catheter migration should not be forgotten. Every top-up given down an epidural catheter that might be dangerous if accidentally injected intravenously or intrathecally should really be regarded as a test dose and should be fractionated if time permits, so as not to produce systemic toxicity or a dangerously high block.

It is difficult – if not impossible – to design a test dose that will detect subdural, extra-arachnoid placement with any reliability. The possibility of subdural catheterisation must always be borne in mind and suspected when an unusual block pattern emerges.

Management options

Subarachnoid placement

This is usually relatively easy to detect, and it is only necessary to choose a dose of local anaesthetic that will produce a recognisable but safe block. Lidocaine 45–60 mg or bupivacaine 7.5–12.5 mg is suitable; lidocaine has the advantage of a slightly faster onset of block, but many practitioners prefer bupivacaine on the grounds that this will be the drug used for the main dose. Signs of sensory block in the lower lumbar segments and motor block of the legs should be sought after 3 minutes with lidocaine or 5 minutes with bupivacaine. This test is regarded as close to 100% specific and sensitive.

Intravenous placement

Most tests rely on the use of sympathomimetic drugs to produce changes in maternal heart rate and/or blood pressure when administered intravenously. Adrenaline 15 µg has been recommended for this purpose. Intravenous injection of adrenaline has been shown to have a low positive predictive value (55–75%) and it has been associated with significant side effects. Even when an adrenaline-free bupivacaine test dose is used, 12% of patients will demonstrate a rise in heart rate that would count as a positive response. The sensitivity is also low but can be improved by ensuring that the heart rate is measured between contractions and by using the change in peak heart rate (as measured over a 2-minute period before and after the test injection), rather than a simple change from a random baseline rate, as the basis of the test.

Subjective symptoms have also been used to detect intravenous placement, and some test-dose regimens rely on this. Fentanyl 100 µg produces obvious sensations of drowsiness within 1 minute when given intravenously, and lidocaine 45–60 mg may cause tingling in the perioral region. These methods are far from reliable, and the increased sensitivity of pregnant women to local anaesthetic toxicity should always be borne in mind when using the systemic effects of lidocaine as a test.

Best practice

It is important to consider the possibility of a misplaced epidural catheter before every top-up. Careful aspiration via the catheter before administering a dose of local anaesthetic and a continuous high index of suspicion are vital adjuncts to an effective test-dose policy.

Since no single regimen has been proven to be superior, many obstetric anaesthetists therefore recommend abandoning a formal test dose, instead fractionating all epidural doses. The current practice of using low concentrations of local anaesthetic (usually 0.1–0.125% bupivacaine) means that accidental intravenous or subarachnoid administration is unlikely to produce any serious adverse maternal or fetal effects.

Midwives should be trained to recognise the early signs of local anaesthetic toxicity and fractionate all doses, to ensure safety if the catheter migrates through a dural tear.

Key points
- A test dose should be safe, with high sensitivity and specificity; high specificity is difficult to achieve when the condition being sought is uncommon.
- Accidental subarachnoid placement is relatively easy to detect with a test dose, while intravenous placement is more difficult to detect.
- Subdural placement cannot be reliably detected with a test dose.
- Catheter migration can occur, and every epidural top-up should be regarded as a test dose.

Further reading
Camorcia M. Testing the epidural catheter. *Curr Opin Anaesthesiol* 2009; **22**: 336–40.
Guay J. The epidural test dose: a review. *Anesth Analg* 2006; **102**: 921–9.

Spinal analgesia

Single-shot spinal analgesia is rarely used alone for labour, since its duration is usually much shorter than that of labour itself. However, it may be useful in the later stages of labour when delivery is felt to be imminent, or to provide rapid onset of analgesia in a mother who is desperate and losing control, thus enabling her to cooperate while an epidural catheter is inserted.

Use of an intrathecal catheter to allow repeated boluses (or infusion) of local anaesthetic or other mixtures is an attractive concept, since the advantages of spinal block (rapid onset, profound block) are potentially combined with those of epidural block (flexibility, titrated effect). In addition, it may be used for rapid extension of the block for caesarean section, which may be desirable in high-risk parturients such as those with morbid obesity, significant cardiopulmonary disease or spinal abnormalities. In practice, however, continuous spinal block is uncommon in the UK.

Problems and special considerations

The main considerations for a single-shot spinal are the risk of postdural puncture headache and the choice of solution, given the requirement for maximal analgesia while minimising motor block and other side effects (see Chapter 29, *Combined spinal–epidural analgesia and anaesthesia*).

Modern intrathecal catheters are very fine (e.g. 28–32 G) and thus may be difficult to handle and insert. They are usually supplied in a kit with a spinal needle; originally these needles had cutting tips, but they are now available with pencil-point tips in an attempt to reduce the incidence of postdural puncture headache. However, even with fine catheters, 22–26 G spinal needles are required. Some catheters include a removable wire to make them stiffer for insertion.

A continuous catheter technique may also be used with a standard epidural kit (e.g. 16 G or 18 G catheter), either because specialist kits are unavailable or when an accidental dural puncture has occurred during attempted epidural block. A reduced incidence of headache after placement of an intrathecal catheter has been claimed when this is done, possibly related to inflammation around the dural puncture site, which leads to faster healing; however, this is uncertain since the evidence is mostly observational.

The main factor that has led to the withdrawal of microspinal catheters in the USA and that has contributed to the technique's unpopularity in the UK is the association between their use and the development of subsequent cauda equina syndrome. This is thought to be caused by a combination of factors, including the use of lidocaine (more common in the USA), the known neurotoxic effect of high concentrations of lidocaine on neural tissue experimentally (more so than bupivacaine), the pooling of drug around the sensitive nerves of the cauda equina associated with very fine catheters placed caudally, and the use of excessive doses of drug in an attempt to extend an inadequately extensive block (resulting in more pooling around the nerves).

Management options

Management after a single-shot spinal is discussed elsewhere (see Chapter 34, *Spinal anaesthesia for caesarean section*).

For continuous techniques, once the catheter has been inserted, it should be clearly labelled, since accidental injection of an epidural-style dose may be disastrous. For labour analgesia, a dose can be given as for a combined spinal–epidural (see Chapter 29, *Combined spinal–epidural analgesia and anaesthesia*). Subsequent analgesia may be provided with repeated boluses of 0.5–1.5 ml bupivacaine 0.1–0.25% ± fentanyl 10–20 μg as required. Infusions (e.g. 0.1–0.25% bupivacaine ± fentanyl at 1–5 ml/hour) have also been used. Unless the technique is commonly used in a particular unit, it is prudent for all top-ups to be given by an anaesthetist, since midwifery and other staff are likely to be unfamiliar with it.

For caesarean section, incremental doses of bupivacaine ± opioid may be given to achieve the required level of block, as slowly as is felt appropriate for the clinical circumstances.

Whatever the indication, directing the catheter caudally should be avoided, as should repeated injections of concentrated solutions of local anaesthetic if the block is inadequate. Greater than normal doses of local anaesthetic should not be given.

Key points

- Single-shot spinal analgesia is rarely used alone for labour but may be useful when delivery is imminent, or to provide rapid onset of analgesia before siting an epidural.
- Continuous spinal techniques are acceptable for both labour and operative delivery.
- Advantages include good quality of block and ability to titrate the dose.
- Disadvantages include difficulty handling the catheters, risk of postdural puncture headache, potential for infection, cauda equina syndrome, cost and mistaking the catheter for an epidural one.

Further reading

Cohn J, Moaveni D, Sznol J, Ranasinghe J. Complications of 761 short-term intrathecal macrocatheters in obstetric patients: a retrospective review of cases over a 12-year period. *Int J Obstet Anesth* 2016; **25**: 30–6.

Loubert C, Hinova A, Fernando R. Update on modern neuraxial analgesia in labour: a review of the literature of the last 5 years. *Anaesthesia* 2011; **66**: 191–212.

Palmer CM. Continuous spinal anesthesia and analgesia in obstetrics. *Anesth Analg* 2010; **111**: 1476–9.

Combined spinal–epidural analgesia and anaesthesia

The combined spinal–epidural (CSE) technique was first described over 60 years ago. Although it is commonly assumed that CSE means a needle-through-needle technique, there are theoretically several ways of instituting CSE:

1. Insertion of an epidural needle into the epidural space, insertion of a long spinal needle through the epidural needle into the subarachnoid space, and finally insertion of an epidural catheter through the epidural needle after the spinal needle has been removed. This is the most commonly used technique in the UK.
2. Insertion of an epidural needle (and usually an epidural catheter) into the epidural space followed by separate insertion of a spinal needle into the subarachnoid space, either at the same or at a different lumbar interspace. This is favoured by a minority of UK anaesthetists.
3. Insertion of a spinal needle into the subarachnoid space followed by insertion of an epidural needle and catheter. This is rarely practised other than when the pain of labour is so severe that the mother is felt to be unable to lie or sit still long enough for epidural insertion.

CSE offers the certainty and speed of onset of spinal analgesia or anaesthesia and the flexibility and continuity of an epidural catheter. For the needle-through-needle technique, successful aspiration of cerebrospinal fluid (CSF) upon insertion of the spinal needle confirms correct placement of the epidural needle, which may be reassuring in difficult cases.

Problems and special considerations

Anaesthetists should be entirely familiar with the management of both spinal and epidural analgesic and anaesthetic techniques before considering CSE. Either a needle-through-needle or separate-space technique can be used, according to the equipment available and the anaesthetist's preference. The separate-space technique has the advantage of not requiring special needles but the disadvantage of inflicting two sets of injections upon the woman, and additionally carries the theoretical risk of damage to the epidural catheter by the spinal needle if the epidural procedure is performed first and at a lower vertebral interspace. The needle-through-needle technique involves only a single injection but requires long (approximately 120 mm) and more expensive spinal needles, either singly or as part of specialised CSE kits.

Any standard Tuohy needle can be used, although most of the leading needle manufacturers produce kits containing specially matched spinal and epidural needles for needle-through-needle CSE. Some of these include locking devices for fixing the two needles together so that once CSF is obtained the spinal needle cannot move in or out during subarachnoid injection, which might help reduce the incidence of inadequate block; however, these devices may reduce the 'feel' as the spinal needle is advanced through the dura. Typically, an 18 G or 16 G Tuohy needle and a 25 G or 27 G spinal needle are used, as for separate epidural and spinal techniques. It is essential to check that the spinal needle will project beyond the end of the epidural needle by an adequate amount to achieve dural puncture (usually 12–15 mm). Some kits include epidural needles with a hole at the curved tip, through which the spinal needle passes (in order to maintain an axial direction rather than following the curve of the tip), but there is no evidence that this confers any advantage.

Management options

Analgesia

The use of CSE for labour analgesia varies. Some maternity units employ the technique routinely, others never. The advantages include rapid onset of pain relief (usually within 5 minutes) and absence of significant motor block in most cases. There is also evidence to suggest that the presence of a hole in the dura (even without injecting drugs intrathecally) may improve epidural analgesia. Despite these benefits, a Cochrane review concluded that there is no difference in maternal satisfaction between women who have received CSE in labour and those who have received low-dose epidural analgesia. The major disadvantage is the additional potential for complications introduced by deliberate dural puncture, and the cost implications of using an additional needle/kit. In addition, while the onset of analgesia is rapid, it may not be complete, especially if the standard low-dose epidural mixture is used (see below), and an early epidural top-up may be required.

The original regimen for the spinal component recommended in the UK was 25 µg fentanyl and 2.5 mg bupivacaine (1 ml of 0.25% solution), made up to a volume of 2 ml with saline. Further experience has suggested that smaller doses of fentanyl (5–15 µg) may be adequate; 3–5 ml of the standard 'low-dose' epidural mixture (bupivacaine 0.1% with fentanyl 2 µg/ml) may also be suitable. These combinations will provide approximately 60–90 minutes' analgesia, in most cases with little motor blockade. (Spinal opioids alone are very rarely used in the UK, although they may be considered in some high-risk women with coexisting medical disease. In the USA and continental Europe sufentanil is widely used.) When further analgesia is needed, a low concentration of bupivacaine with fentanyl is given via the epidural catheter, either by intermittent bolus top-ups, an infusion or patient-controlled epidural analgesia (PCEA).

In labour, the abrupt reduction in the level of circulating catecholamines that may follow administration of intrathecal opioids, and the abolition of their tocolytic effect, may cause uterine hypertonicity and transient fetal bradycardia. The effect on the fetus may be compounded by maternal hypotension secondary to sympathectomy, which may lead to a reduction in placental perfusion. However, with close blood pressure monitoring and support after initiation of analgesia, such changes rarely persist.

Those who do not routinely use CSE analgesia point to the above disadvantages and to the fact that epidural analgesia is usually effective within a few contractions. However, many anaesthetists would consider CSE for women who request regional analgesia late in the first stage of labour, or for those needing regional analgesia for instrumental delivery.

Anaesthesia

The use of CSE for caesarean section combines the speed of onset and reliability of spinal anaesthesia with the ability to extend the block and provide postoperative analgesia through an epidural catheter. There are three different techniques of CSE for caesarean section:

1. The spinal injection is performed using a 'full' spinal dose of local anaesthetic, and the epidural catheter is used as a back-up in the event of inadequate anaesthesia, to extend the block if surgery is prolonged and to provide postoperative analgesia.

2. A smaller volume of local anaesthetic (e.g. 1 ml heavy bupivacaine 0.5%) is used intrathecally, with the intention of producing a limited spinal block (usually to about T8–10). Anaesthesia is then extended gradually with local anaesthetic via the epidural catheter. This technique allows a more controlled and controllable extension of block, which may be advantageous in women with systemic disease (e.g. cardiac, respiratory or neurological).

3. A small dose of local anaesthetic (e.g. 1 ml heavy bupivacaine 0.5%) is given intrathecally and the epidural catheter is then placed as usual. Saline (8–10 ml) is then injected through the epidural catheter to extend the height of the block suitable for surgery, by compression of the dural sac. It is thought that this technique (epidural volume extension, EVE) may result in less cardiovascular instability and motor block, and a reduced requirement for local anaesthetic. However, although it found some evidence of earlier recovery from motor block, a recent systematic review and meta-analysis (which included studies on non-obstetric patients) found no significant difference in the maximum sensory height achieved or in hypotension with or without EVE. The physical compressing effect of epidural solutions on the spread of spinal anaesthesia, however, means that should the subarachnoid block be inadequate, small epidural boluses (< 5 ml) of local anaesthetic may be effective in topping up the block.

Complications

It has been claimed that there is a higher failure rate of the subarachnoid component of CSE than with single-shot spinal anaesthesia. This may be the result of dislodgement of the spinal needle when using the needle-through-needle technique, such that not all of the drug is deposited in the intrathecal compartment, or failure to penetrate the dural sac if there is deviation from the midline. However, this does not appear to be a problem as experience with the technique is gained.

CSE carries similar risks to both spinal and epidural injection alone. A number of early reports of meningitis following CSE suggested that there might be an increased risk of this complication with CSE compared with a single-shot spinal; however, since CSE is widely used this could equally be an artefact of reporting. There have also been reports of neuropraxia and neurological damage with CSE, presumed to be related to needle length and design. A particular concern relates to the difficulty in identifying the correct lumbar interspace – which can be a problem even for experienced anaesthetists – and the risk that the chosen level may be above the termination of the spinal cord. In such a case, there should be no extra risk from epidural analgesia in labour, for example, so long as an accidental dural tap does not occur, but if CSE is used there is a risk of neurological damage from the spinal needle. The 3rd National Audit Project of the Royal College of Anaesthetists (NAP3) found that the incidence of permanent harm associated with obstetric CSEs was approximately six times greater than with epidurals, and approximately three times greater than with spinals (see Section 2, Part IV, *Anaesthetic Problems*).

It must be remembered that the epidural catheter is untested at the time of insertion, which may have implications in high-risk parturients who might require operative delivery. There is also the risk of an 'epidural' dose passing into the subarachnoid space, which might be increased by the presence of a dural hole (though this complication remains a rarity despite widespread use of CSE). Although rare, epidural catheter insertion or migration into the subdural or subarachnoid space has been reported with CSE techniques in obstetric patients.

Key points

- Needle-through-needle combined spinal–epidural (CSE) requires only a single injection but is more expensive than separate-space techniques.
- CSE analgesia provides pain relief usually within one or two contractions but is a more invasive and complex technique than epidural alone.
- CSE anaesthesia combines the advantages of spinal anaesthesia (speed of onset and quality of anaesthesia) with the ability to extend the level and duration of anaesthesia via the epidural route.

Further reading

Groden J, Gonzalez-Fiol A, Aaronson J, Sachs A, Smiley R. Catheter failure rates and time course with epidural versus combined spinal–epidural analgesia in labor. *Int J Obstet Anesth* 2016; **26**: 4–7.

Heesen M, Weibel S, Klimek M, *et al.* Effects of epidural volume extension by saline injection on the efficacy and safety of intrathecal local anaesthetics: systematic review with meta-analysis, meta-regression and trial sequential analysis. *Anaesthesia* 2017; **72**: 1398–411.

Simmons SW, Taghizadeh N, Dennis AT, Hughes D, Cyna AM. Combined spinal–epidural versus epidural analgesia in labour. *Cochrane Database Syst Rev* 2012; (10): CD003401.

Spinal and epidural opioids

Epidural opioids are widely used in combination with local anaesthetics to provide analgesia both during labour and following caesarean section and other procedures. Spinal opioids have also been used to enhance surgical anaesthesia and to provide postoperative analgesia, and more recently to provide analgesia for labour (in combined spinal–epidural techniques). Spinal and epidural opioids alone do not provide adequate pain relief for the late first stage and second stage of labour.

All opioids have significant maternal side effects, ranging from mild nausea to life-threatening respiratory depression. These side effects may occur following administration of opioids by any route, although the published literature has tended to focus on adverse effects associated with neuraxial administration. In the UK, fentanyl is the opioid most commonly used to provide labour analgesia, with diamorphine or fentanyl used for intra- and postoperative analgesia. Epidural morphine is less commonly used because of the greater risk of late respiratory depression, although spinal morphine appears to be safe in low-risk parturients.

Sufentanil is widely used in the rest of Europe and in North America, but is not available in the UK. Other drugs such as pethidine and hydromorphone have also been used for obstetric neuraxial blocks.

Site of action

Opioids act at the opioid receptors in the substantia gelatinosa of the spinal cord. Drugs injected into the epidural space have to penetrate the dura to reach the site of action. Ease of dural penetration will depend on lipid solubility and molecular weight, with highly lipid-soluble molecules (such as fentanyl) entering the subarachnoid space most readily. Once the opioid has reached the cerebrospinal fluid (CSF), the more lipid-soluble drugs will fix readily in the spinal cord, whereas less lipid-soluble drugs (such as morphine) remain in the CSF and are carried in a cranial direction with CSF flow, reaching the lateral ventricles in around 6 hours or longer. This accounts for the slow onset of action, higher incidence of nausea, vomiting and pruritus, and late respiratory depression seen with morphine.

The epidural space is highly vascular in the pregnant woman, and there is significant systemic uptake of epidurally administered opioids (with similar blood concentration curves to those seen after parenteral administration). In addition, some opioid is bound to fat in the epidural space and does not reach the spinal cord. The ratio of epidural to spinal dose of opioid is thus in the order of 5–10:1.

Commonly used epidural and spinal bolus doses are:

- **Fentanyl:** epidural 50–100 µg, spinal 15–25 µg

- **Diamorphine:** epidural 2–3 mg, spinal 200–500 µg
- **Morphine:** epidural 3–4 mg, spinal 75–100 µg

Benefits

Several studies have confirmed that epidural administration of opioids alone provides analgesia for early labour but is inadequate for the later stages of labour. However, the combination of local anaesthetic and opioid is synergistic, allowing improved quality of analgesia, reduced consumption of local anaesthetic, reduced motor block and reduction in opioid side effects. Typical combinations used consist of 0.1–0.125% bupivacaine with 2–2.5 µg/ml fentanyl.

Improved maternal mobility increases maternal satisfaction with labour analgesia, and improvement in rates of spontaneous vaginal delivery compared with the traditional, higher-dose and opioid-free techniques (e.g. 0.25–5% bupivacaine alone). The mechanism of local anaesthetic–opioid synergy is unclear.

Epidural and intrathecal opioids are claimed to provide superior postoperative analgesia, although there are so many variables involved, and different measures of analgesic outcome, that it is difficult to assess this reliably.

Side effects

Side effects of both epidural and intrathecal opioids are dose-dependent and are more severe for less lipophilic drugs such as morphine. With the exception of urinary retention (which is not dose-related), all the side effects seen after neuraxial administration of opioids may occur following parenteral administration (although itching is only common when opioids are given epidurally or intrathecally). A unique side effect is the potential for reactivation of herpes simplex labialis 2–5 days after the epidural administration of morphine. Several theories have been proposed, but the exact mechanism is uncertain.

Use of an opioid receptor antagonist such as naloxone reliably reverses the side effects of epidural and intrathecal opioids, but reversal of analgesia may occur. This has encouraged symptomatic treatment of individual side effects, for example using antihistamines such as chlorphenamine 4 mg orally or 10 mg parenterally for itching. Low doses of propofol (10 mg) and ondansetron have been reported to reduce opioid-induced itching, but the evidence for benefit is inconclusive.

Respiratory depression

The incidence of respiratory depression with neuraxial opioids in obstetric patients is reported to be less than 1%, although methods of detection and definitions vary. Fentanyl has the shortest duration of action following epidural or subarachnoid administration (approximately 4 hours) and the lowest potential to cause respiratory depression, although cases have been reported. Epidural morphine is well recognised as being associated with a small risk of respiratory depression for up to 12–24 hours after administration, but will also provide analgesia for a similar period of time. Diamorphine has an intermediate duration of action, and there have been no reported cases of delayed respiratory depression, although early cases have occurred – usually in combination with other sedatives.

The potential for this life-threatening side effect of centrally administered opioids has led to a general prohibition on the concomitant use of strong opioid and sedative drugs by any other route. It has also caused considerable controversy about the intensity and duration of monitoring and nursing care required for patients who have received epidural or spinal opioids. Respiratory depression manifests itself as increasing sedation (due to carbon dioxide retention) rather than reduced respiratory rate; therefore, in the absence of facilities for prolonged high-dependency nursing (which few obstetric units possess), it is sensible to nurse the mother in a postnatal bed that can be readily observed from the central nursing station, and in the company of other mothers, rather than in a side room. This is particularly recommended in women with additional risk factors such as obesity, and in those who have received or will receive additional parenteral opioids or other drugs with depressant effects, e.g. magnesium. Many obstetric anaesthetists consider that the small but real risks of late respiratory depression associated with neuraxial morphine outweigh the benefits of using it in preference to diamorphine or fentanyl, although there are many studies confirming the safety of spinal morphine.

If naloxone is required to reverse respiratory depression, it is important to use either repeated doses or an infusion, because of the prolonged action of the opioid compared with its antagonist.

Gastric emptying

This is delayed after epidural or intrathecal boluses of opioids, although there is some evidence that low-dose infusions of fentanyl do not impair gastric emptying.

Placental transfer

Although centrally administered opioids cross the placenta, this occurs in a dose-dependent manner. Administration of an epidural bolus of fentanyl 100 µg 20 minutes before delivery results in umbilical artery concentrations well below those needed to cause neonatal respiratory depression. Similarly, although opioids can be found in breast milk after maternal epidural administration, the amounts are negligible.

Key points

- There is synergy between neuraxial opioids and local anaesthetics.
- Side effects occur following all routes of administration.
- Side effects are dose-dependent, with the exception of urinary retention.
- Morphine has a slower onset, longer duration of action and increased incidence of side effects compared with fentanyl. The action of diamorphine is intermediate.

Further reading

American Society of Anesthesiologists Task Force on Neuraxial Opioids. Practice guidelines for the prevention, detection, and management of respiratory depression associated with neuraxial opioid administration. An updated report by the American Society of Anesthesiologists Task Force on Neuraxial Opioids and the American Society of Regional Anesthesia and Pain Medicine. *Anesthesiology* 2016; **124**: 535–52.

Armstrong S, Fernando R. Side effects and efficacy of neuraxial opioids in pregnant patients at delivery: a comprehensive review. *Drug Saf* 2016; **39**: 381–99.

Kwok S, Wang H, Sng BL. Post-caesarean analgesia. *Trends Anaesth Crit Care* 2014; **4**: 189–94.

Marroquin B, Feng C, Balofsky A, *et al.* Neuraxial opioids for post-cesarean delivery analgesia: can hydromorphone replace morphine? A retrospective study. *Int J Obstet Anesth* 2017; **30**: 16–22.

Sultan P, Halpern SH, Pushpanathan E, Patel S, Carvalho B. The effect of intrathecal morphine dose on outcomes after elective cesarean delivery: a meta-analysis. *Anesth Analg* 2016; **123**: 154–64.

Chapter

31

Preoperative assessment

Preoperative assessment before obstetric surgery may be required during the third trimester, usually in the high-risk parturient at an anaesthetic antenatal clinic, in the hours preceding surgery in the elective or semi-elective case, or shortly before an emergency procedure in the non-prepared anxious mother. It may also occur before early obstetric procedures such as cervical cerclage. Preoperative assessment in non-obstetric surgery is discussed in Chapter 8, *Incidental surgery in the pregnant patient.*

Problems and special considerations

Women may be anxious about anaesthesia and surgery when pregnant, particularly in the non-planned setting.

Women may wish their partners to be involved in all stages of delivery, and their presence during the preoperative assessment allows them also to be informed of ensuing events.

When the anaesthetist and patient do not speak the same language fluently, a medical translating service should be involved rather than relying on family translation.

Management options

In the elective or semi-elective setting, time can be given to a relaxed preoperative assessment. In addition to questions asked in a routine non-obstetric preoperative assessment, medical issues related to this and previous pregnancies or deliveries (in particular, neuraxial or general anaesthesia) should be discussed. The airway should be carefully assessed, given the increased incidence of a difficult airway in the obstetric population (see Chapter 38, *Failed and difficult intubation*). Once information has been gathered, a clear description of planned events, proposed management and risks should take place (see Chapter 169, *Consent*); postoperative analgesia should be discussed. If pre-assessment has occurred in the antenatal clinic, there may be time to seek further information if necessary. National Institute for Health and Care Excellence (NICE) guidelines recommend that a preoperative haemoglobin should be checked but that a group and save is unnecessary before routine elective caesarean delivery; local policy should be followed. Locally written information about obstetric anaesthesia should be given if available; alternatively, women can be directed to reputable internet sources such as labourpains.com. An opportunity to ask questions and address concerns must be given.

In the urgent setting, focused, closed questions can be useful to gather salient information. Some information should have been imparted by the attending midwife, such as gestation, parity, labour progress and indication for surgery. A focused assessment in the urgent setting may include:

- Have you had any problems in this pregnancy such as high blood pressure or diabetes?
- Do you have any medical problems unrelated to pregnancy, for example asthma or heart problems?
- Do you take any regular medications? Are you allergic to any medications?
- Have you had any problems with any kind of anaesthetic before?
- Has your epidural been working well for you?
- When did you last eat anything?

The airway should always be assessed, regardless of the urgency of the situation, and results from a recent full blood count and group and save status should be seen. Haemodynamic status must be noted. The anaesthetist should then describe planned anaesthetic technique and in what circumstances this might be deviated from, and any additional steps that might occur, for example plane blocks for analgesia after general anaesthetic.

Local protocol should be followed regarding preoperative drug administration; ranitidine and metoclopramide can often be administered before surgery. The preoperative visit must be carefully documented in the patient's notes.

Most hospitals also run an anaesthetic clinic at which parturients with particular risk factors are seen. Referral criteria are hospital-specific; common reasons include obesity, underlying medical conditions, back surgery, previous anaesthetic problems or known obstetric issues such as abnormal placentation or triplet delivery. Patients are usually seen in the early third trimester (or earlier, depending on severity of condition), which allows time to seek further information if necessary, for example details of previous anaesthesia or back surgery, or to arrange further investigations as indicated. Any encounter with the parturient may be seen as an opportunity to provide anaesthetic antenatal education.

Key points

- The preoperative assessment must be seen as a key interaction for information gathering and provision, and for developing trust between the anaesthetist and the patient.

Chapter 32

Operative vaginal delivery (Instrumental delivery)

Vaginal delivery may be facilitated by the use of forceps or a suction cup (ventouse). Which instrument is used depends on the clinical situation and the operator's skill. The Royal College of Obstetricians and Gynaecologists (RCOG) classification of instrumental deliveries is given in Table 32.1. Low- and mid-cavity positions may be further subdivided into a rotational delivery if the fetal head is more than 45 degrees from the occipito-anterior position.

In the UK, 10–13% of deliveries are performed with forceps or ventouse, but the figure varies considerably from one unit to another and is greatly affected by individual policies with respect to the maximum allowable duration of the second stage, the use of oxytocin to augment contractions, and criteria for caesarean section.

In general, instrumental delivery can be indicated by maternal factors (exhaustion, failure to descend, illness precluding Valsalva manoeuvre) or fetal factors (fetal distress, prematurity). The commonest indication is prolongation of the second stage, often defined as longer than 2 hours for a primigravida (3 hours with an effective epidural) or 1 hour for a multigravida (2 hours with an epidural).

An instrumental delivery may be associated with maternal and fetal trauma. Measures to reduce its incidence, such as continuous maternal support and delayed pushing for women with epidurals, are therefore recommended.

Table 32.1 Classification of instrumental delivery

Classification	Description
Outlet	Fetal head has reached labia or pelvic floor
Low	Fetal head is 2 cm below the ischial spines but has not reached the pelvic floor
Mid-cavity	Fetal head is 1/5 palpable from the abdomen, and below the ischial spines
High	Fetal head is 2/5 palpable and above the ischial spines (instrumental delivery not recommended; caesarean section advised)

Adapted with permission from Royal College of Obstetricians and Gynaecologists. *Operative Vaginal Delivery*. Green-top Guideline 26. London: RCOG, 2011.

Problems and special considerations

Instrumental delivery and regional analgesia

There is no doubt that, in most centres, there is a higher rate of instrumental delivery in mothers who opt for regional analgesia. Although it is very difficult to exclude potential confounders (e.g. it is likely that women who need epidural analgesia are those with other factors that predispose to instrumental delivery, such as slow progress, malpresentation, multiple gestation, relative cephalopelvic disproportion), and most randomised trials of epidural analgesia have been complicated by considerable crossover between groups (mostly from non-epidural to epidural), meta-analysis suggests an increased likelihood of instrumental delivery with epidural techniques (relative risk ~1.4). This must be weighed against the improved quality of analgesia compared with alternatives, the beneficial effect of epidural analgesia on fetal acid–base balance, and the ability to avoid general anaesthesia in many cases should caesarean section be required.

Analgesia

Analgesia produced by low-dose epidural solutions may be adequate for low-outlet ('lift-out') forceps or ventouse delivery, but mid-cavity forceps delivery requires dense surgical anaesthesia. A good pelvic block is essential, and the perineum should be tested before inserting the instrument. For anything other than an outlet forceps or ventouse, the sensory block should extend up to T10, and a block suitable for caesarean section should be considered, depending on the likelihood of failure and the speed at which progression to surgery is likely to be required (see below). It is advisable for the anaesthetist to be present when anything other than the most straightforward instrumental delivery is being performed, in order to assess the existing block, consider the options, and give (and monitor the effects of) an appropriate top-up.

'Trial' of forceps

When it is anticipated that instrumental delivery may be difficult, this should be considered as a 'trial' of instrumental delivery, and provision should be made for immediate conversion to caesarean section. A systematic review has suggested a failure rate of 9% with attempted forceps delivery and 14% with vacuum devices, though a failed forceps delivery is more likely to result in a caesarean section. The procedure should be carried out in the operating theatre, and regional anaesthesia should be adequate for rapid operative delivery. Attempted instrumental delivery is more likely to fail if the mother's body mass index (BMI) exceeds 30 kg/m^2, if the baby is large, or if the head is in the occipito-posterior position or mid-cavity or above. A trial of instrumental delivery should be abandoned if there is no evidence of descent with traction during each contraction, or if delivery is not imminent following three effective attempts by an experienced obstetrician.

Management options

For deliveries other than outlet forceps and ventouse, with a functioning epidural in situ, it is usually an easy matter to intensify the block by administering 10–20 ml of 0.5% levobupivacaine, 0.75% ropivacaine or 2% lidocaine with adrenaline (± bicarbonate), depending on the anticipated difficulty with delivery and the urgency, and local protocols.

Pelvic spread may be encouraged by sitting the mother up, and it is therefore important to establish the block before putting the legs into stirrups. Maternal pushing may be compromised by sensory and motor blockade, so effective coaching by the midwife and partner is often required.

When no epidural is in place, spinal anaesthesia is most appropriate, using ~1.5 ml of hyperbaric 0.5% bupivacaine in the sitting position, ± 10–15 µg fentanyl. However, if caesarean section is anticipated, a spinal or a combined spinal–epidural technique, using the same dose as required for surgical anaesthesia, may be more appropriate.

Pudendal block may be performed by the obstetrician if there is no anaesthetist available, although it has a high failure rate and needs at least 10–20 minutes to become effective. Pudendal block may also be used to supplement an existing epidural with sacral sparing, and infiltration of the perineum with local anaesthetic is a useful adjunctive technique before performing an episiotomy.

In all cases, care must be taken to ensure that aortocaval compression is avoided, for example by tilting the mother's pelvis with a wedge.

Aftercare

It should be remembered that the extensive episiotomy that usually accompanies instrumental delivery, coupled with the inevitable tissue trauma, often results in significant pain in the immediate postpartum period. Non-steroidal anti-inflammatory drugs (NSAIDs) should be used prophylactically if there are no contraindications, and epidural opioids are often required. At present there is insufficient evidence to support routine antibiotic prophylaxis, though local policy should be followed. Significant postpartum haemorrhage can result from cervical or vaginal tears, and this may exceed that at a caesarean section, and so vigilance regarding blood loss is essential. The need for thromboprophylaxis must be re-assessed after an operative vaginal delivery.

Key points

- A good pelvic block is essential for operative vaginal delivery, and should be confirmed by testing.
- Conversion to caesarean section may be required.
- Anaesthesia should be established before elevating the legs.

Further reading

Anim-Somuah M, Smyth RM, Cyna AM, Cuthbert A. Epidural versus non-epidural or no analgesia for pain management in labour. *Cochrane Database Syst Rev* 2018; (5): CD000331.

Liu EH, Sia AT. Rates of caesarean section and instrumental vaginal delivery in nulliparous women after low concentration epidural infusions or opioid analgesia: systematic review. *BMJ* 2004; **328**: 1410.

Royal College of Obstetricians and Gynaecologists. *Operative Vaginal Delivery*. Green-top Guideline 26. London: RCOG, 2011. www.rcog.org.uk/en/guidelines-research-services/guidelines/gtg26 (accessed December 2018).

Chapter 33

Caesarean section

The caesarean section (CS) rate in much of the developed world has increased markedly in recent decades. In England the rate has stabilised since about 2007 (Figure 33.1). The rates are similar in the devolved countries; in Wales and Scotland the CS rate is currently about 1–2% higher, and in Northern Ireland about 5% higher, than in England. There is wide variation between units. There has been general concern over increasing CS rates and the associated complications, notwithstanding the benefits that CS might have in individual cases. Since CS is such an important procedure in obstetrics, and anaesthetic-related maternal deaths commonly involve emergency CS, it is important that obstetric anaesthetists have an understanding of the practical aspects relating to obstetric indications and techniques.

Classification and delivery time

Traditionally, CS was classified as elective (i.e. a date is given beforehand) or emergency (the rest). The latter group is thought by many obstetricians and obstetric anaesthetists to be too broad, since it includes cases in which immediate delivery is required (e.g. severe fetal compromise or cord prolapse) as well as cases in which there is little urgency (e.g. early spontaneous labour in a mother with a breech scheduled for elective CS the next day). This led to the reclassification of CS into four categories (Table 33.1), and this classification has been adopted by all the major UK bodies involved in this field.

Although intended as an audit tool (e.g. to monitor outcomes and allocation of staff), the classification has been used to guide management (e.g. second operating theatre opened for

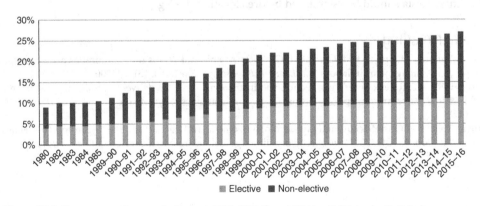

Figure 33.1 Caesarean section rates in England, 1980–2016 (from NHS Hospital Episodes Statistics).

Table 33.1 Classification of caesarean section

1	Immediate threat to life of woman or fetus
2	Maternal or fetal compromise which is not immediately life-threatening
3	Needing early delivery but no maternal or fetal compromise
4	At a time to suit the woman and maternity team

The category is assigned at the time of decision to operate; e.g. an episode of fetal compromise caused by aortocaval compression responding to therapy, followed some hours later by caesarean section for failure to progress, would be graded as category 3, not 2. Similarly, a case booked as an elective procedure for malpresentation could eventually be classified as category 3 if the mother goes into labour before the chosen date of surgery. Also applies whether or not the woman is in labour.

category-1 cases). However, attempts to link the categories to acceptable maximum times to delivery (e.g. 30 minutes for category 1) are hampered by the unwillingness of obstetricians to commit themselves to 'acceptable' delays for categories 2 and 3 in case of a bad outcome. In addition, maximum times to delivery are controversial and not based on good science: the often-quoted maximum of 15–30 minutes for fetal compromise is derived largely from work in the 1960s in which animal fetuses were exposed to varying durations of intrauterine hypoxia and the degree of subsequent fetal damage assessed. Most cases of cerebral palsy are now known to be related to factors arising before labour.

A number of audits within maternity units have found that meeting the particular standard set is extremely difficult to achieve in practice because of delays at each stage of the process (e.g. calling the anaesthetist/anaesthetic assistant, moving the mother to the operating theatre, preparing the surgical equipment, etc.). Finally, the defined time period itself varies: the time from decision to skin incision, from decision to delivery, and from informing the anaesthetist to skin incision or delivery have all been quoted in various recommendations or guidelines.

Analysis of data from the Royal College of Obstetricians and Gynaecologists (RCOG) Sentinel audit of CS in the UK in 2000 suggests that poorer maternal and neonatal outcomes were associated with decision-to-delivery intervals exceeding 75 minutes, but not intervals of 31–75 minutes. Recent guidance from the Joint Standing Committee of the RCOG and the Royal College of Anaesthetists (RCoA) reiterated that all maternity units in the UK should be using the same classification for CS, that every individual woman in labour should be considered to have a continuum of risk, and that the 30-minute interval should be considered as an 'audit standard' and not the 'gold standard' in which to deliver a baby in an emergency. Updated guidance from the National Institute for Health and Care Excellence (NICE) states that category 1 and 2 CS should be performed 'as quickly as possible' and that for category 2, within 75 minutes 'in most situations'. Further, delivery times of 30 minutes for category 1, and both 30 and 75 minutes for category 2 CS, should be used as audit standards for the unit and not to judge performance for any individual CS.

Indications

CS may be performed for the benefit of the mother, the fetus or both (Table 33.2), although in practice maternal indications will ultimately affect the fetus adversely if not relieved, and

Table 33.2 Indications for caesarean section

Previous caesarean section
  Elective
  Following trial of labour
  Other

Maternal disease
  Worsening pre-existing disease, e.g. cardiac
  Associated with pregnancy, e.g. pre-eclampsia

Placenta praevia or abruption

Maternal exhaustion/choice

Obstructed labour/failure to progress

Malpositions

Multiple pregnancy

Fetal compromise

Cord prolapse

vice versa. For elective CS, 39 weeks is commonly chosen as the optimum gestation, reflecting a balance between the benefit to the neonate of a longer gestation and the greater risk of spontaneous labour and emergency surgery. An elective CS may also be the chosen mode of delivery by the mother, once she has been informed of the risks and benefits, and offered counselling if appropriate.

Procedure

For lower-segment CS, skin incision is usually low transverse (i.e. in the L1 dermatome) but may be midline. Once exposed, the rectus sheath is split longitudinally and stretched laterally and the peritoneum incised. The uterus is incised transversely in its thin lower segment. A 'classical' CS involves a midline incision, and the uterus is incised longitudinally in its upper segment. Classical CS is associated with a greater risk of haemorrhage, infection and ileus but is quicker to perform and easier than lower-segment CS. It may be indicated if the lower segment is poorly formed, e.g. in premature delivery, and in placenta praevia, transverse or unstable lie or uterine fibroids.

Uterine incision is accompanied by removal by suction of amniotic fluid if the membranes have not ruptured (mothers and partners may find the noise alarming if unexpected). Delivery of the baby may be difficult if the head has descended well into the pelvis, and may require forceps. If the placenta has already started to separate, the uterus may contract around the baby's head, especially if CS is in the second stage of labour. Increased inspired concentration of volatile agent has been used to relax the uterus during general anaesthesia. Glyceryl trinitrate 50–100 µg intravenously or sublingually, repeated as necessary, has also been used to good effect and is suitable during regional anaesthesia.

The time between induction of general anaesthesia and delivery (the I–D interval) may affect fetal wellbeing, since if it is very short, the induction agent may be present in the fetus at high levels; and if it is very long, fetal accumulation of inhalational agents may occur.

The time from uterine incision to delivery (the U–D interval) is thought to be more important, since placental disruption may occur once the uterus is incised; fetal acidosis is unlikely if the U–D interval is less than 3 minutes.

Following delivery of the baby, oxytocin (Syntocinon) is given (typically 5 U slowly intravenously, though there is evidence that smaller doses, between 0.5 U and 3 U, may be effective). Rapid injection of larger doses may cause severe tachycardia, hypotension and electrocardiogram changes suggestive of myocardial ischaemia and may be no more effective than smaller doses. Uterine contraction may be aided by vigorous rubbing of the uterus; an oxytocin infusion may be required (e.g. 40 U in 500 ml saline at ~125 ml/h), especially after prolonged augmented labour, multiple delivery, in the presence of polyhydramnios and with a previous history of postpartum haemorrhage or multiple deliveries. Increasingly, this infusion is requested as routine prophylaxis rather than treatment of uterine atony for all cases by the obstetricians. An analogue of oxytocin, carbetocin (typically 100 µg intravenously), is longer-acting and may be a suitable alternative; evidence to date suggests a reduced incidence of postpartum haemorrhage and need for postoperative infusion or further oxytocics.

Once the baby and placenta have been delivered, the uterus is checked for tears and then sutured. Many obstetricians prefer the ease of access conferred by exteriorising the uterus, although this may be accompanied by discomfort and nausea/vomiting during regional anaesthesia, bradycardia and an increased incidence of air embolism. The obstetrician should always check with the anaesthetists before performing this manoeuvre.

Problems and special considerations

Surgical problems relating to the procedure itself include difficulty caused by adhesions (especially following previous CS or other abdominal surgery), haemorrhage, surgical trauma to the baby, difficulty delivering the baby with the risk of fetal hypoxia or physical trauma, difficulty delivering the placenta and damage to neighbouring structures. There may be large veins on the anterior wall of the uterus, and wide transverse incisions may extend to the uterine angles when the baby is delivered, leading to severe bleeding. Usual blood loss is ~400–700 ml (increased with general anaesthesia) but is notoriously difficult to estimate accurately. There is an increased risk of placenta accreta in women who have had previous CS, especially if the placenta overlies the previous scar.

Anaesthetic problems include those of general or regional anaesthesia generally. Pain during CS under regional anaesthesia has replaced awareness under general anaesthesia as the main reason for litigation associated with CS. Chest pain and/or electrocardiographic changes may occur; their cause is unknown (although small air emboli or coronary artery/oesophageal spasm have been suggested) and they may occur independently of each other. Elevations of maternal troponin I levels have also been reported. Shoulder-tip pain may occasionally occur, probably related to blood irritating the diaphragm. Other possible problems related to the procedure include air or amniotic fluid embolism and allergic phenomena.

Postoperative problems are as for any surgery and include infection and thromboembolism. Prophylactic antibiotics have been shown to reduce infection; although they are traditionally given after delivery to avoid exposing the fetus to the drug, and in case a severe maternal allergic reaction should occur, NICE guidelines suggest administration before skin incision. Heparin is given prophylactically to women at high risk of thromboembolism in some units and to all women in others. If the former, the RCOG guidelines should be followed. NICE guidelines suggest that observations (including assessment of pain and sedation) should be half-hourly for 2 hours after CS, then hourly, up to 12 hours after intrathecal diamorphine. Postoperative analgesia is discussed in Chapter 41.

Management options

The choice of anaesthetic technique depends on the degree of urgency, whether an epidural catheter is already in place, specific obstetric factors (e.g. complicated surgery anticipated) or anaesthetic issues (e.g. known difficult intubation, previous back surgery), the personal preference of the anaesthetist and the wishes of the mother (see Chapters 34–36).

Absolute figures are unavailable, but recent surveys have shown that over 90% of CS are performed under regional anaesthesia in the UK, reflecting the above preferences and the widely perceived greater safety of regional over general anaesthesia for CS. Particular concerns are the possibly inadequate exposure of anaesthetic trainees to general anaesthesia for CS, the greater tendency of trainees to use general anaesthesia (especially for emergency CS) than more experienced consultants, and the anxiety caused when this occurs. There is also concern that the incidence of failed intubation in obstetrics is increasing, and that this may be related to the above factors.

Key points

- The caesarean section rate in the UK is ~25–30%.
- Indications may be maternal, fetal or both.
- Complications include shoulder-tip, abdominal or chest pain, air or amniotic fluid embolism, haemorrhage, surgical trauma and awareness.

Further reading

Lucas DN, Yentis SM, Kinsella SM, et al. Urgency of caesarean section: a new classification. J R Soc Med 2000; 93: 346–50.

National Institute for Health and Care Excellence. Caesarean Section. Clinical Guideline 132. London: NICE, 2004. https://www.nice.org.uk/guidance/cg132 (accessed December 2018).

Royal College of Obstetricians and Gynaecologists, Royal College of Anaesthetists. Classification of urgency of caesarean section: a continuum of risk. Good Practice 11. London: RCOG, 2010. www .rcog.org.uk/classification-of-urgency-of-caesarean-section-good-practice-11 (accessed December 2018).

Yentis SM. Whose distress is it anyway? 'Fetal distress' and the 30-minute rule. Anaesthesia 2003; 58: 732–3.

Spinal anaesthesia for caesarean section

Continuous audit by the Obstetric Anaesthetists' Association (OAA) suggests that half to two-thirds of caesarean sections (CS) in the UK are currently done under single-shot spinal anaesthesia.

Problems and special considerations

Rapid onset of widespread vasodilatation coupled with the effect of aortocaval compression means that hypotension is an almost inevitable accompaniment to spinal anaesthesia unless specific precautions are taken. Left uterine displacement, frequent blood pressure measurement and instant availability of intravenous fluid and vasopressors are prerequisites for the safe use of this technique.

Careful assessment of the level of block is essential before starting the operation. Despite an apparently adequate block, pain may still occur, although this is less likely than if an epidural anaesthetic has been used. Mothers should be warned of this possibility in advance, and adequate treatment, even to the extent of inducing general anaesthesia, must be offered.

The incidence of postdural puncture headache (PDPH) is related to the size and type of needle used. Pencil-point and conical-tip needles, such as the Sprotte and Whitacre, are associated with a much lower rate of headache than Quincke needles with a cutting tip, so much so that a 24 G pencil-point needle is probably better than a 27 G Quincke needle.

Meningitis and encephalitis are extremely rare. However, once the dura mater has been penetrated, the cerebrospinal fluid (CSF) is particularly susceptible to contamination, and it is considered mandatory to use a completely aseptic technique, including the wearing of mask, gown and gloves.

Management options

Suitability of the technique

In experienced hands, spinal anaesthesia can be almost as fast as general anaesthesia, and there are few occasions when the urgency of the situation means that there is no time for this technique. If the mother already has an effective epidural in situ then, time permitting, this should be topped up in preference to establishing a new block. If time is short, a single-shot spinal has been suggested as an alternative to general anaesthesia in a mother with an epidural in situ. If spinal supplementation of an existing epidural block is thought appropriate, it may be necessary to use a reduced dose if an epidural top-up has recently been given, as there have been case reports of very high blocks in these circumstances.

Spinal anaesthesia is contraindicated in patients with hypovolaemia, coagulation disorders (whether iatrogenic or pathological) and systemic sepsis. Although regional anaesthesia was traditionally avoided previously if massive blood loss was expected, such as in placenta praevia, many anaesthetists would now use a spinal block in this situation. There is some evidence to suggest that blood loss and the need for blood transfusion is reduced if regional anaesthesia is used in these circumstances.

Although traditionally favoured as being better for the baby than general anaesthesia, there is evidence that spinal anaesthesia may be associated with greater neonatal acidosis than after epidural or general anaesthesia, possibly related to the rapidity of onset and cardiovascular changes. However, the rapid onset and more profound block compared with epidural anaesthesia, and the greater maternal safety profile compared with general anaesthesia, make spinal anaesthesia the technique preferred by most obstetric anaesthetists for CS.

Preoperative preparation

Preoperative assessment may be compromised by the urgency of the case, but should include assessment for difficult intubation, since general anaesthesia may be needed if the block is unsatisfactory. An explanation of the technique should be given, and the mother should be warned about the risks of hypotension with associated nausea and vomiting, and intraoperative sensations of tugging or stretching. The possibility of pain during the operation must be mentioned, although she should be reassured that this is unusual and will be treated if necessary with intravenous opioids, inhaled nitrous oxide or even general anaesthesia. Most mothers prefer their partners to be present for the delivery, and it is good practice to involve them in these discussions so that they are aware of what may happen.

Preparation

Standard monitoring is mandatory, and good intravenous access is essential. Most anaesthetists prefer to perform spinal anaesthesia with the patient on the operating table, since this minimises the need for movement after the local anaesthetic has been administered. Sitting and lateral positions are both acceptable, although there is evidence that the former may be easier if the bony landmarks are difficult to palpate. The block tends to develop more rapidly in the lateral position, probably owing to the slope of the vertebral canal in this position in women (the hips are wider than the shoulders, causing a downward slope towards the head, unlike in men, in which the opposite tends to occur).

Administration of the spinal anaesthetic

Full asepsis should be used, and an interspace below L3 should be chosen to ensure that the needle tip is well below the termination of the cord. A pencil-point or conical-tip needle is standard practice in obstetrics nowadays. Once free-flowing CSF has been identified, the chosen dose of local anaesthetic should be administered over 10–20 seconds. 'Dry tap' or pain during insertion or injection should be a signal to withdraw the needle and try again.

Drugs

Hyperbaric bupivacaine 0.5% is the most commonly used local anaesthetic for spinal anaesthesia in the UK. A dose of 10–15 mg (2–3 ml) is typically used for de novo spinal anaesthesia, although low-dose techniques (< 10 mg) have been used in an attempt to reduce hypotension and nausea/vomiting – though at the expense of less reliable anaesthesia. Fentanyl 15–20 µg, preservative-free morphine 75–100 µg, or diamorphine 0.3–0.4 mg is usually added for postoperative analgesia. However, caution must be observed when using intrathecal morphine, as there have been case reports associated with delayed respiratory depression. This is thought to be less likely with intrathecal diamorphine, and there have been no case reports to date of delayed respiratory depression in the obstetric population with diamorphine.

Spinal anaesthesia-induced hypotension may be seen in almost three-quarters of women undergoing CS in the absence of preventive measures, and carries the risk of undesirable maternal and fetal effects, especially if it is prolonged. A preload of 1000–2000 ml was traditionally used before the spinal dose was given. However, 'co-loading' (giving 400–800 ml fluid together with a prophylactic vasopressor) is now widely used, and this avoids excessive fluid administration. Colloid solutions have been shown to be more efficacious than crystalloids at preventing hypotension, but they are more expensive and there is a small risk of allergy. A vasopressor must be to hand, and phenylephrine is now the vasopressor of choice as it has been shown to cause less fetal acid–base disturbance than ephedrine, although the latter may be administered in the presence of bradycardia or in women with certain cardiac conditions in whom its β-agonistic effects may be beneficial. Recent consensus guidelines recommend that phenylephrine is given as a prophylactic infusion, with an aim to preserve maternal systolic blood pressure at or above 90% of the baseline reading. Infusions may be associated with more cardiovascular stability, but the doses given greatly exceed those when bolus injections are used.

After the injection, the mother should be moved quickly but carefully into a left-wedged supine position, ensuring that there is no head-down tilt, and the blood pressure checked at 1–2-minute intervals. Some practitioners prefer to turn the mother into a full lateral posture, avoiding the wedged supine position until just before draping and incision. Some prefer to tip or turn the woman to the right side for a few minutes, before turning her to the left-tilted position, in order to obtain a more symmetrical block.

Testing the block

To minimise the risk of pain, the block should extend up to T5 on both sides when testing to touch, and this is now considered the gold standard. A block to light touch extending to T5 has been shown to be associated with a low incidence of intraoperative pain and a reduced need for intraoperative supplementation, compared with the same extent of block to pinprick or cold sensation. Although a complete block below the upper level is fairly certain when spinal anaesthesia is used, it is good practice to check that the sacral segments are covered and that the mother cannot straight leg raise against gravity. A recalcitrant block can be extended by using a variety of techniques such as turning from side to side, coughing, a Valsalva manoeuvre or judicious head-down tilt. The extent of the block and the modality used for testing must always be recorded.

Failed or inadequate spinal anaesthesia after an apparently uncomplicated injection is usually caused by technical errors such as displacement of the spinal needle (leading to partial or total loss of the intrathecal drug) or under-dosage, or occasionally by the presence of anatomical abnormalities in the subarachnoid space. Subsequent management and the decision to re-attempt neuraxial blockade or to administer general anaesthesia would largely be determined by maternal and fetal risk factors and the urgency of the clinical situation. In patients with partially effective spinal anaesthesia and an existing level of neuraxial block, a combined spinal–epidural might enable titration of the dose and reduction of the risk of a high block with repeat intrathecal injection.

During the operation

The patient should be watched for premonitory signs of hypotension, such as pallor, yawning or nausea. Bradycardia may indicate a high block affecting the sympathetic cardiac accelerator fibres, or be related to the use of phenylephrine. The mother may complain that her chest 'feels heavy'; this sensation is common when the intercostal muscles are affected, and reassurance should be offered. Complaints of discomfort or pain may occur despite an initial satisfactory block and must be managed promptly and effectively (see Chapter 49, *Breakthrough pain during caesarean section*).

After the operation

Positional changes may cause sudden cranial spread of the block even at this late stage. Standard postoperative monitoring and observations must be ensured (see Chapter 33, *Caesarean section*). The sitting position may be carefully adopted if the blood pressure is stable. The mother should not be moved to the ward until there is cardiovascular stability and the block is receding. Anaesthetic follow-up for symptoms of PDPH or persistent block should continue for 48 hours.

Key points

- Pencil-point or conical-tip needles should be used to minimise the risk of postdural puncture headache.
- Hypotension is almost invariable and may be actively prevented by the prophylactic use of vasopressors.
- The extent of the block must be tested and recorded, and the patient should be warned of the risk of pain.

Further reading

Arzola C, Wieczorek PM. Efficacy of low-dose bupivacaine in spinal anaesthesia for Caesarean delivery: systematic review and meta-analysis. *Br J Anaesth* 2011; **107**: 308–18.

Butwick AJ, Columb MO, Carvalho B. Preventing spinal hypotension during Caesarean delivery: what is the latest? *Br J Anaesth* 2015; **114**: 183–6.

Heesen M, Klöhr S, Rossaint R, Straube S. Prophylactic phenylephrine for caesarean section under spinal anaesthesia: systematic review and meta-analysis. *Anaesthesia* 2014; **69**: 143–65.

Kinsella SM, Carvalho B, Dyer RA, *et al.* International consensus statement on the management of hypotension with vasopressors during caesarean section under spinal anaesthesia. *Anaesthesia* 2018; **73**: 71–92.

Langesæter E, Dyer RA. Maternal haemodynamic changes during spinal anaesthesia for caesarean section. *Curr Opin Anaesthesiol* 2011; **24**: 242–8.

Chapter

35

Epidural anaesthesia for caesarean section

Although no longer most anaesthetists' technique of choice for elective caesarean section (CS), the popularity of epidural analgesia for pain relief in labour means that many women presenting for emergency CS have an epidural in situ. A greater understanding of methods to enhance the speed of onset and quality of epidural block has reduced the need for general anaesthesia in this group of mothers. Extension of the block is the technique of choice, unless epidural analgesia during labour has been of poor quality or there is a very urgent indication for delivery within 5–10 minutes.

Problems and special considerations

Poor block with breakthrough pain is more common with epidural anaesthesia than with spinal anaesthesia, and a careful assessment of block is therefore particularly important in this group. The block should be 'mapped out' to ensure that there are no missed segments or patchy areas, and the extent of block should be carefully recorded. The mother must be warned of the risk of pain before starting the procedure, and the anaesthetist should be prepared to supplement the block with further top-ups, intravenous analgesia or even general anaesthesia. Pain during CS is the commonest failure cited in negligence suits against obstetric anaesthetists in the UK.

Hypotension is slower in onset and normally less severe than with spinal anaesthesia, but vasoconstrictors may still be required, and great care should be taken to avoid aortocaval compression.

The possibility of migration of the epidural catheter, whether into the subdural, intrathecal or intravenous compartments, must be borne in mind, especially when large, concentrated doses of local anaesthetic are being used. Doses should be fractionated or given by slow injection and the level of block regularly checked. It is unacceptable to leave a mother for any reason once the process of establishing the block has started. See also Chapter 27, *Epidural test doses.*

Management options

Suitability of the technique

Extending a pre-existing epidural block for anaesthesia for CS is not as fast as general anaesthesia. Thus, for a very urgent CS, spinal or general anaesthesia remains the technique of choice. However, with appropriate top-up solutions given over 2–3 minutes (see below), surgical anaesthesia may be produced within 5–10 minutes – though there is considerable variation in onset times between patients. Further, slow injection of a bolus conflicts with the precautions mentioned above about fractionating doses. The risks and benefits to the mother and fetus of epidural versus general anaesthesia in these circumstances must be carefully considered, and these can be among the most difficult clinical decisions taken by anaesthetists.

A 'fresh' spinal anaesthetic is preferable to attempting to top up a poorly functioning epidural catheter, since the chance of inadequate anaesthesia during surgery is greater if analgesia has been poor during labour. Also, if extension of the epidural proves to be inadequate and a spinal anaesthetic is then chosen, the spread of the spinal dose may be more unpredictable after large volumes of solution have already been injected epidurally.

Contraindications to epidural anaesthesia are discussed in Chapter 26, *Epidural analgesia for labour*.

Preoperative preparation

This is as discussed in Chapter 34, *Spinal anaesthesia for caesarean section*. It is particularly important in women having an epidural top-up to mention the risk of intraoperative pain and to have a plan to deal with this should it occur. The reported need for general anaesthesia after an epidural top-up is ~2–4%; therefore an intravenous H_2-antagonist should be given if the mother has not received it during the last 6–8 hours. Many anaesthetists do not routinely give the mother oral sodium citrate (though it should be immediately available) since it has an unpleasant taste, it only lasts ~30 minutes, and the likelihood of general anaesthesia is small. Prophylactic vasopressors are rarely needed, but should be available, and a large-bore intravenous cannula must be inserted to allow rapid fluid infusion. Before giving an epidural top-up, it is important to test the block that is already present; while the top-up required does not need modifying as a result in most cases, failure to do so will allow a pre-existing unexpectedly extensive block, which might indicate subdural or subarachnoid migration of the catheter, to go undetected.

Choice of drugs

Bupivacaine 0.5% was the mainstay for many years for epidural CS, but large doses (often in excess of the recommended upper limits) are frequently required, and resuscitation from systemic toxicity is less likely to succeed than with other local anaesthetics. Lidocaine 2% has a faster onset for elective cases, especially if pH-adjusted, but adrenaline must be added to minimise systemic absorption; this also enhances its efficacy. Slow bolus injection (including through the needle) has been shown to produce more rapid and reliable block (with lower final volumes) than boluses of 5 ml repeated every 5–10 minutes, but with attendant risks if the injection is misplaced.

For emergency CS, the use of a bolus dose of 15–20 ml concentrated local anaesthetic solution (e.g. (levo)bupivacaine 0.5% or ropivacaine 0.75%), given over 2–3 minutes, can convert labour epidural analgesia to a block suitable for surgery within about 15–20 minutes in most cases. Lidocaine with adrenaline and bicarbonate (e.g. 20 ml lidocaine 2%, 0.1 ml 1:1000 adrenaline and 2 ml 8.4% bicarbonate) has been shown to produce surgical anaesthesia in approximately half this time, though approximately 1 minute may be 'lost' by mixing the drugs, and care must be taken to avoid drug errors (although lidocaine and bicarbonate are stable when mixed, the adrenaline degrades within a few hours of addition).

The use of 2-chloroprocaine 3% has been reported as having a very short onset time, but reports of back pain and neurological damage, shortly after its introduction several decades ago, have led to a very restricted availability (e.g. the USA and a handful of countries in continental Europe), though the modern preparation is free of the preservatives that have since been implicated in causing these complications. Another potential problem with chloroprocaine is that its effects wear off rapidly and so supplementation with further epidural local anaesthetic is required to avoid intraoperative pain.

Opioids (e.g. fentanyl 50–100 µg, diamorphine 2–3 mg, morphine 3–4 mg) are commonly added, either during the initial topping up or towards the end of the case. The evidence that addition of fentanyl might speed the onset of block and/or improve analgesia is weak, especially if the mother has been receiving regular epidural fentanyl in labour and the epidural has been working well.

Administration of the epidural anaesthetic

In most cases, the epidural catheter is already in situ; if this is the case, then it has been argued that the epidural may be topped up in the delivery room before transfer, thus saving what may be important time. This practice is controversial, however, since the delivery room is not an ideal place for dealing with extensive block, severe hypotension or local anaesthetic toxicity. The anaesthetist must, of course, remain with the mother from the point of topping up an epidural with concentrated solutions, wherever this is done, and ensure adequate monitoring. If he/she is 'trapped' in the delivery room then he/she is unable to check and prepare the required drugs and equipment in the operating theatre.

Testing the block

The principles should be as for spinal anaesthesia (see Chapter 34), though an epidural block is more likely to have missed segments or be unilateral than a spinal block, so the extent of sensory loss should be carefully assessed. The epidural catheter allows further doses to be given, and appropriate positioning of the patient, although not as effective as with spinal anaesthesia, may encourage spread into recalcitrant areas. In emergency cases when the epidural has been topped up, it may be more difficult to determine sensory block resulting from the top-up if the mother already has a sensory block from the labour epidural. In such circumstances, the development of a profound motor block in the legs is very reassuring that the top-up is becoming effective.

During the operation

Hypotension is less common than with spinal anaesthesia, but blood pressure should be carefully monitored and treated expeditiously. Inadequate block may become apparent during peritoneal incision, and exteriorisation of the uterus, a manoeuvre much favoured by certain obstetricians, may be poorly tolerated. A delicate surgeon can make all the difference if the block is borderline, and good communication between medical staff is rarely more important. Nausea and vomiting associated with vagal stimuli such as exteriorisation of the uterus or peritoneal manipulation can be treated with glycopyrronium 200–600 µg.

After the operation

If opioids have not been given, an epidural dose of e.g. diamorphine may be given in combination with rectal non-steroidal analgesics, if not contraindicated, at the end of surgery. The same precautions regarding discharge from recovery and monitoring should be followed as for spinal anaesthesia (Chapter 34). The epidural catheter lends itself to further low-dose local anaesthetic or opioid top-ups or infusion, but this can only be done if there are facilities and staff to care for the patient safely. Postoperative monitoring is discussed in Chapter 33, *Caesarean section*, and postoperative analgesia is discussed in Chapter 41.

Key points

- The full extent of the block must be tested before giving an epidural top-up for caesarean section.
- Pain during the operation is more common than with spinal anaesthesia, and the patient must be warned.
- Slow bolus epidural injection may produce a faster block of good quality, but may be more hazardous than fractionated injection.

Further reading

Allam J, Malhotra S, Hemingway C, Yentis SM. Epidural lidocaine–bicarbonate–adrenaline vs. levobupivacaine for emergency Caesarean section: a randomised controlled trial. *Anaesthesia* 2008; **63**: 243–9.

Lam DT, Ngan Kee WD, Khaw KS. Extension of epidural blockade in labour for emergency Caesarean section using 2% lidocaine with epinephrine and fentanyl, with or without alkalinisation. *Anaesthesia* 2001; **56**: 790–4.

Lucas DN, Ciccone GK, Yentis SM. Extending low-dose epidural analgesia for emergency Caesarean section: a comparison of three solutions. *Anaesthesia* 1999; **54**: 1173–7.

Malhotra S, Yentis SM. Extending low-dose epidural analgesia in labour for emergency Caesarean section: a comparison of levobupivacaine with or without fentanyl. *Anaesthesia* 2007; **62**: 667–71.

Sanders SD, Mallory S, Lucas DN, *et al.* Extending low-dose epidural analgesia for emergency caesarean section using ropivacaine 0.75%. *Anaesthesia* 2004; **59**: 988–92.

General anaesthesia for caesarean section

There has been a general trend away from general anaesthesia in many countries over the past few decades because of the associated potential morbidity and mortality, with about 90% of caesarean sections in the UK now performed under regional anaesthesia. General anaesthesia is usually reserved for those women who adamantly refuse a regional technique, for those in whom such a technique is contraindicated (e.g. by medical disease), or if there is lack of time. Conversion to general anaesthesia for inadequate regional anaesthesia may occur. In the UK, audit standards of up to 1% conversion rates have been recommended for elective sections and up to 2.5% for unplanned caesareans.

Problems and special considerations

The incidence of failure to intubate the trachea is approximately 1 in 300–500 in the obstetric population, compared with a 10-fold lower incidence in the general surgical population (see Chapter 38, *Failed and difficult intubation*).

For pulmonary aspiration of gastric contents, see Chapter 59, *Aspiration of gastric contents*, and Chapter 14, *Gastric function and feeding in labour*.

For hypovolaemia, see Chapter 78, *Major obstetric haemorrhage*. The extent of blood loss in fit young people is usually underestimated. Induction of general anaesthesia in an unresuscitated hypovolaemic mother may precipitate catastrophic cardiovascular collapse. Tachycardia should alert the anaesthetist to the possibility of hypovolaemia, although the significance of tachycardia may be difficult to assess in an extremely anxious mother who may also be in pain.

The risk of awareness during general anaesthesia for caesarean section is thought to be minimal if modern techniques are used (see Chapter 60, *Awareness*) but is considered higher than in the general population. Many cases of supposed intraoperative awareness are in fact episodes occurring during recovery from anaesthesia, but claims of intraoperative awareness are difficult to refute if the anaesthetic record is inadequate, and thus meticulous anaesthetic record keeping is vital. However, in the recent National Audit Project (NAP5) into awareness, the vast majority of reported cases of accidental awareness in obstetric patients were thought to be certain or probable cases of awareness, and occurred at induction. Some authorities recommend that all mothers are warned preoperatively of an extremely small risk of intraoperative awareness as part of the consent process, and that this warning is recorded in the preoperative assessment.

General anaesthesia is associated with a tendency towards longer immediate recovery, more pain (see Chapter 41, *Postoperative analgesia*), more postoperative nausea and vomiting, and more neonatal depression than regional anaesthesia. In addition, the parents do not experience the moment of birth as they do with spinal or epidural anaesthesia.

Management options

Preoperative assessment

The time available for preoperative anaesthetic assessment may be brief but vital aspects should not be omitted, especially any previous anaesthesia, drug allergy, recent oral intake, indication (and urgency) for caesarean section, and the mother's airway.

Therapy to raise intragastric pH and minimise intragastric volume is given. It is usual to administer ranitidine (other drugs, e.g. omeprazole, may also be used) preoperatively, either orally or parenterally, depending on timing. This will be of benefit for extubation, another high-risk period associated with general anaesthesia. Metoclopramide is also given in many units. Some obstetric units advocate the administration of antacid prophylaxis routinely to every woman in labour, but this is controversial. 0.3 M sodium citrate (30 ml) is administered immediately before preoxygenation and induction of anaesthesia to neutralise any gastric contents.

Induction of anaesthesia

It is customary to induce anaesthesia for caesarean section in the operating theatre. The obstetric anaesthetist should check the anaesthetic machine in the obstetric theatre at least once a day. Most units will have a tray of emergency general anaesthetic drugs either prepared or ready to be drawn up quickly for emergency cases. A suitably trained anaesthetic assistant must be present before induction of general anaesthesia. There should be an airway trolley equipped with a range of differently sized tracheal tubes, intubation aids, laryngoscopes and equipment for dealing with failed intubation. The uterus must be displaced off the aorta and vena cava either manually (uncommon in the UK), by a wedge placed under the woman's right hip, or by laterally tilting the operating table.

A large-bore intravenous cannula (14 G or 16 G) that is connected to a freely running infusion must be in place before induction of anaesthesia.

Adequate preoxygenation must always precede induction of anaesthesia, regardless of the urgency. It is crucial to ensure a tight fit of the facepiece and, if a circle system is being used, at least 12 l/min of oxygen. The standard recommendation is preoxygenation for 3 minutes or 4–5 vital capacity breaths, although a better guide is the difference between the inspired and expired oxygen content, indicated on the gas monitor (in ideal conditions, with no leak, both should exceed 90% when de-nitrogenation is complete). Some units now routinely employ transnasal high-flow humidified oxygen for preoxygenation and apnoeic oxygenation during intubation of obstetric patients.

Monitoring of the mother should include blood pressure, capnography, electrocardiography, pulse oximetry and end-tidal volatile concentration.

The patient should be draped and catheterised while preoxygenation is happening, to minimise duration of fetal exposure to anaesthetic agents. Traditionally, rapid-sequence induction of anaesthesia with thiopental and suxamethonium would be standard practice in the UK, but this is now the subject of debate. Although use of all induction agents has been described in the literature, the use of propofol has been particularly discussed since recent

NAP5 and Confidential Enquiries into Maternal Deaths (CEMD) reports. The NAP5 report suggested that awareness might be associated with the use of thiopental (especially if relatively small doses are given to obese women), whereas the CEMD report commented on thiopental overdosing in unwell parturients. This has led to calls to replace thiopental with propofol for caesarean section, advocates of propofol citing familiarity with dosing, less potential for drug errors and reduced time for preparation for its use. On the other hand, advocates of thiopental cite familiarity in the obstetric setting, understanding of fetal effects, and haemodynamic stability associated with its use. Propofol has been associated with a slightly less favourable neonatal acid–base profile, though the clinical significance of this is disputed. Whichever drug is chosen, anaesthetists must be confident in its use and dosing in the variety of clinical situations seen with the obstetric population. A normal induction dose for the healthy parturient would be 5 mg/kg thiopental or 2.5 mg/kg propofol; these doses may need to be reduced for the mother who is unwell or has hypovolaemia or a fixed cardiac output, while they might need increasing in obesity. More than just an induction dose of hypnotic agent may need to be given, especially if intubation is difficult and the time to achieve adequate brain levels of volatile agent is prolonged.

Suxamethonium 1–1.5 mg/kg is the most commonly used neuromuscular blocking agent in the obstetric population. Use of rocuronium has been advocated instead of suxamethonium, on the basis that intubation conditions will be maintained for long enough to achieve intubation if the latter is unsuccessful on the first attempt. The traditional counter-argument has always been that the intubation conditions produced by suxamethonium are the best, within the shortest time, and if intubation fails, the return of muscle power favours earlier self-ventilation. However, with the introduction of sugammadex, rocuronium (1 mg/kg) may become the drug of choice, since sugammadex (16 mg/kg) has been shown to reverse the effects of rocuronium within 2–3 minutes (compared with the offset of suxamethonium of up to 10 minutes in late pregnancy). As sugammadex is a relatively new drug, familiarity with its use is still limited, especially in obstetrics; furthermore its cost is high and the incidence of anaphylaxis associated with its use is still not known.

Opioids are traditionally withheld until after delivery of the baby, to avoid neonatal effects. However, the NAP5 report suggested that 'appropriate use of opioids' should be employed to avoid accidental awareness, and administration of opioids such as fentanyl as part of the induction of anaesthesia, even in rapid-sequence induction, has also been advocated in guidelines for difficult intubation in obstetrics.

The induction agent may be supplemented with hypotensive agents and/or opioid analgesics in mothers with pre-eclampsia or cardiac disease, in order to reduce the sympathetic response to intubation (see Chapter 86, *Hypertension, pre-eclampsia and eclampsia*).

Cricoid pressure is applied before consciousness is lost and maintained until the airway is secured and tracheal intubation confirmed (see Chapter 37, *Cricoid pressure*).

Every obstetric anaesthetist should be familiar with both failed intubation and failed ventilation drills, and should mentally rehearse these before every induction of general anaesthesia in the obstetric patient. Every obstetric theatre should have monitoring equipment that includes measurement of end-tidal carbon dioxide, and there should be access to specialised airway equipment, e.g. for cricothyroid access and a fibreoptic endoscope.

An agent to counteract hypotension, such as phenylephrine or metaraminol, must be to hand (although hypotension is usually less marked than with neuraxial anaesthesia).

Perioperative and postoperative management

Traditional practice is to use 50% nitrous oxide in oxygen plus a volatile anaesthetic agent (e.g. isoflurane) to ventilate the lungs, reverting to conventional mixtures of 70% nitrous oxide in 30% oxygen after delivery of the baby, aiming for a total MAC of about 1.0 depending on the situation (though the use of nitrous oxide in general is becoming less frequent, and general anaesthesia using an air/oxygen mixture is increasingly used). The volatile agent should be continued throughout anaesthesia. In severe fetal compromise, 100% oxygen with a corresponding increase in the inspired concentration of volatile agent may be chosen. Some authorities advocate a higher MAC of up to 1.3 until opioids have been given; this can be rapidly reduced if uterine contractility is affected.

A short-acting non-depolarising neuromuscular blocking drug should be used when the suxamethonium has worn off, and if the surgeon is fast it may not be necessary to use further neuromuscular blockers after the initial dose of suxamethonium. Deaths have occurred from inadequate reversal of neuromuscular blockade following the use of long-acting drugs; this and the risk of awareness during emergence from anaesthesia make the use of neuromuscular blockade monitoring mandatory.

Oxytocin (Syntocinon) is usually given as a slow intravenous bolus of 5 U at delivery of the baby (although lower doses of 0.5–3 U may be adequate), often followed by an intravenous infusion of 40 U in 500 ml saline at ~125 ml/hour. Antibiotics were traditionally administered after delivery of the baby, but current National Institute for Health and Care Excellence (NICE) recommendations are for administration before skin incision.

Adequate analgesia should be given following delivery of the baby. A combination of a long-acting opioid such as morphine (7.5–15 mg) and a non-steroidal anti-inflammatory drug (NSAID) such as diclofenac is used in many units. It is important to obtain preoperative consent to rectal administration of drugs. Intravenous paracetamol is also routinely given intraoperatively.

At the end of surgery, residual neuromuscular blockade is reversed and the mother is usually turned into the left lateral position before the trachea is extubated. It is important to remember that the risk of aspiration is also present at extubation and possibly during the initial phase of recovery from anaesthesia. Extubation of the trachea should not be performed until there is evidence of return of protective reflexes.

The mother must be nursed in a properly equipped recovery room by trained staff before returning to the postnatal ward. Deaths have occurred because of inadequately staffed and equipped recovery facilities.

Patient-controlled opioids are popular for postoperative analgesia, and NSAIDs appear to be particularly effective in combating 'afterpains' of uterine involution. NSAIDs should not be used in women with severe pre-eclampsia or severe asthma. Bilateral ilioinguinal block, transversus abdominis plane blocks and rectus sheath blocks have also been used. Further aspects are discussed in Chapter 41, *Postoperative analgesia*.

Heparin should be given according to local protocol.

Current evidence suggests that a woman may breastfeed her baby as soon as she has adequately recovered from the general anaesthetic.

Key points

- All obstetric patients requiring general anaesthesia should be considered high-risk.
- Emergency general anaesthesia is associated with increased morbidity and mortality.
- Failure to intubate the trachea is ~10 times more common in the obstetric population than in the general surgical population.

Further reading

Dahl V, Spreng UJ. Anaesthesia for urgent (grade 1) caesarean section. *Curr Opin Anaesthesiol* 2009; **22**: 352–6.

Lucas DN, Yentis SM. Unsettled weather and the end for thiopental? Obstetric general anaesthesia after the NAP5 and MBRRACE-UK reports. *Anaesthesia* 2015; **70**: 375–9.

Sia AT, Fun WL, Tan TU. The ongoing challenges of regional and general anaesthesia in obstetrics. *Best Pract Res Clin Obstet Gynaecol* 2010; **24**: 303–12.

Chapter 37

Cricoid pressure

The cricoid cartilage is the only cartilaginous part of the upper airway to be a complete ring, and so pressure on its anterior aspect results in compression of the upper oesophagus/hypopharynx against the vertebral body of C6 posteriorly. First described by Sellick in 1961 (hence 'Sellick's manoeuvre'), cricoid pressure is widely used as a means of preventing passive regurgitation (and thus aspiration) of gastric contents during induction of general anaesthesia in at-risk patients. It is thus a standard technique in obstetric anaesthesia, although precisely when the period of risk begins and ends is controversial. In addition, whether cricoid pressure is actually necessary has also been questioned, since it is not routinely practised in many continental European countries without apparent increases in morbidity and mortality, and there is some evidence that it does not completely occlude the oesophagus when applied.

Method

As originally described by Sellick, the assistant's forefinger is placed over the cricoid cartilage and firm pressure is exerted posteriorly, with the thumb and middle finger supporting on either side. In the two-handed technique, the assistant's second hand is placed behind the patient's neck, resisting any flexion of the cervical spine as cricoid pressure is applied. However, it is unclear whether the two-handed technique has any consistent advantage, and it does mean that the assistant has both of his/her hands occupied should the anaesthetist need any more equipment.

The optimal time to start exerting pressure is somewhat controversial, since cricoid pressure is uncomfortable when the patient is awake, whereas regurgitation may occur if it is applied too late. As a compromise, many advocate gentle pressure (10 N) until consciousness is lost, with firmer pressure (30 N) thereafter (as Sellick originally described), although there is evidence that gentle pressure itself may cause relaxation of the lower oesophageal sphincter. Estimates of the force required to prevent regurgitation range from 10 N to over 40 N.

Although the use of cricoid pressure is standard practice, it may hinder tracheal intubation, first because the assistant's hand may obstruct insertion of the laryngoscope blade into the mouth and second because if incorrectly applied (it has been suggested that this is more likely in obstetrics because of lateral tilt) it may distort the laryngeal anatomy. If pressure is excessive, it may also flex the neck (or hyperextend it if two-handed cricoid pressure is used). It is therefore important that anaesthetic assistants are properly trained in its application; studies have demonstrated considerable variation in assistants' ability but also considerable improvement following training. Video laryngoscopy may aid the assistant in providing optimum cricoid pressure, and improve the view of the glottis.

In cases of failed intubation, release of cricoid pressure should be considered, especially if mask ventilation or placement of a laryngeal mask airway is considered, as these may be hindered by cricoid pressure. If not hindering ventilation, cricoid pressure should be maintained until the patient wakes (i.e. maintained throughout surgery if the decision is made to proceed with a supraglottic airway). If regurgitation occurs once cricoid pressure has been reduced, the assistant should be ready to reapply pressure if required while oropharyngeal suction and head-down tilt are introduced. Release is also advocated if there is active vomiting, since oesophageal rupture has been reported; however, cricoid pressure should only be released on the anaesthetist's instruction.

Key points

- Cricoid pressure should be applied as consciousness is lost.
- A force of 10–40 N is required.
- Incorrect application may impede intubation.
- Assistants should be properly trained in its application.

Further reading

Algie CM, Mahar RK, Tan HB, *et al.* Effectiveness and risks of cricoid pressure during rapid sequence induction for endotracheal intubation. *Cochrane Database Syst Rev* 2015; (11): CD011656.

Benhamou D, Vanner R. Controversies in obstetric anaesthesia: cricoid pressure is unnecessary in obstetric general anaesthesia. *Int J Obstet Anesth* 1995; **4**: 30–3.

El-Obarney M, Connolly L. Rapid sequence induction and intubation: current controversy. *Anesth Analg* 2010; **110**: 1318–25.

Lerman J. On cricoid pressure: 'may the force be with you'. *Anesth Analg* 2009; **109**: 1363–6.

Chapter 38

Failed and difficult intubation

Over the last 30 years the number of maternal deaths associated with failed intubation has declined, though it remains one of the main reasons for advising regional, rather than general, anaesthesia for obstetric procedures. It is important to remember that patients do not die from failed intubation; they die from hypoxia or acid aspiration if the failed intubation is unrecognised or the corrective measures are inadequate. Pressure to achieve tracheal intubation may lead to prolonged attempts during which hypoxia occurs.

Problems and special considerations

Tracheal intubation is more difficult in obstetric anaesthesia, and the incidence of failed or difficult intubation is usually quoted as approximately 1 in 300–500 obstetric general anaesthetics, 10 times higher than for non-obstetric general anaesthetics. There are many reasons for difficulties with intubation and the increased risk of developing hypoxia (Table 38.1). Laryngoscopy and placement of a tracheal tube may thus be more difficult, while hypoxaemia develops more rapidly than in general surgical patients. This is compounded by the anaesthetist being under considerable stress during induction of anaesthesia.

The consequences of failed intubation in obstetrics are serious for both maternal and fetal health. Obstetric anaesthetists have been encouraging the use of regional anaesthesia,

Table 38.1 Causes of increased incidence of problems relating to tracheal intubation in obstetric anaesthesia

Anatomical	Difficulty inserting laryngoscope	Large breasts Weight gain/increased fatty tissue Oedema (especially pre-eclampsia) Complete dentition Cricoid pressure
	Poor laryngoscopic view	Weight gain/increased fatty tissue Laryngeal oedema Cricoid pressure causing distortion Swollen mucosa
Physiological	Increased risk of aspiration Increased oxygen demand Reduced lung capacity	
Iatrogenic	Incorrectly applied cricoid pressure Urgency leading to haste Inexperience of staff	

to reduce the number of general anaesthetics administered. As a result, the percentage of general anaesthetics has decreased, although the absolute number may not have fallen dramatically. However, there are now many obstetric units where very few general anaesthetics are given – and this, although a commendable trend, has led to a reduction in training opportunities, not only for trainees but also for trainers. It has been suggested that simulation courses may help address the issue of reduced training in general anaesthesia for obstetrics, but although simulation has been shown to improve practical skills, it is yet to be validated as a training tool.

Management options

If general anaesthesia is to be administered then it is important to do the following:

- Attempt to predict difficult intubation
- Use an anaesthetic technique that will minimise the risk of failing
- Have a failed intubation drill

Prediction of difficult intubation

Prediction of difficult intubation is attempted using the same clinical examination as in the non-pregnant patient:

- Mallampati score
- Coexisting neck pathology
- State of dentition
- Mouth opening
- Thyromental distance

Unfortunately, even in combination these tests have low predictive value (i.e. relatively few of the cases predicted as being difficult will actually be difficult), partly because of the poor function of the tests and partly because difficult intubation is uncommon, even in obstetric cases. Mallampati scores have been shown to change during pregnancy and even during labour.

Anaesthetic technique

The delivery suite theatre should be well equipped for a difficult intubation, and the equipment should include a variety of aids to intubation as well as equipment to aid oxygenation if a problem arises. A video laryngoscope may be a useful piece of equipment in the obstetric setting, and the majority of obstetric units now have some form of device in their difficult airway trolley. Skilled assistance for the anaesthetist is essential.

The anaesthetist should ensure that the patient is well positioned and that adequate doses of induction agent and neuromuscular blocking drug are given after a full 3 minutes' preoxygenation or 3–5 vital capacity breaths. Proper fitting of the facemask is important to ensure efficient preoxygenation. The correct application of cricoid pressure by a trained assistant is important, since badly applied cricoid pressure can make laryngoscopy difficult (see Chapter 37, *Cricoid pressure*).

Although suxamethonium has long been considered the standard neuromuscular blocking drug, it has been suggested that with the availability of sugammadex, rocuronium may be more suitable for obstetrics, since it avoids some of the side effects of suxamethonium while providing a longer period of optimal conditions, with the possibility of rapid and reliable reversal by sugammadex should this be required. However, this remains controversial; many anaesthetists may not be familiar with the appropriate dose of sugammadex (16 mg/kg actual body weight), which may take several minutes to draw up, and not all units have sugammadex readily available because of its high cost. Sugammadex can, however, reverse 1 mg/kg rocuronium in 3 minutes, compared with the ~9 minutes that suxamethonium may take to wear off.

In order to avoid a catastrophe there should be a plan that comes into effect as soon as failure to view the larynx or to intubate the trachea becomes evident. It is at this point that a previously rehearsed 'failed intubation drill' should commence.

Failed intubation guideline

A national obstetric-specific difficult airway guideline was developed in the UK by the Obstetric Anaesthetists' Association (OAA) and the Difficult Airway Society (DAS) in 2015. This should replace the multiplicity of failed intubation drills that previously existed, allowing a consistent approach to a fraught situation (Figures 38.1, 38.2, 38.3, 38.4). The prime focus is to maintain oxygenation.

Figure 38.1 OAA/DAS master algorithm: obstetric general anaesthesia and failed intubation. Reproduced with permission from Mushambi MC, Kinsella SM, Popat M, *et al.* Obstetric Anaesthetists' Association and Difficult Airway Society guidelines for the management of difficult and failed tracheal intubation in obstetrics. *Anaesthesia* 2015; **70:** 1286–306.

Figure 38.2 OAA/DAS algorithm 1: safe obstetric general anaesthesia. Reproduced with permission from Mushambi MC, Kinsella SM, Popat M, *et al.* Obstetric Anaesthetists' Association and Difficult Airway Society guidelines for the management of difficult and failed tracheal intubation in obstetrics. *Anaesthesia* 2015; **70:** 1286–306.

The key factors in the OAA/DAS failed intubation guidelines are:

- Assessment of the airway and preparation for difficulties.
- Up to three attempts at intubation, optimising conditions, equipment and experience. If necessary, cricoid pressure should be altered or released, since oxygenation takes precedence over protection from aspiration.
- Communicating with the team and declaring an emergency early.
- Maintaining oxygenation through a facemask or second-generation supraglottic airway if necessary. Nasal oxygen may also be applied.
- Performing a front-of-neck procedure, and if oxygenation is still not established moving to maternal life support with a perimortem caesarean section.
- Deciding whether to wake or proceed once oxygenation and anaesthesia have been established and maintained.

These guidelines recognise that it may be particularly difficult in obstetrics to decide whether to proceed with surgery, given the presence of two patients with conflicting interests. It is important to remember that the primary duty of the anaesthetist is to the mother; thus, the initial course of action is to allow the mother to wake up, irrespective of the risk to the fetus, and to proceed with a regional anaesthetic. Exceptions to this would be if the mother herself requires the surgery as a life-saving procedure (e.g. major haemorrhage) or if the person

Figure 38.3 OAA/DAS algorithm 2: obstetric failed tracheal intubation. Reproduced with permission from Mushambi MC, Kinsella SM, Popat M, *et al.* Obstetric Anaesthetists' Association and Difficult Airway Society guidelines for the management of difficult and failed tracheal intubation in obstetrics. *Anaesthesia* 2015; **70**: 1286–306.

Figure 38.4 OAA/DAS algorithm 3: can't intubate, can't oxygenate. Reproduced with permission from Mushambi MC, Kinsella SM, Popat M, *et al.* Obstetric Anaesthetists' Association and Difficult Airway Society guidelines for the management of difficult and failed tracheal intubation in obstetrics. *Anaesthesia* 2015; **70**: 1286–306.

Table 1 – proceed with surgery?				
Factors to consider	WAKE ◀		▶	PROCEED
Before induction	Maternal condition	• No compromise	• Mild acute compromise	• Haemorrhage responsive to resuscitation	• Hypovolaemia requiring corrective surgery • Critical cardiac or respiratory compromise, cardiac arrest
	Fetal condition	• No compromise	• Compromise corrected with intrauterine resuscitation, pH < 7.2 but > 7.15	• Continuing fetal heart rate abnormality despite intrauterine resuscitation, pH < 7.15	• Sustained bradycardia • Fetal haemorrhage • Suspected uterine rupture
	Anaesthetist	• Novice	• Junior trainee	• Senior trainee	• Consultant / specialist
	Obesity	• Supermorbid	• Morbid	• Obese	• Normal
	Surgical factors	• Complex surgery or major haemorrhage anticipated	• Multiple uterine scars • Some surgical difficulties expected	• Single uterine scar	• No risk factors
	Aspiration risk	• Recent food	• No recent food • In labour • Opioids given • Antacids not given	• No recent food • In labour • Opioids not given • Antacids given	• Fasted • Not in labour • Antacids given
	Alternative anaesthesia • regional • securing airway awake	• No anticipated difficulty	• Predicted difficulty	• Relatively contraindicated	• Absolutely contraindicated or has failed • Surgery started
After failed intubation	Airway device/ ventilation	• Difficult facemask ventilation • Front-of-neck	• Adequate facemask ventilation	• First generation supraglottic airway device	• Second generation supraglottic airway device
	Airway hazards	• Laryngeal oedema • Stridor	• Bleeding • Trauma	• Secretions	• None evident

Criteria to be used in the decision to wake or proceed following failed tracheal intubation. In any individual patient, some factors may suggest waking and others proceeding. The final decision will depend on the anaesthetist's clinical judgement.
© Obstetric Anaesthetists' Association / Difficult Airway Society (2015)

Figure 38.5 OAA/DAS table 1: proceed with surgery? Reproduced with permission from Mushambi MC, Kinsella SM, Popat M, *et al*. Obstetric Anaesthetists' Association and Difficult Airway Society guidelines for the management of difficult and failed tracheal intubation in obstetrics. *Anaesthesia* 2015; **70**: 1286–306.

making the decision to continue is of sufficient experience and seniority. Factors that may influence this choice have been listed in the guidelines to help inform decision making (Figure 38.5).

Proceeding with a caesarean section under general anaesthesia using a laryngeal mask airway or facemask risks aspiration and airway obstruction during the procedure; this has been reported to occur in nearly 10% of failed obstetric airways. While a literature review has shown that the tendency has been towards proceeding with surgery since the late 1990s, trainees should be reassured that they will always be supported if they wake a mother up after a failed intubation. If surgery proceeds, a senior anaesthetist and obstetrician should facilitate a quick procedure, and extubation/waking should be planned. Consideration should be given to whether immediate waking is appropriate or transfer to an intensive care unit for delayed extubation more appropriate; before waking, the stomach should be emptied with a large-bore gastric tube, neuromuscular blockade must be fully reversed, and intravenous antacids should be administered if not already given (Figure 38.6).

Table 2 – management after failed tracheal intubation	
Wake	**Proceed with surgery**

• Maintain oxygenation
• Maintain cricoid pressure if not impeding ventilation
• Either maintain head-up position or turn left lateral recumbent
• If rocuronium used, reverse with sugammadex
• Assess neuromuscular blockade and manage awareness if paralysis is prolonged
• Anticipate laryngospasm/can't intubate, can't oxygenate
	• Maintain anaesthesia
	• Maintain ventilation - consider merits of:
	  □ controlled or spontaneous ventilation
	  □ paralysis with rocuronium if sugammadex available
	• Anticipate laryngospasm/can't intubate, can't oxygenate
	• Minimise aspiration risk:
	  □ maintain cricoid pressure until delivery (if not impeding ventilation)
	  □ after delivery maintain vigilance and reapply cricoid pressure if signs of regurgitation
	  □ empty stomach with gastric drain tube if using second-generation supraglottic airway device
	  □ minimise fundal pressure
	  □ administer H_2 receptor blocker i.v. if not already given
	• Senior obstetrician to operate
	• Inform neonatal team about failed intubation
	• Consider total intravenous anaesthesia

After waking	

• Review urgency of surgery with obstetric team
• Intrauterine fetal resuscitation as appropriate
• For repeat anaesthesia, manage with two anaesthetists
• Anaesthetic options:
  □ Regional anaesthesia preferably inserted in lateral position
  □ Secure airway awake before repeat general anaesthesia	

© Obstetric Anaesthetists' Association/Difficult Airway Society (2015)

Figure 38.6 OAA/DAS table 2: management after failed tracheal intubation. Reproduced with permission from Mushambi MC, Kinsella SM, Popat M, *et al*. Obstetric Anaesthetists' Association and Difficult Airway Society guidelines for the management of difficult and failed tracheal intubation in obstetrics. *Anaesthesia* 2015; **70**: 1286–306.

Key points

- The patient does not die from failure to intubate the trachea but from failure to stop trying to intubate.
- Oxygenation must be maintained at all times.
- The failed intubation drill should be regularly rehearsed.

Further reading

Kinsella SM, Winton AL, Mushambi MC, *et al*. Failed tracheal intubation during obstetric general anaesthesia: a literature review. *Int J Obstet Anesth* 2015; **24**: 356–74.

Mhyre JM, Healy D. The unanticipated difficult intubation in obstetrics. *Anesth Analg* 2011; **112**: 648–52.

Mushambi MC, Kinsella SM, Popat M, *et al*. Obstetric Anaesthetists' Association and Difficult Airway Society guidelines for the management of difficult and failed tracheal intubation in obstetrics. *Anaesthesia* 2015; **70**: 1286–306.

Quinn AC, Milne D, Columb M, Gorton H, Knight M. Failed tracheal intubation in obstetric anaesthesia: 2 yr national case–control study in the UK. *Br J Anaesth* 2013; **110**: 74–80.

Awake intubation

Awake intubation might be considered in obstetric practice in two situations: management of the mother with a known airway problem, and acute management of the failed intubation after allowing the mother to wake. The need for awake intubation is considerably reduced by the greater proportion of procedures (mainly caesarean sections) performed under regional, rather than general, anaesthesia. Indeed, regional anaesthesia is often considered the technique of choice in both the above situations. Conversely, some authorities would consider a known difficult airway as an indication for awake intubation, since the airway may otherwise be at risk during an inadequate or extensive regional block, and having to deal with a difficult intubation in an uncontrolled manner mid-caesarean is especially hazardous and stressful.

Problems and special considerations

The basic techniques used are the same as for the non-pregnant patient, and fibreoptic intubation is considered the gold standard, although other techniques have also been described. Nerve blocks and transtracheal injection may be difficult because of the increased subcutaneous tissue deposition of pregnancy. Nasal vascular engorgement and a tendency to nosebleeds are common in pregnancy, and so the oral route is often preferred, but nasal intubation is an acceptable route. If the awake procedure follows a failed intubation, there may be considerable airway bleeding and oedema resulting from trauma. In the past, the risk of aspiration of gastric contents has made obstetric anaesthetists wary of obtunding the protective reflexes with local anaesthesia for awake intubation, but this is felt to be safe if excessive sedation is avoided.

There is concern in the UK about the level of training in awake intubation techniques, especially in obstetric patients. Video laryngoscopes are becoming more readily available, and familiarity with their use is increasing, which may lower the threshold for intubation under general anaesthesia in cases suspected to have a difficult airway. Video laryngoscopes have been shown to improve both laryngoscopic view and success at first attempt at intubation of a predicted difficult airway in the non-obstetric population, though studies in obstetric patients are lacking. The time taken to intubate may be longer than with direct laryngoscopy, which may be of concern in the obstetric population. A video laryngoscope may be a more useful tool in the middle of a failing intubation than the fibreoptic 'scope.

Management options

If not already given, H_2-receptor antagonists ± antacids should be administered, and secretions reduced, e.g. with intramuscular or intravenous glycopyrronium 100–300 μg up to an hour in advance. If the nasopharyngeal route is chosen, a local anaesthetic with vasoconstrictor must be used.

During the procedure, the same attention to avoidance of aortocaval compression and to fetal monitoring and wellbeing is required as for any procedure in the labour ward. Particular efforts are required to reassure the mother and her partner, since the situations in which awake intubation is required are especially stressful.

Once the trachea has been intubated and the tube's cuff inflated, general anaesthesia can be induced. It should be remembered that there is a risk of airway obstruction following tracheal extubation, which should be performed only when the mother is awake and in the left lateral position. A bougie or airway exchange device may be placed through the tracheal tube before extubation to facilitate reinsertion of the tube should this be required. Impaired protective reflexes may persist for an hour or more after local anaesthetic techniques have been used in the airway.

Key points

- The indications for awake intubation in obstetrics are controversial.
- The principles of awake intubation are similar to those in non-pregnant women.

Further reading

Baker PA, Weller JM, Greenland KB, Riley RH, Merry AF. Education in airway management. *Anaesthesia* 2011; **66**: 101–11.

Lewis SR, Butler AR, Parker J, Cook TM, Smith AF. Videolaryngoscopy versus direct laryngoscopy in adult patients requiring tracheal intubation. *Cochrane Database Syst Rev* 2016 (11): CD011136.

Popat MT, Srivastava M, Russell R. Awake fibreoptic intubation skills in obstetric patients: a survey of anaesthetists in the Oxford region. *Int J Obstet Anesth* 2000; **9**: 78–82.

Scott-Brown S. Russell R. Video laryngoscopes and the obstetric airway. *Int J Obstet Anesth* 2015; **24**: 137–46.

Removal of retained placenta and perineal suturing

With active management, ~98% of placentas are delivered within 30 minutes of vaginal delivery of the infant. The World Health Organization states that the length of time before making a diagnosis of retained placenta should be left to the judgement of the clinician. Risk factors for retained placenta include a previous retained placenta, uterine abnormalities, gestational age less than 28 weeks and stillbirth. However, it often follows a rapid uncomplicated delivery.

Perineal tears range from small, superficial and uncomplicated ones, to tears involving the deep structures of the anal sphincter (Table 40.1). Small perineal tears occur in up to three-quarters of vaginal deliveries, but tears involving the anal sphincter occur in ~1% of vaginal deliveries.

Third- and fourth-degree tears are more common with instrumental deliveries, nulliparity, Asian ethnicity, large babies, malposition, shoulder dystocia and a prolonged second stage of labour.

Both retained placenta and third/fourth-degree tears may result in postpartum haemorrhage and require transfer to the operating theatre and effective anaesthesia.

Problems and special considerations

The need for anaesthesia and surgery at this stage of childbirth is frequently unanticipated by the mother and her partner, and it may be a significant psychological blow.

A retained placenta prevents the uterus from contracting effectively, so there may be excessive bleeding from any areas of separation. Occasionally, retained placenta is

Table 40.1 Classification of perineal tears adopted by the Royal College of Obstetricians and Gynaecologists

First degree	Injury to perineal skin and/or vaginal mucosa
Second degree	Injury to perineum involving perineal muscles but not involving the anal sphincter
Third degree	Injury to perineum involving the anal sphincter complex
Grade 3a	< 50% of external anal sphincter thickness torn
Grade 3b	> 50% of external anal sphincter thickness torn
Grade 3c	Both external anal sphincter and internal anal sphincter torn
Fourth degree	Injury to perineum involving external anal sphincter and internal anal sphincter (the anal sphincter complex) and anorectal mucosa

complicated by uterine inversion (either partial or complete; see Chapter 77, *Uterine inversion*). Unless the uterus is rapidly replaced manually, the mother will become severely hypotensive and may become bradycardic. A similar clinical picture may be seen with so-called 'cervical shock', in which there is increased vagal tone caused by trapping of the placenta in the cervix.

Severe perineal tears may require lengthy repair and can be associated with significant blood loss, which may go relatively unrecognised.

Management options

Urgency of intervention depends on the degree of blood loss. For a retained placenta, early conservative management is appropriate if bleeding is not excessive and vital signs are stable. An intravenous infusion of oxytocics may be started if the uterus is atonic, and putting the baby to the breast for suckling sometimes stimulates delivery of the placenta. Turning the woman into the left lateral position is anecdotally reported to assist spontaneous placental delivery, and emptying the bladder may also be helpful. If the uterus is very bulky, there is still a risk of aortocaval compression in the supine position.

Choice of anaesthetic technique in both situations should be based on assessment of the relative risks of general and regional anaesthesia. Intravenous access via a large cannula (at least 16 G) with a freely flowing infusion is mandatory before starting any anaesthetic technique. If epidural analgesia has been used for labour it is usually possible to extend this for surgery. There is usually no reason to separate mother and baby if regional anaesthesia is used, and there should be no delay in initiating breastfeeding. Adequate fluid replacement is essential, particularly as the sympathetically induced vasodilatation accompanying regional blockade will aggravate any existing hypovolaemia. Suitable solutions for topping up the epidural catheter are similar to those used for instrumental delivery. An upper extent of block to T6–8 is required for retained placenta, since uterine manipulation may be considerable; lower blocks may be suitable for perineal repair.

In the absence of epidural analgesia, spinal anaesthesia should be instituted, unless the mother is significantly hypovolaemic (see below). It is often more comfortable for the mother to have spinal anaesthesia induced in the lateral rather than the sitting position. A dose of 1.5–2 ml 0.5% heavy bupivacaine with 15–20 µg fentanyl is usually adequate.

If there is evidence of hypovolaemia and continuing bleeding despite adequate resuscitation, general anaesthesia should be used. The mother is assumed to have a full stomach and the same technique as for caesarean section should be used, including antacid prophylaxis and rapid-sequence induction of anaesthesia (see Chapter 36, *General anaesthesia for caesarean section*). Blood should be cross-matched and preferably two large (14 G) intravenous cannulae inserted, and the case managed as for any obstetric haemorrhage. If there is uterine inversion, general anaesthesia may be required to aid replacement of the uterus, unless the mother is stable and regional analgesia is already present.

Postoperative analgesia should be considered, especially for women with extensive perineal repairs. Intrathecal or epidural opioids, together with regular paracetamol and non-steroidal anti-inflammatory drugs, may be required. For third- and fourth-degree tears, broad-spectrum antibiotics and laxatives are recommended.

Key points

- There is a risk of massive bleeding from retained placenta. Repair of perineal tears may be lengthy and associated with significant blood loss.
- Resuscitation should take place before induction of anaesthesia.
- Spinal or epidural anaesthesia is appropriate in haemodynamically stable patients.
- General anaesthesia (with cricoid pressure and tracheal intubation) is indicated in hypovolaemic patients.

Further reading

Royal College of Obstetricians and Gynaecologists. *The Management of Third- and Fourth-Degree Perineal Tears*. Green-top Guideline 29. London: RCOG, 2015. www.rcog.org.uk/en/guidelines-research-services/guidelines/gtg29 (accessed December 2018).

Postoperative analgesia

Adequate pain relief following caesarean section is particularly important, because the mother needs to be sufficiently comfortable to care for her baby. She is also at increased risk of thromboembolism, and effective analgesia enables early mobilisation and facilitates bonding of the mother with the infant. Poorly controlled pain may be a risk factor for the development of chronic pain and may result in adverse psychological sequelae in the mother.

It is also important to remember that women having other procedures (e.g. repair of perineal tears) may be in considerable discomfort or pain afterwards.

Problems and special considerations

Psychological considerations are important. The mother who has been delivered by elective caesarean section under regional anaesthesia, with preoperative preparation and discussion about postoperative analgesia, cannot be directly compared with the mother who has been delivered by emergency caesarean section under general anaesthesia after many hours of labour and a failed trial of forceps delivery. (In the worst scenario she may also have received an episiotomy.)

Most published studies of post-caesarean analgesia are, for logistical reasons, performed in women having elective caesarean section, and the results should therefore be interpreted cautiously.

The ideal analgesic should of course be extremely effective, universally applicable, cheap to use and free from unwanted side effects, which include the risk of adverse outcomes in breastfed neonates (see Chapter 162, *Drugs and breastfeeding*). The ideal analgesic does not exist, and the demand for freedom from unwanted effects is particularly important in obstetric patients.

It is important to remember that unwanted effects include the need for intravenous cannulae and infusions, urinary catheters and additional monitoring equipment. Safety is vital in a patient population that is young and fit with newly born dependants. Other side effects that may be acceptable to an elderly general surgical population (e.g. pruritus, nausea and sedation) are unacceptable to women wishing to care for babies.

The use of various opioids by the subarachnoid or epidural routes has become routine, but the level of nursing care required by women who have received this method of analgesia remains controversial. The relative risk and timing of respiratory depression associated with different opioids variy, but none can be considered completely safe in this respect. Equally, all centrally administered opioids cause nausea, vomiting and pruritus, although to differing degrees. Although there can be no doubt that high-dependency care, either in a high-dependency unit or given in a normal postnatal ward by one-to-one or one-to-two patient supervision, is ideal, many obstetric units are unable to provide this. Protagonists of spinal opioids point out that all opioids, given by any route, have the capacity to cause respiratory depression, and that no special precautions are taken after the administration of intramuscular opioids. Various compromises are made at a local level.

Women undergoing non-caesarean procedures can experience considerable postoperative pain (e.g. perineal) but may find that this is not always appreciated by the medical and midwifery staff, who may focus on mothers who had caesarean section.

Management options

A combination of paracetamol, non-steroidal anti-inflammatory drugs (NSAIDs) and opioids is used in the majority of women to provide analgesia following caesarean section. Analgesics prescribed regularly are more likely to be given than those prescribed 'as required', but midwives should be educated about the assessment and management of postoperative pain and encouraged to give analgesics as prescribed. Published research, including a recent Cochrane review, has failed to demonstrate clearly the superiority of any one route or of any one drug or drug combination for post-caesarean analgesia.

Caesarean section under general anaesthesia

The most commonly used drugs in this situation are intraoperative intravenous opioids (e.g. morphine 10–20 mg or diamorphine 5–10 mg), an NSAID and either oral or patient-controlled intravenous opioids postoperatively. Regular paracetamol and NSAIDs act synergistically with both strong and weak opioids. NSAIDs have an opioid-sparing effect and may also have a role in the management of the visceral component of pain after caesarean section. Nevertheless, their potentially adverse effects on renal function should be considered in women who are hypovolaemic and in those who have compromised renal function. Similarly, they are contraindicated in women with severe pre-eclampsia because of their effect on platelet function and renal function, and should also be used with caution in women with asthma.

Some studies have suggested a role for adjuvant drugs such as gabapentin or ketamine in women who have risk factors for chronic pain or in those with severe postoperative pain that is difficult to control. The paucity of data on the effectiveness and side-effect profile of these agents in the mother and newborn may, however, limit their usage.

Bilateral ilioinguinal blocks have been shown to improve postoperative pain control, and should be considered for all cases under general anaesthesia. Rectus sheath blocks may also be used, although they are more difficult immediately after caesarean section than in elective gynaecological surgery. Increasingly popular are transversus abdominis plane (TAP) blocks, which may be performed under ultrasound guidance at the end of the surgery. Although TAP blocks have been described as easy to perform, the efficacy of the block is variable and very operator-dependent, and there have been case reports of bowel injury, as well as intraperitoneal and intravascular injection of local anaesthetic. In addition, a systematic review and meta-analysis has concluded that a clinically significant opioid-sparing effect of TAP blocks was demonstrable in parturients who have not received intrathecal morphine for caesarean delivery, but not in those who had.

Other local anaesthetic techniques such as single or continuous wound infiltration have also been described.

In the emergency situation there may be an epidural catheter in place but insufficient time to extend a block for anaesthesia, but this does not preclude use of the catheter for postoperative analgesia using epidural opioids.

Caesarean section under regional anaesthesia

There is common anecdotal evidence that women experience less pain following caesarean section under regional anaesthesia than under general anaesthesia, although this is difficult to substantiate. The pre-emptive action of epidural or spinal anaesthesia remains unproven. Subarachnoid fentanyl (10–20 mg) is used to improve the quality of intraoperative anaesthesia, but its action does not extend significantly into the postoperative period. This has led to the global use of subarachnoid fentanyl and morphine (0.1–0.2 mg), which provides very effective analgesia for up to 24 hours, but is considered by some anaesthetists to be associated with the highest risks of nausea, vomiting, pruritus and respiratory depression. In the UK, subarachnoid diamorphine (200–400 μg) is commonly used, providing analgesia both during surgery and extending 6–8 hours postoperatively.

Epidural or combined spinal–epidural anaesthesia allows greater flexibility for postoperative analgesia. Epidural local anaesthetic alone is unsuitable, since women are unable to mobilise and dislike the sensation of being numb. Fentanyl (e.g. 50–100 μg) is relatively short-acting (3–4 hours) but is reported to have the lowest incidence of side effects; morphine (e.g. 2–4 mg) has delayed onset of action but long duration (18–24 hours) and a higher incidence of side effects, including delayed respiratory depression. Diamorphine (e.g. 2–3 mg) is available in the UK although in few other countries in the world and has an intermediate duration of action and incidence of side effects. Sufentanil is widely used in North America and Europe but is not available in the UK.

Patient-controlled administration of epidural opioids (e.g. fentanyl or pethidine) has been described, but this is uncommon in the UK.

Regardless of choice of opioid, analgesia is improved by the addition of an NSAID (subject to the same precautions outlined above) and by the regular administration of simple analgesics such as paracetamol.

Other procedures

Women having perineal repairs and other procedures should be told that adequate analgesia will be made available should they need it, and the staff looking after them should be encouraged to take their pain seriously. A recent Cochrane review has suggested a beneficial effect of NSAIDs in the control of acute postpartum pain in non-breastfeeding women who have sustained perineal trauma. Neuraxial opioids and regular analgesics may be required, and it may be easiest and kindest to prescribe the same postoperative analgesics as for caesarean section.

Key points

- The mother needs to be alert and comfortable in order to feed, care for and bond with her baby.
- Paracetamol, opioids and non-steroidal anti-inflammatory drugs are the mainstay of postoperative analgesia.

- Opioids, whatever the route of administration, are associated with respiratory depression, nausea and vomiting.
- Opioids administered by the epidural and subarachnoid routes are also associated with pruritus and possible delayed respiratory depression.

Further reading

Abdallah FW, Halpern SH, Margarido CB. Transversus abdominis plane block for postoperative analgesia after caesarean delivery performed under spinal anaesthesia? A systematic review and meta-analysis. *Br J Anaes* 2012; **109**: 679–87.

Carvalho B, Butwick AJ. Postcesarean delivery analgesia. *Best Pract Res Clin Anaesthesiol* 2017; **31**: 69–79.

Mkontwana N, Novikova N. Oral analgesia for relieving post-caesarean pain. *Cochrane Database Syst Rev* 2015; (3): CD010450.

Wuytack F, Smith V, Cleary BJ. Oral non-steroidal anti-inflammatory drugs (single dose) for perineal pain in the early postpartum period. *Cochrane Database Syst Rev* 2016; (7): CD011352.

Enhanced recovery

Enhanced recovery (ER), otherwise called 'fast-track' surgery, is a relatively recent approach to perioperative patient management that is now being applied in obstetric practice. The aim is to facilitate patient recovery and expedite discharge, thereby reducing morbidity and improving outcomes while lessening the strain on healthcare systems. The practice is in congruence with the National Institute for Health and Care Excellence (NICE) recommendations on the management of women for caesarean section (see Chapter 33, *Caesarean section*), which state that women who have an uncomplicated postoperative course may get discharged 24 hours after the procedure.

A successful ER pathway in obstetrics requires collaboration between multiple teams – including the pregnant woman – and the existence of clear protocols to guide perioperative management. The initial phase begins with the antenatal screening of women to enable the selection of appropriate candidates and the identification and optimisation of factors that may delay recovery and hinder early discharge, such as preoperative anaemia. Involvement and education of patients at this stage play a vital role, as they tackle issues that may generate potential delays in leaving hospital, such as difficulty with breastfeeding. Psychological preparedness may also drive the woman's enthusiasm to quicken her recovery.

The goal in the perioperative period is to reduce the burden associated with anaesthesia and surgery and enable the restoration of normal function as soon as possible. This may be accomplished by addressing modifiable factors that may cause physiological derangements such as dehydration, hypothermia, nausea and vomiting. Preoperative fasting time may be reduced by allowing the mother to drink clear fluids up to 2 hours before surgery. Simple intraoperative measures such as warming, temperature monitoring and routine prophylactic antiemesis should be employed. Postoperatively, oral intake may be resumed as soon as is feasible. Effective analgesia may be achieved by the intraoperative use of neuraxial opioids in combination with postoperative multimodal analgesia, which – along with early removal of the indwelling urinary catheter – may enable the patient to mobilise sooner.

Enhanced recovery is thought to confer several benefits that extend to the mother, infant, and medical organisations. In addition to the clinical gains, the accelerated return to normalcy may facilitate bonding between the mother and neonate by allowing early skin-to-skin contact and initiation of breastfeeding. The reduction in the length of hospital stay can contribute to a significant reduction in expenditure and consumption of healthcare resources, although it is believed that this may be limited to some extent by the increased need for post-discharge care in the community.

While not yet a nationally implemented protocol, ER continues to be adopted by an increasing number of maternity units in the UK. Some organisational barriers to its widespread uptake still exist, however: for instance, the need for dedicated elective caesarean lists and the implications for human and financial resources, and the need for a robust system to ensure that follow-up and postoperative care are achieved to a high standard.

Key points

- Enhanced recovery is a collaborative effort that aims to reduce the length of hospital stay after caesarean section and subsequently improve patient outcomes.
- Patient selection and education are key to successful implementation.

Further reading

Corso E, Hind D, Beever D, *et al.* Enhanced recovery after elective caesarean: a rapid review of clinical protocols, and an umbrella of systematic reviews. *BMC Pregnancy Childbirth* 2017; **17**: 91.

Laronche A, Popescu L, Benhamou D. An enhanced recovery programme after caesarean delivery increases maternal satisfaction and improves maternal-neonatal bonding: a case control study. *Eur J Obstet Gynecol Reprod Biol* 2017; **210**: 212–16.

Lucas DN, Gough KL. Enhanced recovery in obstetrics: a new frontier? *Int J Obstet Anesth* 2013; **22**: 92–5.

Wrench IJ, Allison A, Galimberti A, Radley S, Wilson MJ. Introduction of enhanced recovery for elective caesarean section enabling next day discharge: a tertiary centre experience. *Int J Obstet Anesth* 2015; **24**: 124–30.

Chapter

43

Bloody tap

Cannulation of an epidural vessel may occur with either the needle or the catheter during siting of an epidural. The incidence is uncertain since widely varying figures have been quoted (e.g. 5–45%), possibly related to different methods of locating the epidural space, different needles or different definitions. Epidural venous engorgement in pregnant women may increase the likelihood of vessel puncture, and this may be exaggerated further in the sitting position. It is thought to be less likely when the paramedian approach is used, when 5–10 ml fluid is injected before threading the catheter, and possibly when smaller needles and catheters are used.

It is important to recognise bloody tap, because injection of local anaesthetic solution intravenously instead of epidurally may result in systemic toxicity (depending on the drug and dose). In addition, an ineffective epidural block may occur. Continued bleeding from a punctured vessel (e.g. after the epidural has been re-sited) may theoretically lead to an epidural haematoma if coagulation is impaired.

Problems and special considerations

Diagnosis is not usually a problem, especially if the needle has punctured a vessel. Puncture of a vessel by the catheter may be marked by discomfort as the vessel wall is pierced. Blood may then be aspirated from the catheter – although this is not always the case, hence the use of a test dose. Similarly, the absence of a bloody tap does not guarantee correct placement of the catheter. Therefore, it is important to aspirate all epidural catheters before administering any local anaesthetic solution.

Management options

If blood flows from the needle there is no option other than to remove the needle and re-insert it at a different interspace. If blood is obtained again, it may represent a new vascular puncture or blood from the original puncture. If blood is aspirated from the catheter, withdrawing the catheter in 0.5 cm increments, and flushing it with saline after each increment until aspiration is no longer possible, may remove the catheter from the vessel while still leaving enough length in the epidural space for effective anaesthesia. If this is not possible, then it should be re-sited in another interspace.

Key points

- In cases of bloody tap, flushing and incremental withdrawal of the catheter may avoid having to re-site the epidural.
- Bloody tap may not always be present when the catheter is placed intravascularly.

Dural puncture

Dural puncture usually refers to puncture of the dura and the underlying arachnoid mater. It may be deliberate during subarachnoid anaesthesia or accidental during epidural analgesia. The incidence in the latter case is traditionally said to be around 1% in teaching centres, but many authorities consider this to be unacceptably high, with an incidence of 0.5–1% being a realistic target and < 0.5% attainable in experienced hands. Most would routinely include dural puncture in their discussion with patients of the risks associated with regional analgesia.

Most accidental dural punctures are caused by the epidural needle, although it is possible for an epidural catheter to migrate through the dura. In-vitro studies suggest that this can only occur if there has been prior (unrecognised) dural puncture or partial tear of the dura by the needle. While there is a lack of randomised controlled trials that evaluate the efficacy of different techniques for location of the epidural space, the use of continuous loss of resistance to saline has, in animal models, shown superiority over the intermittent technique and is associated with a reduced risk of pneumocephalus compared with loss of resistance to air. Rotating the Tuohy needle once its tip is within the epidural space has been implicated in dural puncture and is now generally considered undesirable.

Problems and special considerations

Diagnosis

Dural puncture is usually heralded by a 'give' as the needle passes through the dura, and passage of cerebrospinal fluid (CSF) through the needle. For subarachnoid block, these two signs may be influenced by the design of the needle. In a combined spinal–epidural technique, it is usually easier to identify the dura by feel, especially in less experienced hands, since the starting position of the spinal needle in relation to the dura is more precisely known.

When a 16–18 G Tuohy needle is accidentally passed into the subarachnoid space, there is usually free flow of CSF, which poses no diagnostic difficulty. However, studies during deliberate dural puncture when placing lumbar drains before neurosurgery have revealed that occasionally free flow is not obtained. Thus, the appearance of slowly dripping clear fluid at the hub of the needle may represent CSF from a dural puncture or backflow of saline injected into the epidural space during a loss-of-resistance technique and may cause confusion, especially during a difficult procedure. In this situation, testing for temperature, glucose and protein content and pH (the last three by using urinary testing strips) will reliably distinguish CSF from saline (even saline that has been injected into the epidural space).

Occasionally, typical postdural puncture headache (PDPH) may be the first evidence that dural puncture has occurred, although this may reflect either inexperience on the part of the operator in not recognising accidental dural puncture or the operator not wishing to 'own up' in the hope that PDPH will not occur.

Adverse consequences

Adverse consequences of dural puncture are PDPH (which occurs in 60–90% of cases of accidental dural puncture in parturients) and its sequelae such as cranial nerve palsies, convulsions, subdural or intracranial haemorrhage, and chronic headache (see Chapter 45, *Postdural puncture headache*).

Management options

The aims of management of accidental dural puncture during establishment of epidural analgesia should include provision of adequate analgesia, safety of the patient and, if possible, reduction of risk from the adverse consequences of the dural puncture.

Traditional immediate management of accidental dural puncture comprises removing the needle and placing an epidural catheter at the adjacent (cranial) interspace, although this carries an additional risk of another unintentional dural puncture. Most units advocate that all subsequent top-ups during labour should be administered by an anaesthetist. The woman, her partner and the attending midwives and/or obstetricians should be informed that accidental dural puncture has occurred.

Other management options include converting the initial block to subarachnoid, which may include inserting the catheter into the subarachnoid space for a continuous subarachnoid block, for example by using 1–2 ml of standard low-dose epidural solution as top-ups or 1–2 ml/hour by infusion. Some observational studies suggest that inserting the catheter has been associated with a reduced incidence of PDPH, and it has been suggested that a possible mechanism is via initiating an inflammatory reaction around the catheter. However, other studies have not found this to be the case. If the catheter is placed intrathecally, it must be clearly labelled and the whole team informed, since there is a risk that it might be mistaken for an epidural catheter.

Studies of the association between pushing during the second stage of labour and an increased incidence of PDPH have yielded conflicting results. Traditionally, women who have had an accidental dural puncture have been advised to accept instrumental delivery to avoid pushing, but this is now generally considered unnecessary.

The performance of prophylactic epidural blood patch (see Chapter 46) is not routinely recommended. Likewise, epidural infusion of crystalloid after delivery (e.g. 1 litre of saline over 24 hours) has not been found to reduce the incidence of PDPH.

The use of epidural or spinal opioids has also been claimed to reduce the incidence of PDPH, although most of the evidence for this is weak apart from one randomised controlled study that has shown a reduction in the incidence of PDPH with epidural morphine. The evidence on the usefulness of drugs such as sumatriptan, pregabalin, ACTH or cosyntropin is inconclusive.

After delivery, there is no benefit in restricting the mother to bed, since this does not prevent PDPH. Similarly, although dehydration can exacerbate PDPH there is no evidence that overhydration has any beneficial effect. The mother should be visited regularly and given full support, and if PDPH occurs she should be offered the various management options available (see Chapter 45, *Postdural puncture headache*). She should also be informed about the possible serious sequelae of dural puncture, but reassured that they are rare.

It is equally important that the anaesthetist is honest with his/her colleagues, since attempting to conceal accidental dural puncture may only serve to delay appropriate management. Each unit should have a clear protocol for managing accidental dural puncture, and there should be a system in place for recording and monitoring such cases, usually involving a senior anaesthetist. Postpartum follow-up at 6–10 weeks is recommended in order to check that symptoms have resolved and to advise about future pregnancies.

Key points
- The incidence of accidental dural puncture should be less than 1%.
- Immediate management includes re-siting the epidural or inserting the catheter into the subarachnoid space.
- All top-ups should be administered by an anaesthetist.
- The mother should be allowed to mobilise freely and advised to avoid dehydration.
- Mothers should be followed up regularly and any headache managed promptly.

Further reading

Apfel CC, Saxena A, Cakmakkaya OS, *et al.* Prevention of postdural puncture headache after accidental dural puncture: a quantitative systematic review. *Br J Anaesth* 2010; **105**: 255–63.

Basurto Ona X, Osario D, Bonfill Cosp X. Drug therapy for treating post-dural puncture headache. *Cochrane Database Syst Rev* 2015; (7): CD007887.

Peralta F, Devroe S. Any news on the postdural puncture headache front? *Best Pract Res Clin Anaesthesiol* 2017; **31**: 35–47.

Chapter

45

Postdural puncture headache

Postdural puncture headache (PDPH) is typified by severe headache that is usually frontal or fronto-occipital, bilateral, worsened by standing or sitting upright and relieved by lying. Atypical clinical presentations that lack a positional component are infrequent but have been described in some women. There may be associated neck stiffness, nausea, tinnitus, visual disturbances and photophobia. It is thought to arise from intracranial hypotension resulting from leakage of cerebrospinal fluid (CSF) through the dural hole, with stretching of the cranial nerve roots and meninges in the upright position. Thus, the incidence and severity of PDPH are greatest following dural puncture with large cutting needles that leave large holes in the dura (60–90% in parturients after accidental dural puncture with a 16 G Tuohy needle), whereas small non-cutting needles are associated with a low incidence (under 1% with 25–27 G pencil-point needles). Parturients are the patient group most susceptible to PDPH.

There may be associated cerebral vasodilatation, leading to similarities being made between PDPH and migraine.

Symptoms usually begin within 1–2 days of dural puncture, although later onset (up to 10 days) has been reported. Headache usually lasts for 1–2 weeks but may occasionally persist for several months.

Problems and special considerations

Symptoms may be severe enough to prevent the mother mobilising and caring for her baby; this is particularly unwelcome in the early postpartum period. Discharge from hospital may be delayed, increasing costs and the risks of hospital-acquired infection and thromboembolism.

Rarely, more sinister sequelae may occur. These include cranial nerve palsies (the sixth cranial nerve being most susceptible, owing to its long intracranial course), convulsions, hearing loss and subdural or intracranial haemorrhage, or cortical vein thrombosis. Nerve damage may persist, even on resolution of the headache.

Diagnosis

A full history should be taken and neurological examination performed, as other differential diagnoses need to be considered (Table 45.1). Neurological referral and neuroimaging may be wise in difficult or refractory cases. PDPH is suggested by a history of dural puncture and typical symptoms, especially the postural element.

In approximately one-third of cases, PDPH may follow apparently unremarkable regional anaesthesia. Possible causes include lack of recognition at the time of dural puncture; failure to report dural puncture for fear of retribution; a possible tear of the

Table 45.1 Causes of postpartum headache

Tension, stress, fatigue, depression
Intracranial hypotension, e.g. postdural puncture headache
Intracranial hypertension, e.g. tumour, haematoma, cortical vein thrombosis, idiopathic
   intracranial hypertension
Migraine
Infection, e.g. meningitis, sinusitis, encephalitis
Pre-eclampsia (including posterior reversible encephalopathy syndrome)
Electrolyte imbalance, hypoglycaemia
Drugs, e.g. ondansetron

dura but not arachnoid at the time of epidural insertion, with rupture of the arachnoid subsequently; and migration of the epidural catheter intrathecally during labour.

It has been suggested that an otherwise typical PDPH that only becomes severe hours after getting up is caused by a very small dural hole with slow leak of CSF, for example after spinal anaesthesia with a very fine needle. A useful confirmatory sign is the lessening of headache produced by gradually compressing the upright patient's upper abdomen. This is thought to displace spinal CSF into the cranium by causing venous engorgement in the extradural space. Magnetic resonance imaging and computerised tomography scanning have been used to diagnose intracranial hypotension and to demonstrate cerebrospinal fluid leaks (in the latter case involving further diagnostic dural puncture), but are not widely used.

Management options

Initial management includes simple analgesics such as paracetamol and non-steroidal anti-inflammatory drugs. Although frequently prescribed, there is no evidence that overhydration or bed rest has a preventive effect. Other medical management includes oral caffeine 150–300 mg every 6–8 hours, which has been shown to improve the symptoms temporarily. Caffeine may cause nausea and vomiting in overdosage and has been implicated in convulsions occurring after dural puncture. A recent Cochrane review concluded that the use of gabapentin, theophylline and hydrocortisone was associated with reduced pain severity scores in patients with PDPH. The use of sumatriptan and ACTH analogue has been described, but the evidence supporting their use is weak.

Invasive procedures involve infusion or injection of various substances such as saline or dextran into the extradural space, firstly to shift CSF from the spine into the skull and secondly to tamponade leakage of CSF through the dural hole and even to seal the hole. These are no longer recommended. However, epidural blood patch (EBP) is now generally accepted as the definitive treatment in persistent PDPH, with reported success rates of 60–70% after one patch and 80–90% after a second blood patch if the headache recurs. Many anaesthetists would now proceed to EBP early (e.g. within 24–48 hours of symptoms) if there is a good history, rather than delay for several days as was common previously (see Chapter 46, *Epidural blood patch*).

Full discussion with, and support of, the patient is of prime importance, since she may be more distressed by apparent indifference to the severity of her symptoms than by the complication itself. She should be regularly visited while in hospital and followed up in the initial period after discharge. The patient should be counselled – preferably by a senior anaesthetist – on the various therapeutic options and on the rare possibility of serious sequelae. It is not known whether EBP prevents these, although this is generally assumed if symptoms resolve. If the woman decides against an EBP, she should be reassured that she may come back at any time should her symptoms persist. Healthcare staff who provide postpartum care for the patient – including her general practitioner – must be made aware of her clinical course, outcome and also of 'red flag' features mandating further medical advice. Postpartum follow-up at 6–10 weeks is recommended in order to check that symptoms have resolved and to advise about future pregnancies.

Key points

- Postdural puncture headache occurs in 60–90% of parturients after accidental dural tap with a 16 G Tuohy needle.
- The postural element is the most important confirmatory feature, but atypical presentations have been reported.
- Initial management includes paracetamol, non-steroidal anti-inflammatory drugs, avoidance of dehydration, ± caffeine.
- Definitive treatment is with epidural blood patch.

Further reading

Arevalo-Rodriguez I, Ciapponi A, Roqué i Figuls M, Muñoz L, Bonfill Cosp X. Posture and fluids for preventing post-dural puncture headache. *Cochrane Database Syst Rev* 2016; (3): CD009199.

Basurto Ona X, Osario D, Bonfill Cosp X. Drug therapy for treating post-dural puncture headache. *Cochrane Database Syst Rev* 2015; (7): CD007887.

Klein AM, Loder E. Postpartum headache. *Int J Obstet Anesth* 2010; **19**: 422–30.

Sachs A, Smiley R. Post-dural puncture headache: the worst common complication in obstetric anesthesia. *Semin Perinatol* 2014; **38**: 386–94.

Chapter 46

Epidural blood patch

Injection of blood into the epidural space as a treatment for postdural puncture headache (PDPH) was first suggested in the 1960s, following the observation that the incidence of PDPH was lower when dural tap followed a bloody tap. In fact, this relationship was later found not to be so, but epidural blood patch (EBP) has become widely accepted as the gold-standard treatment for PDPH, despite early fears about adverse effects.

The mechanism of action of EBP is uncertain. Traditional teaching is that the blood seals the dural hole, preventing further leakage of cerebrospinal fluid. However, an alteration of cerebrospinal haemodynamics by EBP has been suggested, accounting for EBP's immediate effect and the observation that lumbar EBP is effective even following cervical dural puncture.

Problems and special considerations

The optimal timing for the performance of an EBP remains controversial. Previous studies have identified a higher failure rate of EBP in patients in whom the initial procedure was performed within the first 24–96 hours of the onset of PDPH, while other studies have demonstrated a favourable outcome when EBP was performed more than 48 hours after the development of the headache. Nevertheless, the need for a repeat procedure in patients who receive an early EBP may be related to the severity of the headache rather than the timing of the intervention, and it is recommended that the intensity of the patient's symptoms be taken into account when making the decision to perform an early EBP. There are conflicting data on the usefulness of prophylactic EBP (via the catheter after delivery). Problems include the difficulty it might cause with analgesia (e.g. postoperatively), the fact that some women will receive an intervention they may not need, and the possible risk of infection if the catheter is left in place throughout a prolonged labour. Although not routinely recommended, some authors have suggested that the procedure may be considered in patients at high risk of developing PDPH.

Contraindications are those of epidural analgesia generally; in particular the risk of epidural abscess is often quoted if the mother is pyrexial. In that situation, other methods of treating PDPH may be tried; alternatively, prophylactic use of antibiotics has been suggested. Some authorities advocate routine sending of blood for microbiological culture in case bacteraemia is present, although this practice is not universal.

Adverse effects of EBP include those of epidural analgesia (including failure or another dural puncture), back pain, transient nerve root pain and pyrexia. More significant complications such as subdural or intrathecal haematoma with consequent neural compression or arachnoiditis have also been described. Transient bradycardia has been reported, but its significance is uncertain.

Management options

Other causes of postpartum headache should be excluded (see Table 45.1). Two operators are required. While one locates the epidural space in the usual way, the other prepares to draw 20 ml of blood under full aseptic conditions. The blood is injected slowly and the patient is asked to report any unpleasant effects. The interspace at or below the level of the original dural puncture is usually recommended, since injected blood has been shown to track mainly upwards after injection.

One of the controversial issues regarding EBP is the volume of blood to inject. It was thought that the more blood that was injected, the greater the chance of success. Currently, however, the general recommendation is that the volume of blood injected should be individualised, and that injection should cease when the patient reports back pain. This is supported by the findings of a recent retrospective review that demonstrated no added advantage in terms of efficacy (no reduction in the need for a second patch when additional volumes of up to 30 ml of blood were injected).

The patient is usually kept lying for 2–4 hours after EBP (reduced efficacy has been suggested if mobilisation is immediate). The success rate of EBP has been reported as 70–100%; typically, there is complete relief of headache, although some degree of headache may return in up to 30–50% of women. Repeat EBP is sometimes required, rarely more than once. The procedure is performed on an outpatient basis in some units.

The mother should be fully informed of the benefits and risks of EBP (including the lack of proper randomised trials and the possibility of inflicting another dural puncture). A senior anaesthetist should perform the EBP for two reasons: first, the original epidural may have been difficult, and a second dural puncture occurring during EBP would be at best embarrassing; second, the mother has suffered considerable distress and deserves the reassurance of knowing that an experienced anaesthetist is handling her case. Since the headache may return after EBP, she should be invited to contact the anaesthetist if this occurs.

Key points

- Epidural blood patch should be performed by a senior anaesthetist under strict asepsis. 15–20 ml of blood is injected if tolerated.
- The mother is kept supine for 2–4 hours after patching.
- The timing of epidural blood patching should be guided by the severity of the patient's symptoms.
- Treatment is effective in 70–100% of cases, but headache may recur in 30–50%.

Further reading

Booth JL, Pan PH, Thomas JA, Harris LC, D'Angelo R. A retrospective review of an epidural blood patch database: the incidence of epidural blood patch associated with obstetric neuraxial anesthetic techniques and the effect of blood volume on efficacy. *Int J Obstet Anesth* 2017; **29**: 10–17.

Kokki M, Sjövall, Keinänen M, Kokki H. The influence of timing on the effectiveness of epidural blood patch in parturients. *Int J Obstet Anesth* 2013; **22**: 303–9.

Peralta F, Devroe S. Any news on the postdural puncture headache front? *Best Pract Res Clin Anaesthesiol* 2017; **31**: 35–47.

Extensive regional block

Obstetric anaesthetists, in routinely extending neuraxial analgesia up to the level of T4, are accustomed to dealing with regional anaesthetic blocks that other practitioners would regard as excessively high. It is inevitable that occasionally the block will extend beyond the anticipated area, either because of accidental subarachnoid or subdural administration or merely because of the unpredictability of spread in some individuals. Although many such blocks may be quite benign and not cause any cardiovascular or respiratory embarrassment, it is important that they are detected in order to pick up misplacement of the local anaesthetic, which may cause more serious problems later.

'Total spinal block' is strictly defined as a spinal block that results in unconsciousness and central depression of respiratory and myocardial activity, accompanied by massive vasodilatation. Since the same may also result from epidural and subdural blocks, and one should not wait until unconsciousness before acting, the terms 'high regional block' or 'extensive regional block' are preferred. A practical definition of these terms would be a regional block that results in the need for tracheal intubation or other airway intervention. The reported incidence of such blocks is between 1 in ~2000 and 1 in ~13,000, probably reflecting differences in definitions used in the studies from which these figures arise.

Problems and special considerations

The effect and spread of local anaesthetic drugs is enhanced in pregnancy, and this should be borne in mind when planning doses for a spinal or epidural block.

An apparently fixed spinal block may extend further if the patient is moved, even 30 minutes or more after the local anaesthetic has been administered. This particularly applies to rotation through the fully supine position from one side to the other and may be due to dural compression resulting from dilatation of the epidural veins, which act as a collateral circulation during aortocaval compression.

Early features of extensive block include weakness or tingling of the upper arms and shoulders, breathing difficulties, slurred speech and sedation. Symptoms and signs may develop late and insidiously.

Hypotension may be severe and may be associated with reduced placental perfusion and fetal hypoxia or ischaemia. Urgent delivery may be necessary both to relieve maternal hypotension and to protect the fetus.

Airway management following total spinal block is made more difficult in pregnancy because of the increased risk of aspiration and the difficulty in maintaining a clear airway without tracheal intubation.

A woman may find the experience of a high regional block very frightening, despite the anaesthetist's reassurance that her breathing is adequate and she is safe. It is important to be aware of this, and to reassure her continuously; offering general anaesthesia should even be considered for extreme distress.

Epidural analgesia and anaesthesia

Relatively large doses of local anaesthetic drugs are used which, if they find their way into the wrong compartment, can cause a dangerously extensive block.

Prevention is the key, and this is achieved by maintaining a high index of suspicion and regarding every dose of local anaesthetic as subarachnoid until proven otherwise. The potential problems are best discussed under the following headings:

- **Epidural analgesia.** A test dose suitable for distinguishing subarachnoid placement should be used after the epidural catheter is inserted, and the effect should be assessed before further local anaesthetic is given. Each epidural dose should be given sufficiently slowly to allow detection of a spinal block before it spreads to a dangerously high level; doses should be administered at intervals of 5 minutes or longer, with the mother moving between increments. These precautions should be used with every dose in labour, since catheter migration has been known to occur between doses. The use of low-dose local anaesthetic–opioid mixtures reduces the risk to the mother if accidentally given intrathecally; the local anaesthetic concentration should be the lowest for the effect required.

- **Epidural top-up for instrumental or caesarean delivery.** Volumes of up to 20 ml concentrated solution may be injected over 3 minutes, the risk of extensive block being weighed against the need for rapid extension for surgery. Alternatively, 3–4 ml of the top-up solution can be given as a test dose, 3–5 minutes before the main dose. It has been suggested that the top-up can safely be given in the labour room and the patient transferred to theatre while the block is extending, although this is controversial, since the ability to monitor and/or resuscitate may not be ideal before or during transit. It is essential that the anaesthetist is by the patient at all times and ensures adequate monitoring and lateral tilt. Regular testing of the block is mandatory.

- **Epidural after dural puncture with the Tuohy needle.** If an epidural catheter has been re-sited following accidental dural puncture, the risk of high block is increased, both because the local anaesthetic can leak through the puncture and because the catheter can migrate. Epidural doses/infusions should be reduced and given by an anaesthetist.

- **Subdural block.** This is thought to occur in up to 1% of 'epidurals'. It may occur when the epidural catheter is passed into the potential space between the dura mater and the arachnoid, probably after the needle has torn the dura. The block is characteristically slow in onset (20–30 minutes) and spreads cranially much higher than expected, often involving the lower cervical dermatomes. Extensive motor block is, however, uncommon, and hypotension is usually mild. The block tends to spare the lumbar and sacral segments and may be patchy; consequently, pain relief is often poor. If analgesia is acceptable, it is tempting to leave the catheter in situ and to continue to use smaller doses. This technique is not recommended, because of the risk of a top-up rupturing the arachnoid, with subsequent development of an extensive subarachnoid block.

- **Accidental subarachnoid block.** This is rarer than subdural block, largely because the anaesthetist is usually alerted by the free flow of cerebrospinal fluid from the hub of the catheter. The consequences are far more hazardous, however, since the resulting block is very rapid in onset, has a considerable motor component, and is normally associated with severe hypotension.

Spinal anaesthesia

High blocks associated with spinal anaesthesia are related to greater spread rather than deposition of local anaesthetic into the wrong space. This may result from the use of hypobaric solutions, or compression of the dural sac from the outside as a result either of recent epidural top-up or of aortocaval compression, or it may represent an extreme of normal variation as anaesthetists have sought higher and higher blocks in order to avoid pain during surgery. The continuous presence of the anaesthetist and the immediate availability in the operating theatre of the necessary equipment and assistance ensure that further supportive measures are readily available if needed.

Prevention of excessive block is achieved by using the minimum necessary dose of local anaesthetic. Excessive barbotage should also be avoided. Maintenance of the natural kyphosis of the thoracic spine if in lateral tilt, or the use of pillows under the shoulders and head if in the full lateral position, will help prevent hyperbaric local anaesthetic spreading higher than the T4 dermatomes. Head-down tilt is very occasionally needed to encourage a recalcitrant block to spread high enough for surgery, but this should be used with great care and reversed as soon as the desired effect has been achieved. The same precautions apply if the mother is rolled through the full supine position as part of the positioning or if she is coughing or otherwise performing a Valsalva manoeuvre; these can result in sudden cranial spread of the block, and this can even happen at the end of a procedure when the block has been established for some time.

The ideal dose of spinal solution to use after a recent (failed) epidural top-up is uncertain. There have been reports of extensive blocks if normal spinal doses are used, presumably as a result of dural compression, but there have also been reports of normal responses or even inadequate anaesthesia if smaller doses are used.

Management options

It has been suggested that all women receiving regional anaesthesia for an operative procedure should be warned about the risk of a high block. Calm reassurance will be necessary for the woman and her partner in what may be a very distressing experience.

The basics of resuscitation ('ABC') should be remembered. Aortocaval compression should be prevented, and the full lateral position is best if cardiopulmonary resuscitation is not needed.

Oxygen should be given by facemask, and tracheal intubation should be performed early if a raising block progresses; waiting until the patient is unconscious may risk airway obstruction and/or aspiration of gastric contents. Careful use of a hypnotic agent (and neuromuscular blocking drug) will be needed for intubation in the presence of haemodynamic compromise.

Cardiovascular support includes intravenous fluids, vasopressors such as phenylephrine or ephedrine if bradycardic (adrenaline may be needed if hypotension is resistant) and cardiopulmonary resuscitation if cardiac arrest or severe myocardial depression is compromising cerebral oxygenation.

Rapid delivery of the fetus should be considered to protect it from hypotension and to relieve aortocaval compression.

Sedation and ventilation will need to continue until there is evidence that the block has regressed to a satisfactory level, i.e. haemodynamic stability with adequate spontaneous respiratory effort.

A post-incident debrief with the woman and her partner should be provided.

Key points

- All epidural doses should be divided into safe aliquots, if time permits.
- Subdural catheter placement is common and may progress to subarachnoid block.
- Spinal blocks can spread cranially even 30 minutes after administration.
- Careful and regular monitoring of the height of block is required after institution of spinal or epidural anaesthesia.
- Delivery of the fetus may protect it from ischaemia and may also benefit the mother.

Further reading

Jenkins JG. Some immediate serious complications of obstetric epidural analgesia and anaesthesia: a prospective study of 145,550 epidurals. *Int J Obstet Anesth* 2005; **14**: 37–42.
Yentis SM, Dob DP. High regional blockade: the failed intubation of the new millennium? *Int J Obstet Anesth* 2001; **10**: 159–61.

Chapter 48

Inadequate regional analgesia in labour

Although epidural analgesia has an excellent track record for relieving the pain of labour, a proportion of epidurals fail to deliver adequate pain relief. Approximately 10% of women will have initially unsatisfactory blocks, and around 2% of these will be persistently inadequate. Poor blocks may be divided into those involving inadequate spread, and those where spread is apparently adequate but the degree of block is insufficient.

Problems and special considerations

Inadequate spread

This may be one of several types:

- A block that, while bilateral, is less effective on one side of the body than the other, usually due to insertion of an excessive length of catheter into the epidural space.
  The unequal block is thought to result from placement of the catheter tip to one side of the epidural space, and even its escape from the epidural space via a lateral foramen. This may even result in a very limited block involving only one or two dermatomes. Lengths greater than ~5–6 cm are generally regarded as at increased risk of transforaminal escape of the catheter tip, while lengths less than 2–3 cm are more likely to result in the catheter's falling out, especially during a long labour.
- Satisfactory cranial and caudal spread, but limited to one side of the body only. Contrast studies of this type of block have shown that it is associated with distribution of fluid to one side of the epidural space. The most likely explanation is the existence of a dorsal midline septum arising from the posterior aspect of the dura mater, which acts as a barrier to the free spread of local anaesthetic. Unilateral block has also been shown to be more common in cases of scoliosis, and this is also presumed to be due to anatomical barriers to spread of local anaesthetic in the epidural space.
- Missed segment, whereby one or more segments remain unblocked despite normal analgesia above and below. This was more commonly seen when low volumes of concentrated local anaesthetic solution were routinely used during labour, but is relatively uncommon with the higher-volume, low concentrations used in modern techniques. Missed segments were thought to arise from isolation of some nerve roots from the local anaesthetic by longitudinal septa or air used in loss-of-resistance techniques, or from relative resistance of larger nerve roots (typically lumbar) to penetration by local anaesthetic.

- Limited cranial or caudal spread despite attempts to extend it with further doses, for example because of a horizontal septum preventing flow or presumed scarring in patients who have undergone spinal surgery.
- Catheters with single terminal eyes are commonly used in the USA, whereas most UK practitioners prefer multi-holed, blind-ending catheters. Studies have demonstrated a higher incidence of unsatisfactory blocks with the former, mostly due to unilateral blocks and missed segments. This is probably due to a 'streaming' effect, whereby all the solution is directed along a single track, encouraging longitudinal spread at the expense of lateral flow.

Inadequate density of block

A block that is insufficient despite apparently adequate spread may occur when excessively dilute mixtures of local anaesthetic are used, when the intensity of pain is increased (e.g. occipito-posterior position, or placental abruption or impending uterine rupture), or in some women who just seem to have lower pain thresholds. A differential block may also be seen; this may be due to different nerve fibres being affected variably by the local anaesthetic, or to variable central somatosensory integration.

Other maternofetal factors may be associated with an increased incidence of breakthrough pain during labour epidural analgesia. These include nulliparity, a raised maternal body mass index (BMI), a longer duration of labour, a larger fetus and abnormal fetal presentations. Rarely, severe breakthrough pain that does not improve with additional epidural dosing may be an indication of more serious pathology such as uterine rupture.

Management options

The key to managing poor blocks is early detection. All mothers who have had an epidural block in labour should be checked by the anaesthetist within 20–30 minutes of the first dose and the level of analgesia tested with a suitable stimulus. Continued review of the patient and the efficacy of epidural analgesia is mandatory throughout subsequent labour. Any complaint of persistent pain at any time during the labour should prompt further testing and review. Dislodgement or disconnection of the epidural catheter should first be excluded by visual inspection of the insertion site and infusion set. Confirmation of block height and assessment of the distribution of pain may enable the anaesthetist to determine the appropriate management strategy. If an epidural cannot be made to function adequately within an hour of troubleshooting, the anaesthetist and woman should consider the benefit of re-siting it.

Generalised abdominal pain with uterine contractions may indicate an insufficient height of neuraxial block, which should extend to a dermatomal level of T8–10 during the first stage of labour. This may be managed by the administration of an additional dose of the epidural local anaesthetic–opioid mixture (a bolus of up to 20 ml has been suggested). This should preferably be given manually, as this is thought to aid wider spread in the epidural space. Occasionally, a solution containing either stronger local anaesthetic or fentanyl, or both, might be required for intense pain during augmented labour.

Perineal pain that results from failure of epidural analgesia to provide effective blockade of the larger sacral nerve roots that are less penetrable by neuraxial drugs (sacral sparing) may respond to topping up in the sitting position, with either the standard low-dose epidural solution or a higher-concentration local anaesthetic (e.g. 0.25% bupivacaine), or with fentanyl (50–100 µg). Supplementation with a pudendal nerve block may be used if delivery is imminent. A combined spinal–epidural (CSE) should be considered in situations when the pain is resistant to treatment.

A limited unilateral block is usually due to insertion of an excessive amount of epidural catheter, and may be rectified by pulling back the catheter to leave 3–5 cm in the epidural space. Unfortunately, once a 'track' has been established for the local anaesthetic solution, it may persist despite this manoeuvre, and the only solution may be to remove the catheter and re-site it in a different space. Even if the catheter was originally inserted to the optimum distance, the possibility of it being drawn further into the epidural space should not be discounted; this has been shown to happen as a result of traction imposed by movements of the vertebrae and activity of the spinal muscles.

Unilateral block can occasionally be overcome by laying the patient on the affected side and administering large volumes of local anaesthetic, with or without opioid. It is presumed that this encourages spread of the solution up and down the epidural space and thus beyond the boundaries of any midline septum, or allows any breaches in the septum to be exploited. These manoeuvres may be effective but there will often be a marked tendency for the block to affect the 'good' side more than the other. In the more recalcitrant unilateral block, the catheter may need to be re-sited in another interspace. Sometimes, when the above manipulations have been unsuccessful, a paramedian approach may help, since the catheter has been shown to travel a straighter course in the epidural space when inserted via this route. A CSE technique may be used to overcome poor spread or missed segments, and for some anaesthetists this is the technique of choice following a failed epidural, as it allows rapid onset of analgesia and it has been suggested that the epidural catheter is less likely to fail if a needle-through-needle CSE technique has been used compared with a plain epidural technique. Other causes for poor block should not be overlooked.

With a missed segment, the above techniques may also be tried. Sometimes, a stronger solution of local anaesthetic may be effective, and this may also be useful in cases of apparently adequate spread but breakthrough pain within the 'blocked' dermatomes, such as back pain or perineal pain. Addition of opioid is usually employed too. The woman should be warned that re-siting will not necessarily lead to a resolution of the problem if it has been caused by anatomical variation.

Continuous infusion techniques may fail if the syringe pump is not functioning properly, has been incorrectly set up or has become occluded. The commonest reason for a previously satisfactory block failing is the epidural catheter falling out – another good reason for checking the catheter first.

Finally, it should be remembered that an inadequate epidural for labour is likely to be inadequate for caesarean section should one be required in an emergency; in such situations it might be appropriate to consider spinal anaesthesia instead. Furthermore, in women with a high risk of caesarean section, the anaesthetist should have a low threshold for re-siting an epidural if the latter is less than perfect during labour.

Key points

- Blocks should be checked regularly to allow early detection of failure.
- In the event of a poor block, especially when previously satisfactory, the catheter should be checked.

- Poor spread is often caused by an excessive length of catheter in the epidural space. A length of 3–5 cm is usually considered optimum.
- Re-siting the catheter early is often a better option than repeated 'fiddling'.

Further reading

Agaram R, Douglas MJ, McTaggart RA, Gunka V. Inadequate pain relief with labor epidurals: a multivariate analysis of associated factors. *Int J Obstet Anesth* 2009; **18**: 10–14.

Hermanides J, Hollmann MW, Stevens MF, Lirk P. Failed epidural: causes and management. *Br J Anaesth* 2012; **109**: 144–54.

Pan PH, Bogard TD, Owen MD. Incidence and characteristics of failures in obstetric neuraxial analgesia and anesthesia: a retrospective analysis of 19,259 deliveries. *Int J Obstet Anesth* 2004; **13**: 227–33.

Breakthrough pain during caesarean section

Breakthrough pain may be experienced during the course of operative delivery under spinal or epidural anaesthesia. Breakthrough pain during caesarean section must be dealt with promptly, as inadequate pain control may interfere with surgery and may cause considerable distress to the woman and her partner, leading to patient dissatisfaction or complaints. Indeed, pain during caesarean section is thought to be the most common source of successful litigation against anaesthetists. Pre-warning the patient of the possibility of intraoperative discomfort or pain and the need for supplementation or general anaesthesia, and the accurate pre-procedural assessment and documentation of the height of neuraxial block using multiple modalities, are therefore of crucial importance.

Problems and special considerations

Despite the benefits offered by epidural anaesthesia in terms of titratability and extendability, the technique may not provide the same density of block as spinal anaesthesia, and the onset of adequate surgical anaesthesia may be variable. Supplementation of the block or conversion to general anaesthesia (reported rates of the latter are ~1–4%) may thus reflect an unreliable or incomplete block, or the limited time available to wait until the block becomes adequate,

Sensations of tugging, stretching or pressure during caesarean section are common, and women – especially very anxious ones – may find these symptoms distressing even though they are not painful. It may therefore be difficult for the anaesthetist to be sure that the patient is actually experiencing pain, although he/she must recognise that if the patient is distressed, her symptoms must be taken seriously and treatment offered.

Visceral pain may be experienced in the course of the procedure despite painless skin incision and superficial dissection, and may be secondary to traction on the peritoneum or the uterine ligaments, exteriorisation of the uterus, swabbing of the paracolic recesses or even rough manipulation of tissues.

Chest pain is experienced by some patients. The cause is unclear, but proposed explanations include small air emboli, oesophageal spasm, and irritation of the diaphragm by amniotic fluid or blood. The latter may also cause shoulder-tip pain.

Management

Parturients who receive epidural analgesia, especially those at high risk of operative delivery, must be assessed periodically during the course of labour. A dysfunctional epidural catheter that has failed to provide satisfactory analgesia or one that has required frequent supplementation is less likely to produce a reliable block for caesarean section. Regular review enables the identification of such issues and the manipulation or re-siting of the epidural catheter if necessary.

If the patient complains of pain intraoperatively, surgery must be paused momentarily while the anaesthetist takes steps to establish the origin of the pain and attempt to resolve it, although this may be challenging once the uterine incision is performed or when bleeding is excessive and immediate intervention is necessary. The management of the pain will depend to a large extent on the stage of the operation. Pain experienced in the initial stages of the procedure (i.e. at or immediately after skin incision) indicates a poor-quality neuraxial block, and in the absence of an in-situ epidural catheter to allow further top-up is likely to require either the re-administration of regional anaesthesia, which should be done carefully to avoid precipitating a high block, or conversion to general anaesthesia.

The presence of an epidural catheter in situ may allow extension of the block using rapid-onset agents such as lidocaine or ropivacaine, and opioids such as fentanyl or diamorphine. Additional options for supplementation of the regional anaesthetic at this stage include inhalational analgesia with nitrous oxide, incremental doses of systemic opioids such as alfentanil, fentanyl or diamorphine, short-acting benzodiazepines such as midazolam, or ketamine in analgesic doses (10–20 mg boluses). The administration of intravenous agents should be done with caution in order to avoid excessive maternal sedation and potential airway compromise. The use of local anaesthetic infiltration of tissues may also be employed as a rescue technique. The anaesthetist must maintain effective communication with the patient and continue to provide explanation and reassurance.

Severe maternal emotional distress or failure of the above measures to control her pain must prompt the anaesthetist to offer the woman general anaesthesia. If women decline, it may be because they are scared by the knowledge (often provided by the same anaesthetist preoperatively) that general anaesthesia is considered more dangerous than regional anaesthesia. The anaesthetist must be mindful of this, reassuring her and being prepared on occasion to recommend strongly that general anaesthesia may be the best option, rather than merely 'offering' it meekly. Adequate preparation and skilled assistance is of paramount importance, as the procedure may be problematic when performed intraoperatively.

Because of the distress that intraoperative pain may cause, and the risk of psychological trauma and of complaints or litigation, it is crucial that clear records are kept. These must include evidence of:

1. Explanation preoperatively that discomfort or pain is possible, and that the options of supplementation and conversion to general anaesthesia are available
2. Appropriate and adequate regional anaesthetic technique, e.g. method of insertion of a de novo block or top-up of an existing epidural
3. Adequate and thorough assessment of the block before surgery starts
4. Appropriate action if/when pain is felt, e.g. halting surgery, administration of further drugs, offer of general anaesthesia, reassurance/support etc.
5. Provision of postoperative follow-up and explanation(s) and further counselling if the mother wishes

Key points

- Breakthrough pain under caesarean section is multifactorial and may occur despite a seemingly adequate level of surgical anaesthesia.

- Women experiencing pain during surgery may be very distressed and may develop post-traumatic stress disorder.
- A multimodal assessment of the height of neuraxial block for operative delivery is recommended.
- Intraoperative management may include: halting surgery if possible; intravenous, inhalational or epidural supplementation; and conversion to general anaesthesia.
- Effective communication with the patient during the procedure, postoperative follow-up and accurate recording of events are all essential.

Further reading

Bogod D. Pain during caesarean section. *BJOG* 2016; **123**: 753.

Mankowitz SK, Gonzalez Fiol A, Smiley R. Failure to extend epidural labor analgesia for cesarean delivery anesthesia. *Anesth Analg* 2016; **123**: 1174–80.

Chapter 50

Backache

Backache is not a trivial symptom. It is one of the commonest causes of time off work in the UK, and can be particularly debilitating for the nursing mother.

Backache is very common, and a high proportion of women have significant backache before pregnancy, with surveys putting this figure at around 15%. During pregnancy, the prevalence of backache rises to ~50%.

Long-term backache after childbirth (defined as backache lasting longer than 3 months) occurs in about a third of women, and this increases to half if there is a history of backache before or during the pregnancy. The incidence of new, long-term backache in women with no symptoms of backache before or during pregnancy is much lower, at around 5–10%.

Problems and special considerations

Prospective studies have found no significant increase in the risk of backache when epidural analgesia is used in labour, nor an association with motor block. Despite this, there is a popular belief among parturients, midwives and even obstetricians that there is a causative link between epidural analgesia in labour and subsequent backache, largely arising from retrospective surveys of mothers in the late 1980s. Many women who develop intractable backache shortly after an anaesthetist has inserted a needle into their back will, not surprisingly, believe that the two are connected, and commonly refer to their backache as starting 'after the epidural' instead of 'after the baby'.

This is not to say, of course, that a poorly administered epidural cannot cause trauma that might lead to backache, or that backache should be ignored after an epidural. In particular, acute tenderness over the epidural site should always raise the suspicion of an epidural abscess or haematoma, especially when accompanied by pyrexia and signs of nerve root irritation or cauda equina syndrome. Finally, rare coincidental causes such as a tumour should not be overlooked.

Management options

Women with backache often present to the anaesthetist in the antenatal period. Referral to the obstetric physiotherapist, lumbar support, simple analgesia and transcutaneous electrical nerve stimulation (TENS) may all be of help.

While the evidence does not support a causal link between epidural/spinal analgesia/anaesthesia and long-term backache, many women ask about this complication, especially at antenatal classes, and the best approach is to inform them of the high risk of backache associated with pregnancy and childbirth, and to reassure them that these techniques do not appear to increase this risk.

The woman who presents with severe backache or a long history of back trouble in the antenatal clinic should be warned that it is very likely that this will continue after childbirth. Epidural analgesia should not be contraindicated in these cases, but it may sometimes be more painful having an epidural sited in a sensitive back. Care should be taken to avoid unnatural postures that will unduly stress the ligaments, and the patient should be allowed to move freely in labour. Support of lumbar lordosis and prevention of hyperextension at the hips are helpful.

Midwives should be alerted to refer severe, acute, localised backache after epidural insertion to the anaesthetist. Management should include a full neurological examination, and a low threshold for early referral to a neurologist and imaging to exclude haematoma or abscess formation.

Localised tenderness and limitation of movement may be due to a small haematoma in the interspinous ligament or paraspinous muscles, and these will often respond to physiotherapy.

Key points

- Backache is very common after childbirth.
- There is no apparent link between epidural/spinal analgesia/anaesthesia and long-term postpartum backache.
- Tenderness associated with pyrexia should raise the suspicion of abscess.

Further reading

Anim-Somuah M, Smyth RM, Cyna AM, Cuthbert A. Epidural versus non-epidural or no analgesia for pain management in labour. *Cochrane Database Syst Rev* 2018; (5): CD000331.
Han IH. Pregnancy and spinal problems. *Curr Opin Obstet Gynecol* 2010; **22**: 477–81.
Orlikowski CE, Dickinson JE, Paech MJ, *et al.* Intrapartum analgesia and its association with post-partum back pain and headache in nulliparous women. *Aust N Z J Obstet Gynaecol* 2006; **46**: 395–401.

Chronic pain after caesarean section

Chronic post-surgical pain is a common perioperative complication and may be seen in up to 85% of patients undergoing certain types of surgery, for example limb amputation. In the obstetric population, pain is often present after delivery, with a higher incidence after caesarean section than vaginal delivery. Chronic pain may develop; this is usually diagnosed at 2–3 months, when acute pain associated with tissue damage is expected to have passed. Depending on the definition given in terms of duration and source of pain, chronic pain has been reported in 5–25% of women after caesarean section.

Problems and special considerations

The pathogenesis of chronic post-surgical pain is thought to be related to tissue damage and nerve injury, with release of inflammatory mediators (e.g. cytokines, bradykinin and prostaglandins), loss of inhibitory neurones, amplification of sensory input, and spontaneous ectopic discharges causing hypersensitivity and allodynia. Central sensitisation is an important trigger for the development of persistent pain, so anaesthetic and analgesic techniques aimed at attenuating sensitisation may be of benefit.

Certain groups may be at an increased risk for the development of chronic pain after caesarean section; these include women with increased anxiety about childbirth and those with pre-existing chronic pain syndromes. There may also be a genetic predisposition for the development of chronic pain syndromes. Studies report that women who experience severe acute postpartum pain have a 2.5-fold increased risk of experiencing a chronic pain syndrome.

Some studies have shown that women who have a caesarean section under general anaesthetic seem to be at increased risk of chronic pain. This may be related to increased nociceptive afferent transmission perioperatively and worse control of pain in the immediate postoperative period.

Persistent postpartum pain may have far-reaching consequences. It has been associated with a decreased quality of life, impaired activities of daily living and an increased incidence of postnatal depression.

Management options

By identifying those at risk, such as those with pre-existing chronic pain or particular anxieties about childbirth, an antenatal plan can be made in an attempt to reduce the risk; efficacious analgesia such as effective epidural analgesia during delivery can be recommended, and effective post-delivery analgesia provided.

Multimodal analgesia should be offered to all women, particularly those who have a caesarean delivery. This should include simple analgesics, opioids (preferably neuraxial) and local anaesthetic techniques; this is particularly relevant to those who deliver under general anaesthesia. If an epidural is in situ, long-acting opioids should be given at the end of the procedure unless contraindicated. If an epidural is not in situ, local anaesthetic techniques such as transversus abdominis plane (TAP) blocks should be employed. Use of preoperative gabapentin has been shown to reduce acute pain scores at the expense of increased sedation in the obstetric population; there is no evidence of a reduction in chronic pain, but study numbers have been small. There is some suggestion that intrathecal clonidine may decrease the risk of developing chronic pain by reducing hyperalgesia; however, its use is not common and it is not licensed for use in obstetric practice.

Any acute postpartum pain should be addressed proactively. Issues may be actively sought during routine follow-up.

If chronic post-caesarean pain does develop, it should be treated in the conventional way of managing chronic pain. After underlying causes have been ruled out, appropriate multi-modal analgesia should be prescribed, depending on the nature of the pain (e.g. neuropathic versus somatic). Patient education, counselling and anti-neuropathic agents such as amitriptyline or gabapentin may be beneficial. If the severity of pain and impact on life are severe, referral to pain specialists may be required. However, most studies in the obstetric population indicate that chronic pain is often not severe and tends to improve spontaneously with time.

Key points

- Chronic pain after a caesarean section is a common complication.
- Acute postoperative pain is a recognised risk and should be managed promptly.

Further reading

Daly B, Young S, Marla R, *et al.* Persistent pain after caesarean section and its association with maternal anxiety and socioeconomic background. *Int J Obstet Anesth* 2017; **29**: 57–63.

Jin J, Peng L, Chen Q, *et al.* Prevalence and risk factors for chronic pain following cesarean section: a prospective study. *BMC Anesthesiol* 2016; **16**: 99.

Weibel S, Neubert K, Jelting Y, *et al.* Incidence and severity of chronic pain after caesarean section: a systematic review with meta-analysis. *Eur J Anaesthesiol* 2016; **33**: 853–65.

Chapter 52

Horner's syndrome and cranial nerve palsy

Horner's syndrome is the combination of partial ptosis, myosis (small pupil), enophthalmos and hypohydrosis, and represents interruption of the ipsilateral sympathetic supply to the head anywhere along its length. There may also be associated nasal stuffiness and reduced taste sensation on the ipsilateral side (Gustav's sign). Horner's syndrome may occasionally occur during an otherwise unremarkable epidural block.

Palsies of cranial nerves V and VI have been reported following uncomplicated obstetric epidural anaesthesia, although much less commonly than Horner's syndrome. In addition, cranial nerve palsies are well known to occur (albeit uncommonly) following dural puncture, and cases (including cranial nerve VII palsy) have been reported after accidental dural tap during childbirth. An idiopathic lower motor neurone lesion of cranial nerve VII (Bell's palsy) may occur rarely in pregnancy, but there is no evidence that it is related to regional anaesthesia.

Problems and special considerations

The mechanism for Horner's syndrome occurring during apparently normal and non-extensive epidural analgesia and anaesthesia is uncertain. Partial subdural cranial extension of local anaesthetic solution has been suggested, although there may be no other features of atypical block. The sympathetic innervation of the iris is variable and may arise from C8 to T5; in addition, sympathetic fibres are thought to be more sensitive to local anaesthetics than somatic fibres. Increased incidence in pregnancy has been suggested and may be related to the greater susceptibility of pregnant women to local anaesthetics generally or to more extensive central neural blocks in particular.

Cranial nerve palsy is also thought to be related to excessively high blockade; palsy of cranial nerve V is commonly associated with Horner's syndrome. Cranial nerve palsy following dural puncture is thought to be related to stretching of the nerve caused by traction of intracranial contents, and it is usually associated with postdural puncture headache. Other mechanisms that have been implicated in cranial nerve paresis include raised intracranial pressure secondary to infection or thrombosis, and ischaemic neuropathy triggered by systemic hypotension.

Management options

Lesions may go unnoticed or may cause alarm to the patient, her partner or labour ward staff. In addition, if another possibly unrelated complication or event were to occur, or if general anaesthesia was administered subsequently, the pupillary signs especially may cause confusion. For cases occurring during uncomplicated epidural analgesia and anaesthesia, no specific treatment is required other than reassurance, since the signs themselves are harmless and disappear when the epidural block wears off. Once diagnosed, simple observation is all that is required, bearing in mind that the intense interest of medical and midwifery staff may cause more anxiety than the syndrome itself.

Although there are other more sinister causes of Horner's syndrome and cranial nerve palsies, they are rare and do not usually present so acutely or for a limited duration. An association with other symptoms or signs would indicate neurological referral and/or imaging. Palsies associated with dural puncture should be managed as for the headache; it has been suggested that resolution of the palsy is less likely if epidural blood patch is delayed.

There is no evidence that the occurrence of Horner's syndrome or cranial nerve palsy during one labour epidural predisposes the patient to the same thing during subsequent epidurals.

It must not be forgotten that some individuals naturally have unequal pupils or an asymmetrical face; it is therefore worth asking the patient and her partner whether the signs are new.

Key points

Horner's syndrome

- Comprises partial ptosis, myosis, enophthalmos and hypohydrosis.
- May occur during an otherwise unremarkable epidural.
- Is harmless and requires no treatment if related to epidural anaesthesia.

Cranial nerve palsy

- Most commonly involves nerves V or VI, although the incidence is lower than that of Horner's syndrome.
- Requires no treatment if of short duration and associated only with regional anaesthesia.

Further reading

Barbara R, Tome R, Barua A, *et al.* Transient Horner syndrome following epidural anesthesia for labor: case report and review of the literature. *Obstet Gynecol Surv* 2011; **66**: 114–19.

Chambers DJ, Bhatia K. Cranial nerve palsy following central neuraxial block in obstetrics – a review of the literature and analysis of 43 case reports. *Int J Obstet Anesth* 2017; **31**: 13–26.

Hofer JE, Scavone BM. Cranial nerve VI palsy after dural-arachnoid puncture. *Anesth Analg* 2015; **120**: 644–6.

Peripheral nerve lesions following regional anaesthesia

Although spinal and epidural needles and catheters must, by virtue of their mode of action, pass close to nerve roots, the incidence of neurological damage appears to be very low. Surveys have suggested that around 1 in 2000 obstetric epidurals/spinals is complicated by numbness, paraesthesia or weakness in the distribution of a single nerve root that may take several days to a few months to resolve. The incidence of permanent symptoms is approximately 1 in 15, 000.

Problems and special considerations

Nerve root damage

A needle or catheter touching a nerve root is almost certain to cause paraesthesia in the awake patient, usually of a severe, lancinating quality and characteristically described as being like an electric shock in the distribution of the nerve root. Unless transient and mild, paraesthesia should always prompt the anaesthetist to remove the needle or catheter and to reorientate it. Presence or absence of paraesthesia should always be recorded. If damage has occurred, symptoms are usually experienced in the same distribution (Table 53.1).

Peripheral nerve damage

While it is perhaps natural to blame any lower limb neurological deficit on the neuraxial block that preceded it, nerve palsy is more likely to arise as a result of obstetric factors, as witnessed by patients with demonstrable permanent lesions despite not having had epidural or spinal procedures. The incidence of postpartum obstetric nerve palsies is around 1%, the causes and features

Table 53.1 Neurological deficit following nerve root trauma

Root	Sensory loss	Motor weakness
L2	Upper anterior thigh	Hip flexion
L3	Lower anterior and medial thigh	Thigh adduction
L4	Lateral thigh, knee and medial leg	Leg extension
L5	Lateral leg and dorsum of foot	Ankle dorsiflexion
S1	Lateral foot	Ankle plantar flexion

of which are listed in Table 53.2. The potential for nerve damage during childbirth is apparent when one considers the anatomy of the nerves arising in the pelvis (see Figure 10.6), with possible mechanisms of injury including stretching or compression of the nerve .

Neuraxial analgesia may contribute indirectly to the development of nerve injury by eliminating the discomfort caused by prolonged nerve compression in certain positions, which would normally prompt the woman to re-position herself.

Central neurological lesions
Single nerve damage should be distinguished from the more serious central lesions that occur extremely rarely (see Chapter 54, *Spinal cord lesions following regional anaesthesia*; Chapter 55, *Arachnoiditis*; Chapter 56, *Cauda equina syndrome*).

Management options
Prevention is the most important aspect of management. Blocks should be performed with the patient awake (not normally an issue in obstetric practice), and care should be taken to ensure that the interspace chosen is below the level of termination of the spinal cord. Patients should be asked to indicate if they feel paraesthesia, and this should be a signal to the anaesthetist to remove the needle or catheter and start again. Spinal injections should only be given if there is free flow of cerebrospinal fluid, to ensure that the needle tip is not obstructed by nerve tissue. A note should always be made as to the

Table 53.2 Nerve lesions with non-anaesthetic, obstetric causes

Lesion	Presentation	Cause
Lateral cutaneous nerve of thigh	Meralgia paraesthetica – altered sensation over anterolateral aspect of thigh	Antenatal weight gain ± lumbar lordosis. Prolonged pushing in lithotomy position
Femoral nerve	Loss of sensation front of thigh. Quadriceps weakness. Reduced knee jerk	Hyperflexion of thighs, especially squatting or lithotomy position. Instrumental delivery
Peroneal nerve	Foot drop	Pressure from lithotomy poles or prolonged squatting
Lumbosacral trunk	Foot drop. Loss of sensation especially L4–5, S1	Pressure in pelvis from fetal head or forceps
Obturator nerve	Weakness of thigh adductors. Loss of sensation in an area in upper third of medial thigh. Wide-based gait	As for femoral nerve
Conus of spinal cord	Anterior spinal artery syndrome – cauda equina/paraplegia	Obstruction of aberrant blood supply to conus by fetal head during prolonged labour. Herniated disc

presence or absence of paraesthesia during the procedure, as this information can be invaluable later.

Routine follow-up should be carried out assiduously, and midwives should be alerted to notify the anaesthetist if any mother shows signs of slow recovery of sensory or motor function. Careful mapping of the deficit should be carried out at the earliest opportunity to establish a baseline from which improvement can be measured. Other, non-anaesthetic, causes should be considered; the aetiology may be suggested by the distribution and nature of the deficit and by the presence of precipitating factors (see Table 53.2). The benign course of the vast majority of these lesions means that an explanation to the patient can include a reassuring prognosis. Generally, neuropraxias recover in 3–4 months, though occasionally chronic pain may ensue so postpartum follow-up should always be offered.

Except for minor and resolving lesions, further management should generally involve referral to a neurologist or neurophysiologist. Imaging of the thoracolumbar region should be considered in the presence of local or radicular back pain, associated sphincter incontinence, motor or sensory abnormalities in a root or cord pattern, signs of infection, and in patients with progressive symptoms or those with a history of immunosuppression. Nerve conduction studies are often invaluable, as they allow the site of the lesion to be identified and may help in estimating prognosis.

Key points

- Paraesthesia should always be documented and is a sign to withdraw the needle, reorientate it and start again.
- Delayed recovery needs assiduous follow-up to detect neuraxial haematoma or abscess.
- Nerve palsy is usually a result of pregnancy or childbirth and unrelated to regional anaesthesia.

Further reading

Cook TM, Counsell D, Wildsmith J; Royal College of Anaesthetists Third National Audit Project. Major complications of central neuraxial block: report on the 3rd National Audit Project of the Royal College of Anaesthetists. *Br J Anaesth* 2009; **102**: 179–90.

Moen V, Irestedt L. Neurological complications following central neuraxial blockades in obstetrics. *Curr Opin Anaesthesiol* 2008; **21**: 275–80.

O'Neal MA, Chang LY, Salajegheh MK. Postpartum spinal cord, root, plexus and peripheral nerve injuries involving the lower extremities: a practical approach. *Anesth Analg* 2015; **120**: 141–8.

Richards A, McLaren T, Paech MJ, *et al.* Immediate postpartum neurological deficits in the lower extremity: a prospective observational study. *Int J Obstet Anesth* 2017; **31**: 5–12.

Wong CA. Nerve injuries after neuraxial anaesthesia and their medicolegal implications. *Best Pract Res Clin Obstet Gynaecol* 2010; **24**: 367–81.

Chapter 54

Spinal cord lesions following regional anaesthesia

Postpartum neurological lesions are often blamed on peripartum anaesthetic interventions, even though non-anaesthetic causes are much more likely. Obstetric anaesthetists may therefore find themselves involved in the assessment and management of these problems. There are many causes of spinal cord lesions (Table 54.1).

Problems and special considerations

The initial problem is one of diagnosis. Different lesions may present in different ways that may overlap with each other and with other conditions (Table 54.1). Spinal cord lesions are more commonly associated with spinals and combined spinal–epidurals, and it should be remembered that peripheral neuropathies may arise as a result of obstetric interventions, especially those involving the lithotomy position. Spontaneous epidural haematoma or abscess (without neuraxial interventions) may also occur. Although cord lesions generally

Table 54.1 Causes of postpartum spinal cord lesions

Mechanism	Condition	Comment
Compression	Epidural haematoma	Not associated with back pain
	Epidural abscess	Associated with back pain plus evidence of local and/or systemic infection; typically presents several days postpartum
	Prolapsed disc	
	Tumour	
Ischaemia	Severe hypotension	
	Anomalous arterial blood supply plus prolonged labour and hypotension	
	Normal vascular supply and normotension	
Neurotoxicity	Injection of wrong solution	
Trauma	Back injury	Associated with back pain
	Direct damage during regional anaesthesia	May be associated with back pain, although paraesthesia is more common

171

present with upper motor neurone signs and sensory impairment below the level of injury, and peripheral nerve injuries present with lower motor neurone signs, it may be surprisingly difficult to distinguish them clinically (see Chapter 53, *Peripheral nerve lesions following regional anaesthesia*).

Sinister signs such as pyrexia, severe back pain, bilateral distribution, or loss of bladder or bowel function are suggestive of a compressive lesion such as epidural or spinal haematoma or abscess. These conditions are very rare (< 1 in 100,000) but may cause major, irreversible damage unless relieved within hours of presentation. Any suspicion should prompt immediate referral for a neurosurgical opinion. In the case of early lesions, some effects of spinal or epidural blockade may persist for several hours, occasionally over 12 hours (up to 48 hours has been observed, with no apparent cause), obscuring the underlying pathology. Since regression of a block often occurs under observation by non-anaesthetic staff, there may be delay in requesting appropriate medical input. In the case of acute potentially reversible spinal cord damage, for example cord compression caused by haematoma, delay of more than 6–8 hours is associated with an increasing chance of permanent impairment

Similarly, problems that present later, such as epidural abscess, may be missed if associated back pain is dismissed as trivial.

Management options

Anaesthetic-related problems may be reduced by attention to details such as:

- Assessing the coagulation status and pre-existing neurological status before performing regional techniques.
- Aseptic technique and exercising caution to avoid the contamination of needles and catheters with antiseptic solutions.
- Determining appropriate anatomical landmarks during the procedure, and awareness of the existence of anatomical variants and the risk of inserting the needle too high. Ultrasound guidance may help the identification of the correct intervertebral level, particularly when landmarks are difficult to palpate.
- Removal of the needle or catheter if severe paraesthesia or pain is experienced during a regional block.
- Prevention and management of hypotension after anaesthesia.

Maternity units should have local protocols for monitoring recovery from neuraxial blockade, and both patients and clinical staff should be educated on the 'red flag' features that they need to report without delay (e.g. persistent/progressive bilateral sensory/motor deficit, urinary retention/incontinence, faecal incontinence, persistent severe back pain). Any unexpectedly dense or prolonged block should always be observed carefully, especially if other risk factors (e.g. heparin therapy or sepsis) are present. A careful history and examination, and knowledge of the relevant anatomy, are vital to distinguish the various lesions from less severe conditions, and neurological referral is always advisable if there is any suspicion.

Individual conditions are managed as for non-pregnant patients, e.g. surgical decompression for cord compression, plus antibiotics for abscess.

Key points

- Anaesthetists may be involved in the assessment and management of postpartum spinal cord lesions.
- Knowledge of the appropriate anatomy and variations is crucial.
- In acute spinal cord compression, delay in decompression beyond 6–8 hours may result in permanent disability.

Further reading

Chambers DJ, Howells ACL. Neurological complications in obstetric regional anaesthesia. *Anaesth Intensive Care Med* 2016; **17**: 372–4.

Cook TM, Counsell D, Wildsmith JA; Royal College of Anaesthetists Third National Audit Project. Major complications of central neuraxial block: report on the 3rd National Audit Project of the Royal College of Anaesthetists. *Br J Anaesth* 2009; **102**: 179–90.

Moen V, Irestedt L. Neurological complications following central neuraxial blockades in obstetrics. *Curr Opin Anaesthesiol* 2008; **21**: 275–80.

Porter JR, Christie LE, Yentis SM, Durbridge J, Dob DP. Prolonged neurological deficit following neuraxial blockade for caesarean section. *Int J Obstet Anesth* 2011; **20**: 271.

Wong CA. Nerve injuries after neuraxial anaesthesia and their medicolegal implications. *Best Pract Res Clin Obstet Gynaecol* 2010; **24**: 367–81.

Arachnoiditis

Arachnoiditis is a rare condition comprising chronic radicular pain associated with radiologically diagnosed abnormalities, classically filling defects in the subarachnoid space, absence of spinal nerve root sleeves, arachnoid cysts and obstruction to flow of radio-opaque contrast medium. It is important to realise that radiological abnormalities may be present in asymptomatic patients, and a diagnosis of arachnoiditis should not be made on radiological criteria alone. It may occur spontaneously, although it has followed radiation and perispinal injection of irritant substances, such as the oil-based contrast medium that used to be employed for myelography. Antiseptic solutions, powder from surgical gloves and preservatives in drug solutions (e.g. sodium metabisulfite) have been implicated, as have infection and traumatic bleeding. Arachnoiditis has been reported following regional anaesthesia and analgesia, including after epidural blood patch, but it is very rare and the precise aetiology is uncertain (apart from cases following obvious injection of antiseptic solution).

Arachnoiditis may occasionally be confused with cauda equina syndrome; typical features of the two conditions are shown in Table 55.1.

Problems and special considerations

Chronic adhesive arachnoiditis may develop several months or even years after the trigger, so it may be difficult to establish a causal link. Typically, arachnoiditis presents with back

Table 55.1 Typical features of arachnoiditis and cauda equina syndrome

	Aetiology	Features
Arachnoiditis	Inflammation of the arachnoid meningeal layer and subarachnoid space	Meningeal irritation may occur early, although usually presents months or years later
	Progressive fibrosis may cause spinal canal narrowing, ischaemia and permanent nerve damage	May involve the cauda equina, presenting with similar features
		Rarely extends cranially
Cauda equina syndrome	Damage to the lumbosacral nerve roots	Presents soon after regional anaesthesia, with numbness in corresponding myotomes, sphincter dysfunction

pain that worsens with activity, with or without leg pain, paraesthesia or weakness. It is usually steadily progressive and may follow neurological complications of regional anaesthesia.

Management options

Although obstetric regional analgesia and anaesthesia are considered to be extremely safe, it is important to maintain scrupulous attention to aseptic and atraumatic technique and to minimise the use of novel drugs and multiple combinations of drugs. Thus all solutions injected epidurally or spinally should be carefully checked first. Chlorhexidine used for skin asepsis is neurotoxic, and while arachnoiditis has followed accidental injection of large amounts into the neuraxis, introduction of even apparently insignificant traces has been linked (somewhat controversially) with its development. The use of 0.5% chlorhexidine in alcohol is therefore recommended over the 2% solution, and steps to minimise the potential for accidental contamination of equipment or injectate with antiseptic solution should be taken, as per the available guidance.

Once a diagnosis of arachnoiditis is suspected, early involvement of a neurologist is mandatory, with confirmation of the diagnosis by magnetic resonance imaging (MRI) scan. Detailed follow-up and possibly long-term support will be required. There is no specific treatment for arachnoiditis; steroids have been tried, although they are thought to be effective only in the very acute stage of the inflammatory process. Psychological support is important, since the consequences of the condition may be catastrophic.

Key points

- Arachnoiditis is inflammation of the arachnoid and subarachnoid space; it typically occurs months or more after injury.
- Although rare, it may cause permanent neurological damage.
- Meticulous attention must be paid to maintaining aseptic precautions and the avoidance of accidental contamination of regional anaesthetic equipment or drugs with antiseptic solution.

Further reading

Association of Anaesthetists of Great Britain and Ireland, Obstetric Anaesthetists' Association, Regional Anaesthesia UK. Regional anaesthesia and patients with abnormalities of coagulation. *Anaesthesia* 2013; **68**: 966–72.

Association of Anaesthetists of Great Britain and Ireland, Obstetric Anaesthetists' Association, Regional Anaesthesia UK, Association of Paediatric Anaesthetists of Great Britain and Ireland. Safety guideline: skin antisepsis for central neuraxial blockade. *Anaesthesia* 2014; **69**: 1279–86.

Carlsward C, Darvish B, Tunelli J, Irestedt L. Chronic adhesive arachnoiditis after repeat epidural blood patch. *Int J Obstet Anesth* 2015; **24**: 280–3.

Moen V, Irestedt L. Neurological complications following central neuraxial blockades in obstetrics. *Curr Opin Anaesthesiol* 2008; **21**: 275–80.

Cauda equina syndrome

Cauda equina syndrome is a rare condition that is caused by injury to the lumbosacral nerve roots. It has been associated with ultra-fine spinal catheters, especially when hyperbaric lidocaine has been injected, when it is thought to result from poor mixing of local anaesthetic in the cerebrospinal fluid and pooling of anaesthetic in the terminal dural sac, especially if large doses are used to extend an inadequate block. Local anaesthetics are known to be directly neurotoxic in high concentrations, lidocaine more than bupivacaine. The cauda equina nerve fibres may be more vulnerable to damage than other structures because they lack protective sheaths.

Although rare, cauda equina syndrome due to lumbar disc herniation has been reported in the early postpartum period.

Problems and special considerations

Early symptoms may include lower limb neurological deficit and bladder and bowel disturbances. Isolated areas of numbness on the leg and disturbances of perineal sensation are relatively common after delivery, sometimes making diagnosis difficult. Occasionally, obstetric-related neurological deficit may be permanent. Cauda equina syndrome may also be confused with arachnoiditis; for typical features of the two conditions, see Chapter 55, *Arachnoiditis*.

Management options

Scrupulous attention to technique should be used when performing regional analgesia and anaesthesia. Special precautions should be taken when using continuous spinal blockade (e.g. avoiding lidocaine, especially in high concentrations, and not injecting large volumes of hyperbaric solutions). Once the diagnosis is suspected, early involvement of a neurologist is mandatory, since detailed follow-up and possibly long-term support will be required. There is no specific treatment for cauda equina syndrome (other than urgent decompression in cases of acute traumatic compression), although steroids may be tried. Psychological support is important, as the consequences of the condition may be catastrophic.

Key points

- Cauda equina syndrome results from damage to the lumbosacral nerve roots; the condition occurs soon after the insult.
- Although rare, it may cause permanent neurological damage.

Further reading

Cook TM, Counsell D, Wildsmith JA; Royal College of Anaesthetists Third National Audit Project. Major complications of central neuraxial block: report on the 3rd National Audit Project of the Royal College of Anaesthetists. *Br J Anaesth* 2009; **102**: 179–90.

Kowe O, Waters JH. Neurologic complications in the patient receiving obstetric anesthesia. *Neurol Clin* 2012; **30**: 823–33.

Opioid-induced pruritus

Itching can result from the administration of opioids by any route, but it is much more common following epidural and intrathecal opioids than after systemically administered opioids. The reported incidence of itching varies from 0% to 100%, and it is sometimes only discovered as a result of observing the patient or asking direct questions. Severe itching is only a problem in a very small number of cases (possibly as low as 1%). The incidence of itching associated with opioids is higher in the obstetric population, probably owing to an oestrogenic influence at the opioid receptors.

Facial itching predominates after epidural and intrathecal opioids. This is possibly related to migration of opioid in the cerebrospinal fluid to the trigeminal nucleus and the trigeminal nerve roots. More generalised itching occurs with systemically administered opioids and may be due to activation of peripheral opioid receptors and partly to histamine release (especially with morphine). The mechanism of opioid-induced itching is still not completely understood; suggested mechanisms include modulation of the serotonergic pathway and activation of the medullary dorsal horn.

Problems and special considerations

The incidence of pruritus varies considerably between different opioids, being highest with morphine and lowest with the most lipophilic drugs such as fentanyl and sufentanil. Mixed agonist–antagonist drugs such as buprenorphine and butorphanol have been used via the epidural route to reduce the incidence of itching without decreasing analgesia.

Itching following administration of intrathecal fentanyl for caesarean section does not appear to predict that itching will also occur after epidural administration of diamorphine for postoperative analgesia.

Management options

No treatment is necessary for opioid-induced itching unless the mother is distressed. Simple antihistamines may be effective, but this may be through their sedative effect. Naloxone is an effective treatment for pruritus, but reduces the duration of analgesia obtained with neuraxial opioids, although a low-dose continuous infusion (0.4–0.6 mg/h) of naloxone is said to treat itching while maintaining analgesia from intrathecal morphine. A systematic review has suggested that prophylactic 5-HT$_3$ receptor antagonists, such as ondansetron, may reduce the severity of pruritus.

A variety of other treatments have been proposed, including intravenous droperidol, subhypnotic doses of propofol, nalbuphine and intramuscular promethazine. There is little evidence that any are effective.

Key points

- Itching can occur following the administration of any opioid drug by any route, but is most common following the epidural or intrathecal administration of morphine.
- Although the incidence of pruritus may exceed 90%, it is not often distressing for the mother and may not require any treatment other than reassurance.

Further reading

Bonnet MP, Marret E, Josserand J, Mercier FJ. Effect of prophylactic 5-HT$_3$ receptor antagonists on pruritus induced by neuraxial opioids: a quantitative systematic review. *Br J Anaesth* 2008; **101**: 311–19.

Kumar K, Singh SI. Neuraxial opioid-induced pruritus: an update. *J Anaesthesiol Clin Pharmacol* 2013; **29**: 303–7.

Waxler B, Dadabhoy ZP, Stojiljkovic L, Rabito SF. Primer of postoperative pruritus for anesthesiologists. *Anesthesiology* 2005; **103**: 168–78.

Shivering

Although shivering may occur in about 10% of normal labours and following general anaesthesia, it is particularly associated with regional (especially epidural) anaesthesia and analgesia, during which it has been reported to occur in up to two-thirds of cases. The cause is uncertain, but evidence suggests the tremor is at least partly thermoregulatory, accompanied by core-to-periphery heat redistribution due to sympathetic blockade. Centrally mediated shivering and vasoconstriction thresholds also appear to be lowered by neuraxial anaesthesia. Epidural blockade may inhibit the subjective feeling of being cold, even when the core temperature has fallen. Other postulated mechanisms include altered control of peripheral muscles and a central effect resulting from systemic absorption of local anaesthetic or its transport via the cerebrospinal fluid to the brain. In labour, the high levels of circulating catecholamines and general arousal may also be important. Finally, the tendency for maternal temperature to increase after prolonged epidural analgesia may contribute to shivering, although it has also been suggested that shivering may contribute to the increase in temperature. Shivering is also commonly seen after misoprostol, with reported incidences of 50–70%.

Problems and special considerations

In most cases, shivering is mild and benign, although if severe it may increase maternal catecholamine concentrations and metabolic rate, interfere with fetal and maternal monitoring and be alarming to the mother. It also increases maternal oxygen consumption and carbon dioxide production, although this is rarely a problem in practice. Rarely, the mother may be unable to cooperate with medical and midwifery staff during examinations, etc.

Anecdotally, epidural lidocaine (e.g. top-up for caesarean section) has been associated with an increased incidence of shivering compared with other local anaesthetics, but firm evidence is lacking, and this possibility must be weighed against any advantages of lidocaine (e.g. rapid speed of onset).

Management options

If shivering is mild, simple reassurance is often all that is required. Measures that have been studied include warming of epidural, intrathecal and intravenous solutions and administration of intravenous opioids (pethidine 10–30 mg has been shown to be especially effective in the non-pregnant population). Epidural opioids may also reduce the incidence and severity of shivering. Other drugs shown to be effective after general anaesthesia outside of obstetrics include clonidine and doxapram, although these are infrequently used in the maternity suite. Active warming appears to reduce the incidence of shivering during caesarean section under epidural anaesthesia if it commences preoperatively.

Key points

- Shivering is common during epidural analgesia and anaesthesia.
- Simple reassurance is adequate treatment in most cases.

Further reading

Crowley LJ, Buggy DJ. Shivering and neuraxial anesthesia. *Reg Anesth Pain Med* 2008; **33**: 241–52.
Witte J, Sessler DI. Perioperative shivering: physiology and pharmacology. *Anesthesiology* 2002; **96**: 467–84.

Aspiration of gastric contents

Aspiration is one of the three factors consistently associated with maternal deaths related to obstetric general anaesthesia, the others being emergency operation and difficult tracheal intubation. Often, these three factors occur together.

Problems and special considerations

Several risk factors make the pregnant woman more prone to aspiration:

- Reduced efficacy of the lower oesophageal sphincter caused by progesterone
- Reduced gastric emptying if opioids have been given, particularly if systemic
- The physical effect of the gravid uterus on the stomach
- The presence of gastric contents if the mother has eaten (see Chapter 14, *Gastric function and feeding in labour*)

Every mother in the third trimester should be considered at risk of aspiration, although the point during pregnancy at which increased risk occurs, and the point postpartum at which the risk returns to normal, are controversial. Many obstetric anaesthetists would consider 16–18 weeks of pregnancy as representing the onset of the 'at-risk' period, although an earlier cut-off point has also been suggested, especially if there are symptoms of gastro-oesophageal reflux, the mother is obese, or the procedure requires her to be positioned head-down. Similarly, although hormonal profiles alter dramatically within a few hours of delivery, studies of gastric emptying have not produced consistent results, although some have suggested as little as 4–8 hours postpartum as the time required for the risk to return to normal (longer if opioids have been administered). Most would treat women as still at increased risk of gastric aspiration for 48 hours postpartum. However, other general physiological changes of pregnancy may take several weeks to disappear.

Finally, it should not be forgotten that any pregnant woman with an obtunded level of consciousness may be at risk from aspiration, for example during or after convulsions, drug overdose, anaphylaxis, etc. Thus, women identified as high risk may not only be those in whom surgical intervention is planned or expected.

Mortality or morbidity may be related to:

- Impairment of the view at laryngoscopy causing difficulty with intubation.
- Obstruction of the upper airway by solid or semi-solid matter causing complete or partial airway obstruction, hypoventilation and atelectasis.
- Chemical pneumonitis (Mendelson's syndrome), related to the pH and volume of the aspirated material, with a continuum of risk such that smaller volumes are required if the pH is lower. The alveolar inflammatory reaction may be intense, with oedema,

cellular infiltration and the features of acute lung injury. There may be associated hypotension and poor peripheral perfusion if large amounts of fluid have been transferred from the intravascular space into the alveoli. Aspiration pneumonitis may also be caused by particulate antacids, e.g. magnesium trisilicate.

- Aspiration pneumonia, in which aspirated secretions are colonised with bacteria causing infection of the respiratory tract.

Management options

Prevention

Reduction of the volume and acidity of gastric contents. This may be achieved by:

- Withholding oral intake during labour
- Administration of metoclopramide or other prokinetic drugs
- Use of antacids or acid-reducing drugs such as H_2-antagonists and proton pump inhibitors
- Emptying the stomach with a stomach tube before general anaesthesia or by inducing vomiting (rarely used, although it has been suggested that a stomach tube should be routinely passed during general anaesthesia for emergency caesarean section in order to reduce the risk of aspiration after extubation)

The first three measures are used to differing extents in different situations and countries. Thus, for example, all women in a particular unit might be given regular oral antacids and ranitidine throughout labour, whereas only women identified as being at high risk of intervention might be treated in another unit. Similarly, feeding in labour occurs to different degrees on different labour wards (see Chapter 14, *Gastric function and feeding in labour*). Proponents of all-inclusive treatment point to the potentially devastating effect of aspiration, the relative cheapness of therapy and the difficulty of identifying women truly at risk of a general anaesthetic. Supporters of selective treatment cite the low incidence of aspiration overall, the relatively low incidence of general anaesthesia in modern obstetric practice, the cost of therapy compared with no therapy, and resistance from many women and midwives to the 'medicalisation' of normal labour.

A practical breakdown of commonly used pharmacological preventive measures might be as follows (although, as already mentioned, the protocol in use may vary widely between units):

- Normal (i.e. low-risk) labour. Nil, plus local unit oral intake policy, e.g. a light diet, low-fat snacks.
- High-risk labour suggesting an increased risk of surgical intervention (e.g. obstetric complications, multiple pregnancy) or high-risk parturient suggesting an increased risk of aspiration if surgical intervention occurs (e.g. obese, significant reflux). Regular oral ranitidine 150 mg 6-hourly in active labour; following administration of pethidine: ranitidine 50 mg intramuscularly 8-hourly, plus local unit oral intake policy, e.g. clear fluids.
- Emergency caesarean section. Ranitidine 50 mg ± metoclopramide 10 mg slowly intramuscularly or intravenously when the decision for surgery is made, 30 ml sodium citrate 0.3 M orally immediately before induction of general anaesthesia.

- Elective caesarean section. Oral ranitidine 150 mg the night before and repeated the morning of surgery, metoclopramide/sodium citrate as above.

Preventing regurgitation during general anaesthesia. Standard general anaesthetic practice includes a rapid-sequence induction with application of cricoid pressure, although the method of its application and the possibility that cricoid pressure might make laryngoscopy more difficult are controversial areas (see Chapter 37, *Cricoid pressure*). Tracheal extubation should be in the lateral position with the patient awake, following return of full protective reflexes.

Avoidance of general anaesthesia altogether by using regional anaesthesia for operative procedures. This is generally thought to be a major factor in the reduction in maternal mortality associated with anaesthesia that occurred over the 1970s–1990s, although there is no doubt that improvements in training in, and assistance and facilities for, general anaesthesia also occurred during this period.

Diagnosis

Regurgitation may be obvious, either during induction of anaesthesia or intra-/postoperatively. It may or may not be associated with aspiration. It is also possible for aspiration to occur without obvious, massive regurgitation, for example during induction or intraoperatively past the cuff of the tracheal tube. Features include bronchospasm, raised airway pressure, hypoxaemia, tachypnoea, tachycardia and pyrexia; these may present for the first time postoperatively following otherwise uneventful anaesthesia. A high index of suspicion is therefore required. If fluid is aspirated from the pharynx, larynx or tracheal tube, simple litmus paper is useful for identifying its acidity, although this may not always be reliable if antacid therapy has been used.

Treatment

Initial management consists of removing the regurgitated material from the airway by using pharyngeal, laryngeal and tracheal suction and maintaining oxygenation. Tracheal intubation has the advantage of securing the airway and protecting it against further aspiration, as well as allowing ready access to the tracheobronchial tree for suction. Cricoid pressure may prevent further regurgitation during intubation, though this should be released if there is any active vomiting. The head-down lateral position may be appropriate, depending on the particular circumstances of the case, in order to encourage drainage of fluid from the upper airway and discourage further aspiration should regurgitation recur. Bronchospasm may occur, requiring usual management. Although popular in the past, the use of prophylactic steroid and antibiotic therapy in cases where aspiration is suspected is no longer advocated, since this approach has not been shown to reduce mortality and may even increase it. Antibiotics should only be administered for clinical evidence of infection. Solid particles may be removable via bronchoscopy; bronchoalveolar lavage may also be used to dilute the acidic fluid aspirated.

A chest x-ray may be useful to show the presence of large amounts of aspirated material (usually in the right lower lobe if aspiration occurred in the semi-recumbent position, and in the upper lobes if aspiration occurred when supine) and as a baseline, although a normal appearance does not exclude aspiration. In 25% of cases, there are no visible changes seen on x-ray, and any changes tend to lag behind the clinical course by up to 24 hours. Patients suspected of having aspirated should be observed and monitored carefully for at least 12–24 hours, since their condition may worsen considerably during this time. If a patient is unstable, consideration should be given to a delayed extubation once she is clinically improved.

Key points

- Aspiration of gastric contents is a major factor in maternal death associated with general anaesthesia, especially related to emergency caesarean section and difficult tracheal intubation.
- Prevention includes sensible policies on feeding in labour, use of pH-raising drugs and antacids, emptying the stomach, rapid-sequence induction when general anaesthesia is used and avoidance of general anaesthesia by encouraging regional anaesthetic techniques.
- Diagnosis may not always be obvious.
- Treatment includes general supportive measures; antibiotics and steroid therapy are no longer advocated.

Further reading

Gyte GM, Richens Y. Routine prophylactic drugs in normal labour for reducing gastric aspiration and its effects. *Cochrane Database Syst Rev* 2006; (3): CD005298.

Mendelson CL. The aspiration of stomach contents into the lungs during obstetric anaesthesia. *Am J Obstet Gynecol* 1946; **52**: 191–205.

Robinson M, Davidson A. Aspiration under anaesthesia: risk assessment and decision-making. *Contin Educ Anaesth Crit Care Pain* 2014; **14**: 171–5.

Chapter 60

Awareness

Accidental awareness under general anaesthesia (AAGA) is a term referring to a state of unintentional inadequate general anaesthesia, resulting in the patient remembering all or part of a procedure. It is almost exclusively associated with techniques involving the use of neuromuscular blocking drugs, when the patient is unable to move or otherwise attract attention to her plight. Awareness is not an all-or-nothing phenomenon and may range from unpleasant 'dreams' to the extreme situation where the patient is fully conscious and experiencing pain but unable to move.

Problems and special considerations

Before the early 1970s it was common practice to avoid volatile agents altogether and use a 50:50 mixture of nitrous oxide and oxygen; not surprisingly this led to maternal awareness in 12–26% of cases. The addition of a low concentration of a volatile agent (e.g. isoflurane 1%) reduces this to less than 1%, and current evidence suggests a ~0.15% risk of AAGA for caesarean section under general anaesthesia (compared with ~0.02% for the general population).

The recent 5th National Audit Project (NAP5) has furthered our understanding of AAGA and its associations. It has long been known that AAGA is particularly associated with anaesthesia for caesarean section, and AAGA is thought to have a higher incidence in the obstetric population. In NAP5 this was supported by the finding that obstetric general anaesthetics accounted for an estimated 0.8% of the dataset denominator, but 10% of the cases of AAGA. Numerous factors may account for this, including the perceived need to protect the fetus from the sedative effects of the anaesthetic agent, coupled with an exaggerated fear of the adverse effects of volatile agents upon uterine contractility. Fortunately, pregnancy reduces anaesthetic requirements by as much as 40%, or complaints of awareness would probably be more common.

Most obstetric general anaesthetics are for category-1 caesarean sections, which by their nature involve many risk factors that were identified by NAP5 such as a rapid-sequence induction, use of thiopental and neuromuscular blockade, increased risk of a difficult airway and/or obesity, urgency and out-of-hours, non-consultant-led care. Other factors suggested include the omission of sedative or analgesic premedication, and the physiological changes of pregnancy including tachycardia and increased cardiac output.

The need for adequate fetal oxygenation during caesarean section has led to the use of higher inspired concentrations of oxygen (and therefore less nitrous oxide) than for other surgical procedures, and this also has an impact on the depth of anaesthesia. There is little evidence to support the use of more than 30% oxygen for delivery of the unstressed fetus, but when fetal distress is present, 50% or even 100% oxygen has been advocated. The loss of the anaesthetic contribution of nitrous oxide and the second-gas effect mean that higher concentrations of volatile agent should be used throughout these cases, and the initial concentration should be higher still (overpressure) to drive up the alveolar concentration quickly. With the decreasing use of nitrous oxide generally, and its replacement with air as the 'carrier gas' in anaesthetic gas mixtures, the influence of inspired oxygen concentration on the risk of awareness should become less of an issue.

The contribution of opioid drugs to the anaesthetic should not be ignored, and part of the explanation for the high incidence of awareness during obstetric anaesthesia lies in the common practice of withholding these drugs until after the baby is delivered. This also has adverse consequences for cardiovascular stability during tracheal intubation, and there is an increasing tendency to use a modest dose of short-acting drugs such as fentanyl and alfentanil to obviate both of these problems.

Nearly half of those who experience AAGA have been reported to experience long-term psychological morbidity, typified by 'waking dreams', difficulty in sleeping, depression, and fear of hospitals and doctors. Full-blown post-traumatic stress disorder may also occur.

In addition to awareness, inadequate anaesthesia may result in release of catecholamines, which further decrease placental perfusion and promote fetal hypoxia.

Management options

It has been recommended by some authorities (including the authors of NAP5) that patients undergoing general anaesthesia for a caesarean section should be warned about the risk of awareness as part of the consent process, but this is not widely practised. It is advisable to warn the woman that she may wake up with a 'tube in her throat' so that her memory of this is less likely to be confused with intraoperative awareness.

Some incidents of awareness may be clearly traced back to a technical problem with the anaesthetic apparatus, vaporiser faults being the most common. When checking the anaesthetic machine, correct seating of the chosen vaporiser on its mount and adequate filling should be ensured. The anaesthetist should be familiar with the breathing system and ventilator, and should understand how air or oxygen can be entrained into the system and how the inspired concentration of volatile agent can be lower than that set on the vaporiser (e.g. a circle system). A volatile agent monitor is considered mandatory.

There is no guaranteed 'sleep' dose of an induction agent, and the drug must be titrated against the patient's response, bearing in mind that it will be responsible for maintaining anaesthesia throughout the onset of neuromuscular blockade and tracheal intubation. Factors such as obesity will influence the induction dose that is used. Thiopental is probably still considered the drug of choice for induction (see Chapter 36, *General anaesthesia for caesarean section*), and the anaesthetist should have a minimum of 5 mg/kg available in the syringe. Despite its shorter duration of action, propofol was associated with less AAGA than thiopental in NAP5, possibly because of greater familiarity with its use and appropriate dosing. A second syringe of induction agent should be accessible in case of prolonged airway manipulation. One particular risk associated with thiopental is that it is easily mistaken for antibiotic, and vice versa. Concern has been raised that current guidelines advocating administration of prophylactic antibiotics before skin incision could lead to the preparation of two very similar-looking syringes at a time of potential stress, increasing the chance of a drug error; it is advisable that antibiotic syringes should not be present during induction.

Volatile agents with a low lipid solubility will achieve alveolar-inspired equilibrium most quickly. Isoflurane is the best of the 'established' agents, but desflurane and sevoflurane are commonly used as a result of their more rapid onset times. Concentrations representing at least 0.5 minimum alveolar concentration (MAC) should be used during the procedure, and this should be higher if the inspired nitrous oxide concentration is less than 60% (a total MAC of at least 1.0 should be aimed for; a higher MAC of 1.3 may be necessary if opioids have not been given). The effect of these concentrations upon uterine contractility is minimal, and even at 1.5 MAC the uterus should respond normally to oxytocic drugs. An overpressure of 1.5–2 MAC should be employed in the first 2–3 minutes if a more soluble agent is being used.

The patient should be closely watched for signs of lightening anaesthesia (tears, sweating), and the monitors should be observed frequently for evidence of sympathetic overactivity (tachycardia, hypertension). Some practitioners advocate the use of specific monitors of anaesthetic depth, but these have not yet been widely evaluated in obstetrics and none has so far been shown to be any more effective than simply watching vital signs (Table 60.1). A meticulous record should be kept, which should include vaporiser settings and end-tidal volatile concentrations, if available.

Table 60.1 Methods for monitoring depth of anaesthesia

Clinical signs – PRST score (pressure, rate, sweating, tears)
Isolated forearm technique
Lower oesophageal contractility
Skin resistance
Evoked auditory/somatosensory potentials
Electroencephalogram/cerebral function analysing monitor and derivations thereof (e.g. bispectral index, entropy)

A generous dose of a suitable opioid drug should be given directly after cord clamping, and the volatile agent left on until the skin is being sutured. It is better to wait a few minutes at the end of the operation rather than risk awareness.

All mothers undergoing general anaesthesia for caesarean section should be followed up within 24 hours of delivery and questioned about dreaming or sensation during the operation. The psychological sequelae of awareness can be minimised by a sympathetic approach. Midwives should be alert to the possibility of awareness and ensure early referral to an anaesthetist. A suggested management pathway has been created by the authors of NAP5; this includes a meeting between the patient, anaesthetist involved and senior anaesthetist to explore what occurred, analysis of the event to attribute contributing factors, and formal support at 2 weeks and by a clinical psychologist if necessary.

Some patients will mistake their memory of awake extubation for true intraoperative awareness. This risk can be minimised by careful preoperative explanation, but any markers as to the timing of such memory should be sought in order to reassure the patient if possible. Just because true awareness did not occur does not mean that the patient will not be traumatised.

Key points

- Clinical signs are still the best indicator of awareness.
- A clinically effective concentration of volatile agent, suitably monitored, should be used at all times.
- Patients should be warned about awake extubation.
- Complaints of awareness should be treated seriously and sympathetically.

Further reading

Paech MJ, Scott KL, Clavisi O, *et al.* A prospective study of awareness and recall associated with general anaesthesia for caesarean section. *Int J Obstet Anesth* 2008; **17**: 298–303.

Pandit JJ, Cook TM (eds). *Accidental Awareness During General Anaesthesia in the United Kingdom and Ireland: Report and Findings.* NAP5: Fifth National Audit Project. London: Royal College of Anaesthetists and the Association of Anaesthetists of Great Britain and Ireland, 2014. www.nationalauditprojects.org.uk/NAP5report (accessed December 2018).

Platt F, Lucas N, Bogod DG. AAGA in obstetric anaesthesia. In Pandit JJ, Cook TM (eds), *Accidental Awareness During General Anaesthesia in the United Kingdom and Ireland: Report and Findings.* London: RCoA and AAGBI, 2014, pp. 133–43.

Robins K, Lyons G. Intraoperative awareness during general anesthesia for cesarean delivery. *Anesth Analg* 2009; **109**: 886–90.

Air embolism

Subclinical entry of air into the circulation has been shown with Doppler techniques to occur in up to 60% of caesarean sections (possibly more if the head-down position is used or if the uterus is exteriorised), although the significance of circulating microscopic bubbles is uncertain. It has been suggested that chest pain or ST segment depression occurring during caesarean section under regional anaesthesia may be related to air in the coronary circulation, although both are frequently unaccompanied by Doppler demonstration of bubbles. Large amounts of air may cause cardiovascular impairment, but this is less common (up to 2%); the mechanism is obstruction of right ventricular output by the presence of compressible gas within the contracting ventricle. Volumes of 5 ml/kg are thought to be necessary to cause complete cardiovascular collapse. In addition, bubbles may lodge in the pulmonary circulation, increasing dead space, while paradoxical embolism may occur when there is a patent foramen ovale (a probe-patent foramen is found in about 30% of 'normal' hearts on routine autopsy) or other right-to-left shunt.

Although most cases are related to caesarean section, it should not be forgotten that air embolism may occur whenever open veins are above the level of the heart, such as when central venous lines are manipulated with the patient in the sitting position or when the arm in which a peripheral venous cannula has just been placed is held aloft to prevent spillage of blood; both are more likely to occur when staff are inexperienced in the management of intravenous lines, as may (unfortunately) occur on the labour ward. There have also been cases of air embolism associated with epidural catheter insertion, either through a loss-of-resistance technique using air, or through accidental cannulation of the epidural veins. Finally, the danger of accidental intravenous injection of air, for example when pressurising devices are used with air-containing bags of intravenous fluid or when bubbles are allowed into intravenous infusion lines, must not be forgotten. In patients with right-to-left shunts, even small bubbles may have disastrous systemic effects.

Problems and special considerations

The diagnosis may not be clear, especially at first. Clinical features are fairly non-specific and include hypotension, tachycardia, reduced arterial saturation and reduced end-expiratory carbon dioxide concentration (during general anaesthesia), the last because of (1) reduced cardiac output and hence return of carbon dioxide from the tissues, and (2) increased pulmonary dead space. There may be an audible churning sound on cardiac auscultation, although this is usually only present in massive air embolism. Paradoxical embolism may result in systemic infarction of vital organs, especially heart and brain.

The differential diagnosis of air embolism therefore includes any cause of cardiovascular impairment or collapse, at least initially; a high index of suspicion is thus required. In particular, amniotic fluid embolism or thromboembolism may cause the same initial right ventricular outflow obstruction. If it occurs during regional anaesthesia, air embolism may mimic hypotension produced by anaesthesia-induced sympathetic blockade. It may be possible to aspirate bubbles from the right ventricle or atrium via a central venous catheter, but inability to do so does not exclude the diagnosis. Diagnosis may be aided by specialist monitoring, but this is unlikely to be used in obstetric cases. Precordial Doppler or transoesophageal echocardiogram are the diagnostic modalities of choice, but most units do not have the necessary equipment to hand.

Manoeuvres for preventing further embolism and managing the current embolism (as described below) may be difficult to carry out midway through a caesarean section, especially if the patient is awake and distressed. In addition, some of the traditional advice concerning positioning of the patient is self-contradictory (head-up for prevention of further embolism; head-down for its management).

Management options

Methods to reduce occurrence in the first place should be employed. These include minimising the time spent with the operative site above the level of the right atrium for a procedure such as exteriorising the uterus, careful use of intravenous and epidural catheters, and maintaining normovolaemia.

Prevention of further embolism is important as soon as the diagnosis is considered. This includes immediately informing the obstetrician, who should return the uterus to the abdomen if possible, flood the surgical field with saline and look for open veins (the ability to do this will obviously depend to some extent on the stage of surgery). Positioning the patient head-up is generally suggested to raise the level of the heart and increase venous pressure in the pelvis and abdomen.

Damage limitation is generally achieved by reducing the size of the bubble(s); this is done firstly by stopping any nitrous oxide that is being administered and secondly by attempting to remove air from the circulation, or more specifically from the right side of the heart. It may be possible to aspirate air from a routine central venous cannula or catheter; special wide-bore multi-perforated cannulae are manufactured specifically for this task but are not generally available on many labour wards. The head-down position is traditionally required for central venous cannulation, and the left lateral head-down position is advised for isolation of the bubbles away from the right ventricular outflow tract and easier aspiration of air. Both of these positions may compromise the advice given above, and moving to the left lateral position is at best awkward in the middle of surgery.

Further management consists of general supportive treatment (increased concentration of inspired oxygen, vasopressor/inotropic drugs, intravenous fluids) and basic resuscitative measures in an 'ABC' approach as appropriate. If the baby has not yet been delivered, the cardiovascular effects of air embolism will be exacerbated by aortocaval compression; thus lateral displacement of the uterus is especially important and delivery should be expedited.

It has been suggested that caesarean section should always be performed in the head-up position to reduce the incidence of air embolism; however, this has implications for the incidence and effects of hypotension following regional anaesthesia and for the spread of spinal blockade. It has also been suggested that Doppler or ultrasound monitoring (transthoracic or transoesophageal) should always be available during caesarean section, but this is hampered by the lack of equipment and expertise in its use.

Key points

- Subclinical air embolism occurs in up to 60% of caesarean sections as detected by Doppler studies.
- Air embolism may cause cardiovascular collapse if large.
- Management includes general resuscitation, preventing further embolism and removal of air already in the circulation.

Chapter

62

Malignant hyperthermia

Malignant hyperthermia (MH) is a rare genetic condition in which exposure to volatile anaesthetic agents or suxamethonium triggers a hypermetabolic state. Abnormal calcium movement results in generalised muscle rigidity, increased oxygen consumption and increased lactate and carbon dioxide production with hyperkalaemia and myoglobinaemia due to cell breakdown. Even with dantrolene, which prevents the release of calcium from the sarcoplasmic reticulum, mortality remains as high as 5%. The incidence of a fulminant syndrome was 1 in 62,000 general anaesthetics involving suxamethonium and a volatile agent in a previous study. MH is particularly rare in obstetric practice, given the preference for regional anaesthesia.

Problems and special considerations

Women with known susceptibility to MH may present in pregnancy. This is identified through muscle biopsy and the caffeine–halothane contracture test. Women with a positive family history of MH who have not been tested are best treated as susceptible to MH, owing to its autosomal dominant nature.

Alternatively, an undiagnosed case may become apparent on exposure to triggers during the peripartum period. This should be treated as per national and local guidelines. Previous uneventful general anaesthesia does not rule out susceptibility to MH.

Management options

Planning and preparation are key in the approach to the parturient with known suscept-ibility to MH. Antenatal review by a consultant anaesthetist in the high-risk obstetric clinic should occur. Regional techniques are recommended, and a plan should be in place in case elective or emergency surgical intervention is needed. Regional anaesthesia, opioids and nitrous oxide are not associated with MH.

On admission of the patient to the labour ward, the anaesthetist should be informed; this allows further discussion and planning of anaesthetic input. At this point, dantrolene should be readily available.

Regional analgesia is strongly indicated. In the event that general anaesthesia is required for operative intervention, careful consideration of the risk–benefit profile should occur, and local guidelines should be followed. Most departments no longer keep a vapour-free anaesthetic machine for use with MH patients. Instead, the vaporisers and carbon dioxide absorber can be removed from the anaesthetic machine, a new circuit attached and the circuit flushed with high-flow oxygen; duration of flushing is machine-dependent, and studies have indicated this may be between 5 and 104 minutes. If available, an activated charcoal filter may be placed in both the inspiratory and expiratory limbs of the ventilation circuit; this has been shown to render the anaesthetic machine vapour-free in under 3 minutes. In an emergency, hand ventilation using a self-inflating bag or Mapleson C breathing system will always be available. Anaesthesia can be induced with propofol or thiopental depending on personal preference and/or unit policy, but suxamethonium must not be used. A non-depolarising agent such as rocuronium should be used instead; an appropriate sugammadex dose should be calculated before induction and should be available in the event of airway difficulties. Total intravenous anaesthesia can be used to maintain anaesthesia. End-tidal carbon dioxide and temperature should be monitored carefully.

If MH is triggered, local and national treatment guidelines should be followed; this includes dantrolene administration, active cooling and correction of metabolic derangement. Treatment of hyperkalaemia, hypoxaemia, acidosis, hyperthermia and arrhythmias will require additional anaesthetic support, which should be requested immediately. Masseter spasm may prevent laryngoscopy; hand ventilation is usually possible until suxamethonium has worn off. Uterine atony has been described after dantrolene administration; laboratory investigation has suggested this is related to the mannitol it is provided with. Dantrolene may also be associated with neonatal hypotonia.

If the father is susceptible to MH, this may have been passed to the fetus. Triggers that cross the placenta such as volatile agents should be avoided. Although the placenta acts as a relative barrier to suxamethonium, it is probably best avoided.

Key points

- Malignant hyperthermia (MH) is a rare but potentially fatal condition that may be triggered in susceptible women in the peripartum period.
- Regional analgesia and anaesthesia should be encouraged in women susceptible to MH.
- Appropriate preparation and early administration of dantrolene if necessary are key to a successful outcome.
- When anaesthetising the mother of a potentially MH-susceptible fetus, an MH-safe anaesthetic should be administered.

63 Induction and augmentation of labour

Induction of labour (IOL) is the artificial commencement and stimulation of labour and involves the ripening of the cervix, artificial rupture of the membranes (ARM) and stimulation of uterine contractions. It is indicated when delivery of the baby before spontaneous labour occurs is in the best interests of the mother or fetus, or both.

Augmentation of labour is used where the normal progress of labour is slower than expected or when there is rupture of membranes but no uterine contraction.

Induction of labour

The indications for IOL are shown in Table 63.1. Certain factors (e.g. previous caesarean section or breech pregnancy) may increase the risk of complications of IOL (see below), so it should only be offered by a senior obstetrician and after the risks and benefits have been clearly discussed.

Before an induction of labour is offered, a membrane sweep may be performed; this is viewed as an adjunct that increases the chance of spontaneous labour by stimulating prostaglandin release. Once the decision to induce labour has been made, the ease of induction is usually assessed by using the Bishop score, based on the result of pelvic examination. This takes into account the station of the presenting part and cervical features (dilatation, effacement/length, position and consistency). A Bishop score above 8 suggests the cervix is ripe and spontaneous labour or response to induction is likely, whereas a low score

Table 63.1 Indications for induction of labour

Fetal reasons	Prolonged pregnancy
	Fetal growth restriction
	Multiple pregnancy
	Unstable lie
	Infection
	Rhesus disease
	Lethal fetal abnormality
	Intrauterine death
Maternal reasons	Pregnancy-induced hypertension
	Essential hypertension
	Other maternal disease, e.g. renal, malignant
	Antepartum haemorrhage
	Poor obstetric history, e.g. previous stillbirth

indicates that the cervix is unfavourable and spontaneous labour is unlikely. In the latter case, the cervix may be ripened by vaginal dinoprostone (PGE2), which may be repeated at intervals of 12–24 hours depending on the change in the Bishop score. This process may take more than 48 hours. Misoprostol and mifepristone have also been used to induce labour, but currently are usually used only in women who have an intrauterine fetal death.

Surgical IOL (ARM) is performed if the cervix is favourable or following cervical ripening with prostaglandins, or if there are clinical reasons not to use PGE2 such as a uterine scar, severe fetal growth restriction or medical reasons such as asthma. This stimulates labour and allows the colour of the liquor to be assessed and a fetal scalp clip electrode to be applied to monitor the fetal heart, both of which give information about the wellbeing of the fetus. Balloon catheters are not used routinely for IOL but may be used for women with a uterine scar.

Oxytocics are usually an integral part of the management of IOL, and therapy is normally commenced after ARM has been performed.

Augmentation of labour

Augmentation of labour is used when labour is not proceeding at the standard rate (see Chapter 19, *Normal labour*) or when there has been premature rupture of membranes without signs of labour after 12–24 hours. It is usually done by ARM (if intact) and/or oxytocics.

Problems and special considerations

The most common complications of IOL are:
1. Prolapse of the cord.
2. Abruption of the placenta.
3. Acute fetal compromise – particularly when ARM is performed in the presence of polyhydramnios.
4. Hyperstimulation of uterine contractions, causing acute fetal compromise. A PGE_2 pessary may need to be removed or oxytocin stopped and a tocolytic such as terbutaline (250 µg subcutaneously) or glyceryl trinitrate (50 µg intravenous boluses or 200–400 µg sublingually) administered.
5. Postpartum haemorrhage associated with uterine atony.

Complications of augmentation are as above. In addition, there is an increased risk of infection if the membranes have been ruptured for some time.

IOL is often prolonged, and may be particularly tiring and painful, as it increases the strength of the contractions. Therefore epidural analgesia should be discussed as part of the labour management, as well as the above complications. Contractions augmented by oxytocic drugs are also more intense and frequent, and therefore appear to be more painful. There may also be maternal or fetal reasons for the advisability of epidural analgesia, for example pregnancy-induced hypertension.

Induction of labour may not be successful, and since there has been a commitment to deliver the baby these women may need to be delivered by caesarean section.

IOL is often associated with a high-risk pregnancy.

There is an increased risk of precipitous labour and instrumental delivery.

Key points

- Induction and augmentation of labour may employ pharmacological or surgical methods.
- There may be an increased need for anaesthetic involvement, secondary to increased pain, operative delivery or complications.

Further reading

Mozurkewich EL, Chilimigras JL, Berman DR, *et al.* Methods of induction of labour: a systematic review. *BMC Pregnancy Childbirth* 2011; **11**: 84.

Mozurkewich E, Chilimigras J, Koepke E, Keeton K, King VJ. Indications for induction of labour: a best-evidence review. *BJOG* 2009; **116**: 626–36.

National Institute for Health and Care Excellence. *Inducing Labour.* Clinical Guideline 70. London: NICE, 2008. www.nice.org.uk/guidance/CG70 (accessed December 2018).

Chapter 64

Oxytocic and tocolytic drugs

Oxytocic drugs are used to promote uterine contractions, whereas tocolytic drugs relax the uterus. Both groups of drugs are widely used in obstetric practice.

Oxytocic drugs

These drugs may be given: (1) during labour to augment progress; (2) at delivery and in the puerperium to reduce postpartum haemorrhage and aid expulsion of the placenta; and (3) at earlier stages of pregnancy to help empty the uterus, for example following evacuation of retained products of conception or termination of pregnancy. While uterotonics may be life-saving in postpartum haemorrhage (PPH), they must be used with care as they all have significant side effects.

Although the third stage of labour can be managed without oxytocic drugs ('physiological management of the third stage'), it is common practice to give an oxytocic to all women at childbirth, usually on delivery of the anterior shoulder (vaginal delivery) or following delivery of the baby (caesarean section) to hasten delivery of the placenta and reduce the risk of PPH. In most units, the drug used is either a mixture of oxytocin analogue and ergometrine or oxytocin analogue alone, according to local protocols.

Oxytocin analogues

The most widely used is Syntocinon, a synthetic oxytocin; its effects resemble those of natural oxytocin, released from the posterior pituitary gland. Oxytocin causes milk ejection from the lactating breast and acts directly on specific oxytocin receptors in the uterine myometrium, increasing the force and frequency of contractions. In early pregnancy, the uterine receptors are present in small numbers and their sensitivity is low; thus there is little value in giving the drug for operative procedures in early pregnancy, although this is commonly requested by the surgeon. Syntocinon may cause vasodilatation and tachycardia; the latter is especially likely if the intravenous route is used, if large doses (> 5 U) are given by bolus injection, and if other drugs causing tachycardia (e.g. ephedrine) are given concurrently. These effects can be disastrous in patients with fixed cardiac output states such as aortic stenosis.

A potential problem with prolonged Syntocinon therapy during labour is related to its antidiuretic effect, due to its similar structure to vasopressin, which may result in excessive water retention, compounded by excessive fluid administration if infused in weak solution over a long period of time. This has resulted in hyponatraemia and convulsions, hence the recommendation that Syntocinon should be diluted in physiological saline rather than dextrose solutions. The half-life of Syntocinon is approximately 10 minutes, another reason for giving it by infusion at caesarean section. Over recent years, dose-finding studies have been done in relation to Syntocinon because of the recent discovery that it may be associated with coronary artery vasospasm, which has been implicated in intraoperative ECG changes. The current ED_{95} for adequate uterine tone is ~0.3–3 U, with the lower bolus dose being recommended in the elective setting and the higher bolus dose in the emergency setting.

Carbetocin is a longer-acting oxytocin analogue, otherwise similar to Syntocinon. It was introduced as an alternative to Syntocinon in the hope of avoiding the side effects associated with the latter. However, as it is an analogue of oxytocin, the side effects are expected to be similar – though they have not yet been studied in detail. It is more expensive than Syntocinon and not routinely used in most units in the UK. However, its longer duration of action may be advantageous in prophylaxis of PPH, and current evidence suggests it may be more effective at reducing the need for further uterotonics, particularly after caesarean section.

Ergometrine

This acts on smooth muscle generally; thus it may cause vasoconstriction and hypertension (both systemic and pulmonary), coronary artery spasm and increased central venous pressure. It may also cause severe vomiting, and bronchospasm has been reported. It is therefore avoided in women with hypertensive disease. It is commonly given intramuscularly together with oxytocin analogue (Syntometrine; 5 U Syntocinon and 500 μg ergometrine) at vaginal delivery, though Syntocinon 10 U intramuscularly is currently recommended as first-line PPH prophylaxis because of its more favourable side effect profile. Ergometrine may also be given by slow intravenous injection, although side effects are more common so this is usually reserved for major haemorrhage. It increases the force, frequency and duration of uterine contractions.

Prostaglandins

Gemeprost (PGE_1) is given vaginally to soften and ripen the cervix before termination of pregnancy or to induce abortion. Dinoprostone (PGE_2) has also been used for this purpose but is more commonly used to induce labour. Both may cause nausea, vomiting, pyrexia, diarrhoea, bronchospasm and hypertension (especially dinoprostone, which may also cause uterine hypertonus and fetal distress. The occurrence of bronchospasm and hypertension is despite PGE_2's traditionally ascribed broncho- and vasodilator effects).

Carboprost ($PGF_{2\alpha}$) is used in PPH associated with uterine atony if standard oxytocics are ineffective. It is given intramuscularly (250 μg, repeated every 15 minutes up to 2 mg if necessary) and has been injected directly into the myometrium (off-licence); following reports of myometrial ischaemia, this mode of administration has now become obsolete in the UK but is still used in other parts of the world. Carboprost is associated with the same side effects listed above.

Misoprostol has been used for medical termination of pregnancy, induction of labour and prevention/treatment of PPH; it is usually given per rectum (600–1000 μg), but may be given sublingually. The main side effects seen are diarrhoea, shivering and pyrexia, although uterine hyperstimulation has been reported when misoprostol is used for induction.

All the prostaglandins are more effective in late pregnancy, although this is thought to be related to increased sensitivity rather than increased number of receptors.

Tocolytic drugs

Tocolytic drugs may be used to reduce uterine contractions in preterm labour or uterine hyperstimulation during labour, or to relax the uterus in situations such as shoulder dystocia or external cephalic version. There are several different groups of drugs that have been used or studied as tocolytics. As with many areas of obstetric practice, their value (and even efficacy in some cases) is controversial.

β_2-Adrenergic agonists

These act on uterine β_2-receptors, causing relaxation of myometrium. Although these are the most commonly prescribed tocolytics for premature labour, improvement in outcome has not been conclusively proven. The emphasis of therapy has shifted away from long-term prolongation of pregnancy towards allowing enough time for steroids to promote fetal lung maturity before delivery. The most commonly used drugs are terbutaline, salbutamol and ritodrine, and these may be given orally, subcutaneously or by intravenous infusion. They may cause tremor, restlessness, hypotension, tachycardia and pulmonary oedema. The last is thought to arise from fluid overload during the infusion, together with increased pulmonary blood flow resulting from β_2-receptor -mediated pulmonary vasodilatation, often compounded by maternal steroid administration. Careful monitoring of blood pressure, pulse and arterial oxygen saturation is required during therapy. Metabolic effects include hypokalaemia and hyperglycaemia (thus they should be used with caution in women with diabetes). Salbutamol is no longer licensed for tocolysis in the UK for oral use, or for intravenous infusions lasting more than 48 hours.

Both regional and general anaesthesia may be used following β_2-agonist therapy; excessive fluid administration (e.g. during regional anaesthesia) should be avoided and drugs that may cause tachycardia (e.g. ephedrine) used with caution. The drugs may also be given by intravenous bolus (salbutamol or terbutaline 100–250 μg) as part of intrauterine resuscitation of the fetus, for example in severe fetal distress.

Oxytocin antagonists

Oxytocin antagonists (e.g. atosiban) bind competitively to uterine oxytocin receptors, causing dose-dependent reduction in contractions. Atosiban does not affect uterine sensitivity to oxytocin subsequently, and thus does not increase the risk of uterine atony and PPH. It has been shown to be comparable with β_2-agonists in preterm labour and to have fewer side effects (although it may cause nausea, vomiting, tachycardia and hypotension), but it is more expensive. It is usually given as a bolus injection followed by a continuous infusion.

Calcium channel antagonists

Oral calcium antagonists (e.g. nifedipine) are commonly used as tocolytics in preterm labour as they are associated with superior efficacy and fewer side effects than other drugs. However, the safety of calcium channel antagonists has not been rigorously tested and nifedipine is still unlicensed for use as a tocolytic.

Glyceryl trinitrate (GTN)

This acts directly on uterine smooth muscle and has been given intravenously (50 µg boluses) or sublingually (200–400 µg) to produce acute but relatively brief uterine relaxation, for example in cases of uterine hypertonicity, retained placenta and uterine inversion and for external cephalic version. Similar doses have been used in severe fetal distress. Hypotension and headache are the main side effects. The use of GTN delivered by dermal patch has been studied as a means of preventing premature labour following preterm rupture of membranes.

Magnesium sulfate

This acts directly on smooth muscle via calcium ion antagonism; it is rarely used as a tocolytic in the UK, although it is more commonly given for this purpose elsewhere, for example in the USA. (Anaesthetic considerations of magnesium therapy are discussed in Chapter 87, *Magnesium sulfate*.) It is however used for fetal neuroprotection in preterm labour between 24 and 30 weeks' gestation, where its tocolytic action may be a desirable side effect.

Key points

- Oxytocic drugs are used routinely during labour, following delivery, in early pregnancy and in the emergency management of postpartum haemorrhage.
- Tocolytic drugs are used in premature labour and for intrauterine resuscitation of the fetus.
- Drugs of both groups may have implications for the anaesthetist because of their side effects.

Further reading

Mavrides E, Allard S, Chandraharan E, *et al.*; Royal College of Obstetricians and Gynaecologists. Prevention and management of postpartum haemorrhage. *BJOG* 2016; **124**: e106–49.

Meshykhi LS, Nel MR, Lucas DN. The role of carbetocin in the prevention and management of postpartum haemorrhage. *Int J Obstet Anesth.* 2016; **28**: 61–9.

National Institute for Health and Care Excellence. *Preterm Labour and Birth.* NICE Guideline NG 25. London: NICE, 2015. www.nice.org.uk/guidance/ng25 (accessed December 2018).

Vallera C, Choi LO, Cha CM, Hong RW. Uterotonic medications: oxytocin, methylergonovine, carboprost, misoprostol. *Anesthesiol Clin* 2017; **35**: 207–19.

Vercauteren M, Palit S, Soetens F, Jacquemyn Y, Alahuhta S. Anaesthesiological considerations on tocolytic and uterotonic therapy in obstetrics. *Acta Anaesthesiol Scand* 2009; **53**: 701–9.

Premature labour, delivery and rupture of membranes

Labour or rupture of membranes is defined as preterm if it occurs at less than 37 completed weeks' gestation. Preterm prelabour rupture of membranes (PPROM) is diagnosed when rupture of the membranes is not followed by spontaneous uterine contractions before 37 weeks' gestation. When this occurs after 37 weeks, prelabour rupture of membranes (PROM) is diagnosed; the period of latency required before the diagnosis is made varies but is usually up to 8 hours.

About 5–10% of deliveries are preterm in the UK, in about a third of cases without rupture of membranes as the initiating event. Prematurity is a major cause of fetal and neonatal morbidity and accounts for the majority of infant deaths in the developed world; 75% of perinatal mortality occurs in preterm babies. Many epidemiological studies have investigated neonatal morbidity and mortality according to birth weight instead of gestation, although there is evidence that the interplay of these two factors is more important than either one alone. For example, at a given gestation, heavier babies have less morbidity and mortality than lighter ones; similarly, at a given birth weight, mature babies do better than immature ones.

Although several risk factors for preterm delivery are recognised, about half of preterm deliveries have no obvious precipitating cause. Known risk factors include a previous history of prematurity; young maternal age; maternal disease (especially infection), surgery or trauma; uterine abnormality; stress; smoking and use of recreational drugs; multiple gestation; placenta abnormality; and fetal disease.

Problems and special considerations

Diagnosis

Careful obstetric assessment is required to establish the diagnosis of PROM, since it is not always obvious. If pooling of amniotic fluid is not seen, vaginal fluid can be tested for insulin-like growth factor binding protein-1 or placental α-microglobulin-1, chemicals present in amniotic fluid. However, these tests have a high false-positive rate and must be interpreted in the context of the woman's clinical condition. Antibiotics are given to women diagnosed with PPROM. The diagnosis of preterm labour is made according to gestation, the frequency of uterine contractions and changes in cervical dilatation or effacement. In some countries (not routinely in the UK) fetal maturity is assessed by the lecithin–sphingomyelin (LS) ratio, which increases as surfactant production increases and may indicate the likelihood of respiratory distress syndrome.

Maternal problems

Prolonged rupture of membranes may lead to chorioamnionitis with or without systemic features of infection. Thus there may be theoretical risks from regional anaesthesia (see Chapter 139, *Sepsis*, and Chapter 144, *Pyrexia curing labour*).

Administration of tocolytic drugs may result in tachycardia, fluid overload and pulmonary oedema (see Chapter 64, *Oxytocic and tocolytic drugs*). Tachycardia may also be related to maternal sepsis and anxiety; the latter may be considerable because of the mother's fears for her baby.

Any underlying cause of preterm labour or PROM (such as maternal disease) may have implications for the anaesthetic management.

The best method of delivery is controversial, but the operative delivery rate is higher than for term deliveries. Breech presentation is more common. Classical caesarean section may be required if the lower uterine segment is poorly formed (uncommon after 26 weeks' gestation), with a greater risk of haemorrhage and implications for future pregnancies.

Neonatal problems

These can be short- or long-term. The immediate problems for the neonate are respiratory distress (occurring in approximately 50–60% of babies at 26–28 weeks, 20–40% at 30–32 weeks and 5–10% at 34–36 weeks), hypoglycaemia and intracranial haemorrhage. The last may be related to trauma during delivery, although it may also occur postpartum in severe respiratory distress. The neonate is more likely to require resuscitation. Necrotising enterocolitis and patent ductus arteriosus are also more common in premature neonates. Long-term problems include cerebral palsy (in around 20% of babies born at 22–26 weeks, with 7% severe), neurodevelopmental delay and chronic lung disease. If maternal infection is suspected, neonatal screening is performed, since infection may also be present in the baby. Survival rates are approximately 40–45% for babies born at 24 weeks, and 80% for babies born at 26 weeks. It should be remembered that even with modern neonatal intensive care, the neonate has a greater risk of morbidity when born at 35–36 weeks than at 37–38 weeks.

Interpreting cardiotocographic (CTG) monitoring for preterm babies may be difficult, and fetal blood sampling is not performed before 34 weeks' gestation, which may lead to an increase in expedited deliveries.

Management options

'Rescue' cervical cerclage may be offered to women between 16 and 28 weeks of pregnancy with a dilated cervix and exposed, unruptured fetal membranes if there are no signs of infection or contractions (see Chapter 7, *Cervical suture*).

Management of delivery includes finding the cause and ensuring that the timing of delivery is optimised. Steroids are given to the mother to aid maturation of the fetal lungs and are of benefit for up to seven days. Magnesium sulfate for neuroprotection is offered to all women between 24 and 30 weeks' gestation who are in preterm labour, and should be considered in those between 30 and 34 weeks. Since steroids and magnesium require 24 hours to become optimally effective, delivery is usually delayed for this period if possible. Tocolytic drugs are commonly used in an attempt to prevent or stop labour, but their use is controversial, as the evidence suggests that although they may delay labour, they do not improve perinatal outcome. Antibiotics have been shown to reduce the incidence of preterm labour in women with PROM. Delivery is required in the presence of chorioamnionitis or fetal distress, although the precise mode of delivery is controversial. Since the preterm infant is more susceptible to intracranial haemorrhage, the need to prevent trauma during delivery often leads to caesarean section although the benefit of this is unproven.

Anaesthetic options are discussed more fully under the relevant related topics. In general, regional analgesia is often preferable in labour and is considered safe in the absence of systemic features of infection and if antibiotic cover has been provided, since it provides good conditions for a controlled delivery and can be readily extended for instrumental delivery. If caesarean section is required, regional anaesthesia may offer the parents their only chance to see and hear their baby free of tubes and other equipment if the chance of neonatal survival is poor. In addition, neurobehavioural and physiological outcome is better in premature neonates when regional anaesthesia is used than with general anaesthesia. It is important to appreciate the dangers of concurrent tocolytic therapy with any anaesthetic technique. The preterm fetus is especially vulnerable to the adverse effects of maternal hypotension.

Key points

- Between 5% and 10% of deliveries in the UK are preterm.
- Potential maternal problems are those of fever and sepsis, use of tocolytic drugs and the increased requirement for instrumental delivery and anaesthetic intervention.
- Fetal and neonatal problems are those of prematurity, infection and the increased need for neonatal resuscitation.

Further reading

National Institute for Health and Care Excellence. *Preterm Labour and Birth*. NICE Guideline NG 25. London: NICE, 2015. www.nice.org.uk/guidance/ng25 (accessed December 2018).

Simhan HN, Canavan TP. Preterm premature rupture of membranes: diagnosis, evaluation and management strategies. *BJOG* 2005; **112** (Suppl 1): 32–7.

Simhan HN, Caritis SN. Prevention of preterm delivery. *N Engl J Med* 2007; **357**: 477–87.

Chapter 66

Malpresentations and malpositions

Definitions

It is important that obstetric anaesthetists understand the terminology used by their obstetric and midwifery colleagues:

- **Lie:** the relationship of the long axis of the fetus to that of the mother, e.g. longitudinal, transverse, oblique
- **Presentation:** the part of the fetus that is foremost in the birth canal, e.g. cephalic, breech or compound
- **Position:** the relationship of the presenting part of the fetus, using a reference point such as the occiput or sacrum, to the maternal pelvis, e.g. left occipito-anterior (LOA) or right sacral transverse (RST)

Approximately 85% of fetuses at term lie longitudinally, with a cephalic presentation in an occipito-anterior position. A malpresentation is anything that does not fulfil these criteria.

Problems and special considerations

The malpresenting fetus is less likely to deliver spontaneously, and instrumental or operative intervention is often required. Labour is often prolonged and particularly painful. Although it has been suggested that epidural analgesia may increase the likelihood of malpresentation through relaxation of pelvic musculature, impeding rotation, there is little evidence to support this view.

Occipito-posterior position

This is the commonest malpresentation, occurring in over 10% of term pregnancies – though in only 5% of vaginal deliveries, as many turn during labour. Progress of labour and descent of the head may be slow, and the mother often experiences particularly severe pain in the back, which may be resistant to treatment by regional blockade. Manual or instrumental rotation may be attempted to bring the head into a more favourable occipito-anterior position. The likelihood of operative delivery and perineal trauma may be increased.

Breech presentation

This occurs in 3–4% of term pregnancies and can be subdivided into:

- Frank (hips flexed and legs extended over abdominal wall)
- Complete (hips and legs flexed)
- Footling (foot or knee presenting)

The mother with a breech presentation may get the urge to 'push' before the cervix is fully dilated, thus running the risk of trapping the fetal head; this is a particular risk if the labour is preterm. It is becoming increasingly common for women with breech presentation to be delivered by elective caesarean section, especially if primiparous, as this reduces neonatal short-term morbidity and mortality. Perinatal mortality is 2 in 1000 with vaginal breech delivery, 1 in 1000 with vaginal cephalic delivery, and 0.5 in 1000 with caesarean section after 39 weeks. However, appropriate selection of pregnancies and skilled intrapartum care may allow planned vaginal breech delivery to be nearly as safe as planned vaginal cephalic delivery. Maternal complications are least with a vaginal breech delivery, but 40% of planned vaginal breech deliveries will end in emergency caesarean section. External cephalic version (ECV) is routinely offered to women with breech presentation; in this manoeuvre, the obstetrician applies external pressure to rotate the fetus to a vertex (cephalic) presentation (see Chapter 67, *External cephalic version*).

Transverse lie

This occurs in 0.3% of term pregnancies and may be associated with placenta praevia, polyhydramnios and grand multiparity. There is an increased risk of cord prolapse. Spontaneous delivery is impossible unless the lie is converted to longitudinal, which may be achieved by external version provided that placenta praevia has been excluded. Caesarean section is usually necessary, and a vertical uterine incision may be needed to aid delivery.

Face and brow presentations

These are rare presentations, where the head is hyperextended. They are associated with multiparity, prematurity, polyhydramnios and fetal abnormality. A face presentation may deliver vaginally, but caesarean section is often needed.

Prolapsed cord

Cord prolapse occurs in 0.4% of cases when the head is presenting, but this incidence rises to 0.5% in frank breech, 4–6% in complete breech and 15–18% in footling presentations. It is generally more common when the fetus does not fully occlude the pelvic inlet, as in preterm labour, and may follow artificial rupture of the membranes with a high presenting part. If immediate vaginal delivery is not feasible, the presenting part is pushed and held out of the pelvis to prevent cord compression, often aided by steep head-down tilt, while the mother is transferred to theatre for immediate caesarean section. (See Chapter 73, *Cord prolapse*.)

Management options

Good regional analgesia is desirable at an early stage, since intervention is more likely to be required. If there is breakthrough pain, for example with an occipito-posterior position, addition of an epidural opioid such as fentanyl may improve pain relief, although more concentrated solutions of local anaesthetic than those used in 'low-dose' techniques may be required.

If vaginal delivery of a breech presentation is planned, epidural analgesia will help prevent premature 'pushing' and will enable controlled manipulation, extensive episiotomy and application of forceps to the after-coming head. If head entrapment occurs, the anaesthetist may be asked to relax the uterus, for example by using sublingual glyceryl trinitrate. Delivery will often occur in the operating theatre, where an emergency operative delivery can be provided.

For cord prolapse requiring caesarean section, general anaesthesia is usually the quickest option, although extension of a pre-existing epidural block or institution of spinal anaesthesia is also possible (see Chapter 73, *Cord prolapse*).

Key points

- Regional analgesia is particularly indicated in malpresentation.
- Prolapsed cord is often associated with breech presentation and transverse lie, and with preterm delivery.
- Early multidisciplinary communication will help optimise management.

Further reading

Hannah ME, Hannah WJ, Hewson SA, *et al.* Planned caesarean section versus planned vaginal birth for breech presentation at term: a randomised multicentre trial. Term Breech Trial Collaborative Group. *Lancet* 2000; **356**: 1375–83.

Impey LWM, Murphy DJ, Griffiths M, Penna LK; Royal College of Obstetricians and Gynaecologists. External cephalic version and reducing the incidence of term breech presentation. Green-top Guideline 20a. *BJOG* 2017; **124**: e178–92.

External cephalic version

External cephalic version (ECV) is a procedure performed to convert a breech or shoulder presentation into a cephalic one by manipulating the fetus through the mother's abdominal wall and the anterior wall of the uterus. Its reported success rate is 30–80%, and Royal College of Obstetricians and Gynaecologists (RCOG) guidance suggests that overall success rates of 40% for nulliparous women and 60% for multiparous women should be possible.

Problems and special considerations

ECV is usually attempted at 36–37 weeks' gestation; a fetus at earlier gestation is more likely to revert to a breech presentation subsequently since there is more room available, and since the procedure carries a risk of premature delivery a more mature gestation is preferable. On the other hand, the larger the fetus the more difficult it may be to achieve successful version, especially if the presenting part is engaged. If an ECV attempt fails at 36 weeks' gestation, it is extremely unlikely the fetus will turn spontaneously.

Contraindications include multiple pregnancy (although ECV is occasionally used to turn the second twin), antepartum haemorrhage, placenta praevia, ruptured membranes, fetal abnormalities and factors that indicate caesarean section. Previous caesarean section, fetal growth restriction, pre-eclampsia and obesity are controversial relative contraindications. The mother should be nil-by-mouth in case a complication occurs. The fetus is monitored continuously, and with the mother in the tilted supine position, talcum powder is applied to the abdominal wall and rotationary pressure applied to the fetus while attempting to lift the presenting part out of the pelvis. Tocolytic drugs (e.g. β_2-agonists) have been shown to increase the success rate of ECV.

There may be considerable discomfort, particularly if the mother is very tense, which reduces the chance of success. Various manoeuvres have been used in an attempt to improve the success and tolerability of ECV, including sedation (e.g. with benzo-diazepines), nitrous oxide, remifentanil and regional analgesia, with the last being the only method shown to influence success. However, many obstetricians consider the degree of discomfort a useful indicator of when to stop the attempted procedure, and prefer to avoid the use of adjuncts.

In the UK, anaesthetists are rarely involved, although meta-analysis suggests that the success rate can be significantly improved with regional analgesia without an increase in complications. Current RCOG guidelines state that regional anaesthesia should not be routinely offered, but may be considered for a second attempt at ECV or when the mother requires improved analgesia. A maximum of 10 minutes is usually allowed before considering the attempt at version unsuccessful.

Apart from discomfort, complications of ECV include maternal or fetal bradycardia, onset of labour and placental abruption, with about 0.5% of cases requiring immediate caesarean section. Labour after successful ECV is also associated with a slight increase in delivery by instrumental delivery or caesarean section. Because of these possibilities, a clear discussion with the mother and her partner about the options, risks and timings is essential. It should also be remembered that breech presentation is more common in fetuses with other congenital abnormalities and in placenta praevia or uterine abnormalities.

Management options

From the anaesthetic viewpoint, awareness that ECV is being planned is usually the main issue, since anaesthetic input may be required at short notice. However, anecdotal experience suggests that many obstetricians perform ECV in clinics, wards or the delivery suite without routinely informing anaesthetists. If regional anaesthesia is requested, spinal and combined spinal–epidural are both appropriate techniques, with the usual attention paid to maintaining uteroplacental blood flow.

Key points

• External cephalic version has a reported success rate of 30–80%.
• Analgesia or sedation may occasionally be required.
• Regional analgesia improves the success rate but is uncommonly used in the UK.
• Complications include fetal distress, onset of labour and haemorrhage.

Further reading

Hutton EK, Hofmeyr G, Dowswell T. External cephalic version for breech presentation before term. *Cochrane Database Syst Rev* 2015; (7): CD000084

Impey LWM, Murphy DJ, Griffiths M, Penna LK; Royal College of Obstetricians and Gynaecologists. External cephalic version and reducing the incidence of term breech presentation. Green-top Guideline 20a. *BJOG* 2017; **124**: e178–92.

Khaw KS, Lee SW, Ngan Kee WD, *et al.* Randomized trial of anaesthetic interventions in external cephalic version for breech presentation. *Br J Anaesth* 2015; **114**: 944–50.

Lim S, Lucero J. Obstetric and anesthetic approaches to external cephalic version. *Anesthesiol Clin* 2017; **35**: 81–94.

Magro-Malosso ER, Saccone G, Di Tommaso M, Mele M, Berghella V. Neuraxial analgesia to increase the success rate of external cephalic version: a systematic review and meta-analysis of randomized controlled trials. *Am J Obstet Gynecol* 2016; **215**: 276–86.

Multiple pregnancy

The incidence of multiple pregnancy has increased owing to an increase in assisted conception programmes, although twins, triplets and quadruplets also occur naturally. The natural incidence of twins is 1 in 80 pregnancies, triplets 1 in 8000 and quadruplets 1 in 800,000. The obstetric anaesthetist has an important part to play in the management of these deliveries.

Problems and special considerations

The mother carrying a multiple pregnancy experiences all the minor pregnancy complaints in excess. She will be more likely to be very uncomfortable and to suffer from backache, heartburn and varicose veins. Often she will be dyspnoeic at rest or on minor exertion, and she may be unable to lie on her back because of supine hypotension, which may be difficult to relieve except in the full lateral position. She is also more prone to the following risks:

- Anaemia (real and dilutional)
- Pregnancy-induced hypertension
- Gestational diabetes
- Fetal growth restriction
- Malpresentations, including of the second twin after delivery of the first twin
- Premature labour
- Prolonged labour
- Operative interventions for delivery
- Postpartum haemorrhage (because of uterine atony and the large placental site)
- More technically challenging electronic fetal heart rate monitoring
- Intrauterine death

Management options

Many twins and nearly all triplets and quadruplets are booked for delivery by elective caesarean section, although because premature labour is more common, caesarean section is often performed as a non-elective procedure. The indications for twins to be delivered by elective caesarean section include malpresentation of the first twin, previous caesarean section, poor obstetric history (which may include assisted conception) and maternal request. Regional anaesthesia is considered preferable for caesarean section. Great care must be taken when performing regional anaesthesia in these women to ensure that supine hypotension is avoided. If general anaesthesia is required, the reduction in functional residual capacity secondary to the enlarged uterus may be greater than with singleton pregnancies, resulting in more rapid oxygen desaturation during apnoea.

Twins may be delivered vaginally, although the labour and delivery may not be straight-forward and the above factors should be considered. Fetal heart monitoring should be reviewed frequently to ensure both babies are being monitored. Epidural analgesia is recommended; firstly it should provide excellent analgesia for what may be a long labour requiring oxytocic drugs, and secondly – and most importantly – the epidural can be used if there are problems with the second twin. It is important, therefore, to ensure that the epidural is working well throughout labour.

Approximately 40% of twins present vertex–vertex, a further 40% present vertex–non-vertex, and the remaining 20% present both non-vertex. Malpresentation of the second twin may require external or internal version and/or operative delivery, including caesarean section (which may be required urgently in approximately 5–10%, with 60% of all twin pregnancies being delivered by caesarean section). The anaesthetist should be present for the delivery of twins to ensure that the epidural block is adequate for these manipulations. Uterine relaxation with a tocolytic such as glyceryl trinitrate may be required to help facilitate intrauterine manipulation.

The second stage is usually conducted in the operating theatre. If caesarean section is indicated for the second twin, the anaesthetist must be able to extend the epidural block for the operation. Some anaesthetists advocate extending the epidural to produce a block suitable for caesarean section in all cases of twins, in case surgery is required. In rare instances, general anaesthesia may be required for the delivery of the second twin.

The oxytocin bolus must not be given until delivery of the second twin, and an infusion is particularly important post-delivery because of the increased risk of uterine atony.

Key points

- Women with multiple pregnancies are an 'at-risk' group.
- The anaesthetist should be actively involved with the care of these women, whether they are in labour or not.
- Special care is required to avoid aortocaval compression.
- There is increased likelihood of premature or prolonged labour, instrumental delivery and postpartum haemorrhage.

Further reading

Kilby MD, Bricker L; Royal College of Obstetricians and Gynaecologists. Management of monochorionic twin pregnancy. Green-top Guideline 51. *BJOG* 2016; **124**: e1–45.

Melka S, Miller J, Fox NS. Labor and delivery of twin pregnancies. *Obstet Gynecol Clin North Am* 2017; **44**: 645–54.

National Institute for Health and Care Excellence. *Multiple Pregnancy: Antenatal Care for Twin and Triplet Pregnancies.* Clinical Guideline 129. London: NICE, 2011. www.nice.org.uk/CG129 (accessed December 2018).

Vaginal birth after caesarean section

Vaginal birth after caesarean section (VBAC, previously called 'trial of scar') is the term used for the trial of labour in a woman who has a scar on her uterus, usually from a lower-segment caesarean section, but also from a previous hysterotomy or myomectomy.

Problems and special considerations

Risk factors for unsuccessful VBAC are induction of labour, increased maternal age, high body mass index (BMI) and no previous vaginal delivery. A previous vaginal delivery is the single biggest predictor of success.

A trial of scar would be considered if the reason for the scar was not a recurrent obstetric problem, such as cephalopelvic disproportion. The major anxiety is rupture of the uterine scar, particularly during strong uterine contractions. The incidence of uterine rupture in women undergoing a planned VBAC is around 0.2–0.5%, although it is substantially higher after a vertical uterine incision (4–9%), which is seen as a contraindication to VBAC. The risk is thought to be increased if prostaglandins are used for the induction of labour, although oxytocin, which is more controllable, is not usually considered contraindicated.

Uterine rupture may present with an abnormal fetal heart trace in up to 76% of cases. Other associated features may include abdominal pain, tenderness over the uterine scar, maternal haemodynamic compromise, intrapartum bleeding or cessation of labour. If uterine rupture occurs, this is an obstetric emergency and urgent delivery is required.

There is a 25–30% likelihood of a repeat caesarean section if the reason for the previous caesarean section is non-recurrent.

There have been anxieties that epidural analgesia may mask the pain of uterine dehiscence. However, pain is not a constant feature of uterine rupture and may be absent in some cases. In addition, severe pain may be present in the absence of uterine rupture. Finally, the pain of uterine rupture has been reported to 'break through' analgesia provided by modern, low-dose epidural techniques. In fact, many would consider epidural analgesia indicated in VBAC, since it may be readily converted to anaesthesia suitable for caesarean section if required (unless there is uterine rupture, in which case there may not be time to extend the epidural).

Management options

Women undergoing VBAC (and often, their obstetricians) should have the potential advantages and disadvantages of regional analgesia explained to them. Pain that breaks through low-dose epidural analgesia or is present between contractions should raise the possibility of uterine dehiscence.

Key points

- Uterine rupture is the most important complication of VBAC and occurs in ~2–5 cases per 1000.
- Epidural analgesia is not contraindicated, and early insertion is recommended.
- Pain in the presence of a working epidural may be a warning of impending uterine rupture.

Further reading

Cahill AG, Odibo AO, Allsworth JE, Macones GA. Frequent epidural dosing as a marker for impending uterine rupture in patients who attempt vaginal birth after cesarean delivery. *Am J Obstet Gynecol* 2010; **202**: 355.e1–5.

Guise JM, Denman MA, Emeis C, *et al.* Vaginal birth after cesarean: new insights on maternal and neonatal outcomes. *Obstet Gynecol* 2010; **115**: 1267–78.

Royal College of Obstetricians and Gynaecologists. *Birth after Previous Caesarean Birth*. Green-top Guideline 45. London: RCOG, 2015. www.rcog.org.uk/en/guidelines-research-services/guidelines/gtg45 (accessed December 2018).

Scott JR. Intrapartum management of trial of labour after caesarean delivery: evidence and experience. *BJOG* 2014; **121**: 157–62.

Chapter 70

Under-age pregnancy and advanced maternal age

Under-age pregnancy refers to pregnancy in girls under the age of consent (16 years in the UK). The term 'advanced maternal age' applies to parturients aged 35 years or over. Some women are now able to conceive at an even later stage in life; mothers who give birth at the age of 45–49 years are said to be of 'very advanced maternal age', and those at the age of 50 years or over are of 'extreme advanced maternal age'. The UK has one of the highest teenage pregnancy rates in Europe, while the incidence of pregnancy in older women is increasing in the developed world as a result of both maternal choice and infertility treatment.

Problems and special considerations

Under-age pregnancy

Those girls who are under-age when they present in pregnancy can be placed in the following groups:

- Those who have had normal antenatal care and have the full support of their family. This group usually have a parent available to give consent on behalf of the minor if that is felt appropriate, e.g. for epidural analgesia or for anaesthesia.
- Concealed pregnancy. This group may pose a problem with consent. Many will have had little or no antenatal care, and they may present to the hospital for the first time when they are in labour. Many present in advanced labour or to the emergency department with a life-threatening condition such as eclampsia, and there may not be time to find a parent or guardian before instituting treatment. Overall, this is an 'at-risk' group who often need considerable support, including epidural analgesia.

Hypertension, anaemia and poor nutritional status are more common in under-age mothers, and other risk factors may coexist, such as smoking and drug or alcohol abuse. Fetal risks include premature labour, fetal growth restriction, low birth weight and stillbirth.

Advanced maternal age

Miscarriage, fetal chromosomal abnormalities, multiple pregnancy, hypertension, ischaemic heart disease, diabetes, obstetric interventions, neonatal mortality and postpartum haemorrhage are more common in elderly mothers, who feature disproportionately in the reports of the Confidential Enquiries into Maternal Deaths.

Management options

In under-age mothers, it is important to remember at all times that the minor is the patient and must be involved in the decision making. In line with the Mental Capacity Act (in England and Wales), the child may take the decisions for her treatment if deemed competent. This may involve regional analgesia and/or anaesthesia. Ideally, the support and consent of a parent or guardian should be sought, although this may not be practical.

Elderly mothers require no special management other than an appreciation of the increased risks associated with advanced age. These women too should be considered an 'at-risk' group.

Key points

- Both under-age and elderly mothers are at-risk groups and have a higher incidence of complications.
- For minors, parental consent should be obtained when possible; if none is available, treatment should not be denied.
- Elderly mothers should be managed as routine, but the increased risk of complications should be remembered.

Further reading

Laopaiboon M, Lumbiganon P, Intarut N, et al.; WHO Multicountry Survey on Maternal Newborn Health Research Network. Advanced maternal age and pregnancy outcomes: a multicountry assessment. *BJOG* 2014; **121** (Suppl 1): 49–56.

Osmundson SS, Gould JB, Butwick AJ, Yeaton-Massey A, El-Sayed YY. Labor outcome at extremely advanced maternal age. *Am J Obstet Gynecol* 2016; **214**: 362.e1–7.

Abnormal placentation

Abnormal placentation refers to situations in which the placenta is either abnormally situated or abnormally invasive, both of which are conditions associated with an increased risk of haemorrhage and subsequent maternal and neonatal morbidity and mortality.

The placenta usually implants in the fundus of the uterus. Placenta praevia is the term used to describe an abnormally low placenta, implanted in the lower uterine segment. The previously widely used classification of grade 1 (placenta low-lying), grade 2 (reaches the os), grade 3 (asymmetrically covers the os) or grade 4 (symmetrically covers the os) has been replaced with a simpler division into minor (leading edge of the placenta is in the lower uterine segment, but not covering the cervical os) or major (placenta lies over the os). This classification may be further subdivided into anterior or posterior.

A low-lying placenta is noted in about 5% of early ultrasound scans, but most of these have moved into the fundus by the third trimester, and this finding is thus only regarded as significant after 27 weeks' gestation. The incidence at term is ~1 in 200–250. It occurs more frequently in mothers who have previously delivered by caesarean section (incidence is ~10% after four caesarean sections), and is also associated with increased parity, increasing maternal age and multiple gestation.

In addition to the above, the placenta may be morbidly adherent. The incidence is ~1 in 2500 overall, increasing to ~5–9% in placenta praevia, 25–30% in placenta praevia with previous caesarean section, and 40–50% in placenta praevia with two previous caesarean sections. The terms placenta accreta, increta and percreta are used to describe placental penetration through the uterine decidua, into the myometrium, and through the myometrium's serosa, respectively.

Vasa praevia refers to the presence of fetal vessels lying within the membranes over the os, unprotected by placental tissue or the umbilical cord, associated either with a velamentous cord insertion or a multi-lobed placenta. It occurs in 1 in 2000–6000 pregnancies.

Problems and special considerations

There are two main problems caused by abnormal placentation:

1. The physical presence of placental tissue and vessels low down in the uterus, and in major placenta praevia or vasa praevia between the presenting part of the baby and the os, means that compression or rupture of vessels may occur during pregnancy as well as during labour and/or vaginal delivery (in caesarean section, placental tissue may be encountered before the baby can be reached). Thus there is a risk of fetal compromise and severe haemorrhage during pregnancy, labour and/or delivery.

2. The relative lack of muscle in the uterine lower segment compared with the upper segment results in less effective haemostasis when the uterus contracts after delivery; this is compounded by the presence of the placental bed itself and any penetration of the myometrium by the placenta (i.e. accreta/increta/percreta). The incidence of postpartum haemorrhage is therefore also increased.

Diagnosis

Antenatally, transabdominal ultrasound may suggest a low-lying placenta, and its position may be more accurately identified by transvaginal ultrasound. High-resolution ultrasound, magnetic resonance imaging and colour flow Doppler imaging may define the degree of invasion of the placenta, although none is totally accurate. The mother who presents with late bleeding should undergo urgent ultrasonography to determine the position of the placenta. The differential diagnosis is of placental abruption, in which bleeding is normally accompanied by abdominal pain and tenderness (see Chapter 72, *Placental abruption*). If there is uncertainty as to whether vaginal delivery is possible, then an examination in theatre may be performed with a view to proceeding to immediate caesarean section if necessary.

Presentation

Placenta praevia usually presents as painless bleeding, with the first bleed commonly occurring at 27–32 weeks' gestation. Occasionally, bleeding may not be apparent until the mother goes into labour, which is more likely to be preterm. If there has been recurrent bleeding, the mother is usually kept in hospital, with cross-matched blood continuously available. Vasa praevia may present as abrupt onset of bleeding with rupture of the membranes and, since blood loss is entirely fetal, it is associated with a high perinatal mortality.

Mode of delivery

Although lesser degrees of placenta praevia, where the placenta does not encroach on the os, may be managed conservatively, caesarean section is the normal method of delivery. Timing of delivery will depend on the individual circumstances, including antenatal symptoms, maternal and fetal condition, risk of preterm delivery and imaging results. When the mother is actively bleeding, emergency caesarean section and delivery of the placenta may be essential to preserve the life of the mother and the baby. Placenta praevia may interfere with the development of the usually thin lower uterine segment and thus increase blood loss. Occasionally it may be necessary for the obstetrician to divide an anterior placenta praevia in order to gain access to the fetus, and this is usually accompanied by very heavy blood loss. If the placenta is morbidly adherent, placental separation may be difficult or even impossible to achieve, and torrential haemorrhage may occur, which can only be controlled by removing the uterus.

Management options

Immediate resuscitation

Management of the bleeding mother should follow basic principles of resuscitation. Two large-bore peripheral cannulae should be inserted and blood taken for haemoglobin estimation and emergency cross-match. The possibility of disseminated intravascular coagulation should be borne in mind if blood loss is very heavy, and coagulation factors should be replaced (fresh frozen plasma, cryoprecipitate, platelets) according to local haematological guidelines for massive transfusion.

Caesarean section

The presence of one or more consultant anaesthetist(s) and obstetrician(s) is mandatory for caesarean section with placenta praevia; other specialists (e.g. vascular surgeon, urologist) may be required for extreme cases of placenta percreta. Preparations should be made for major blood loss; this might include cell salvage, especially in elective cases.

Placenta praevia has commonly been regarded as an indication for general anaesthesia, because of the risk of heavy, uncontrolled bleeding. Regional anaesthesia has traditionally been contraindicated because of the perceived risk of vasodilating the patient who is, or is about to become, hypovolaemic. However, in recent years, the use of regional anaesthesia in these circumstances has become more acceptable, and many senior anaesthetists would consider a regional technique for caesarean delivery, depending on each individual situation. In addition to the well-known advantages offered by the use of regional anaesthesia, including reduced blood loss, the avoidance of general anaesthesia in this situation enables clinical monitoring of the mother's cerebral function, which is an indication of the adequacy of perfusion. Points that would tend to favour a regional anaesthetic would be a posterior placenta that will not interfere with delivery (although bleeding from a posterior placental bed may be more difficult to control), no or little active bleeding, prior cardiovascular stability, and a low risk of placenta accreta (no previous sections). However, the mother and her partner should be warned about the potential for major haemorrhage and the increased risk of conversion to general anaesthesia. The patient who is bleeding heavily, or who has an anterior placenta or a history of previous caesarean section, may be best managed with general anaesthesia.

Interventional radiology is recommended by the Royal College of Obstetricians and Gynaecologists as an adjuvant in the prophylactic management of placenta praevia and accreta. In the elective situation, balloon catheters may be inserted prophylactically in the internal iliac/uterine arteries (or even aorta) via the femoral arteries before caesarean section, with a view to inflating the balloons should uncontrolled haemorrhage occur. Risks of catheter placement include lower limb ischaemia and fetal bradycardia necessitating emergency delivery.

An alternative is to place femoral artery sheaths through which balloon or embolisation catheters can be passed should they be required subsequently. In the emergency situation, embolisation procedures may be performed after angiography to identify the bleeding vessels, and this may be life-saving. The procedure is not without risks – not least those associated with transferring a potentially unstable patient to the radiology suite. In some facilities, elective caesarean sections may be performed in adequately equipped radiology suites.

Occasionally, when there are signs of acute placental insufficiency, the risks to the fetus of waiting for cross-matched blood must be balanced against the risk to the mother of proceeding without it; these are decisions that must be taken coolly and rationally, with full consultation between the parties.

Key points

- The chances of placenta accreta increase with the number of previous caesarean sections.
- The risk of massive haemorrhage should be assessed when choosing an anaesthetic technique.
- Successful management of the parturient with an abnormally implanted placenta relies on advance planning and interdisciplinary communication, with the involvement of senior clinicians.

Further reading

Fitzpatrick KE, Sellers S, Spark P, *et al.* The management and outcomes of placenta accreta, increta, and percreta in the UK: a population-based descriptive study. *BJOG* 2014; **121**: 62–70.

Jauniaux E, Alfirevic Z, Bhide AG, *et al.*; Royal College of Obstetricians and Gynaecologists. Placenta praevia and placenta accreta: diagnosis and management. Green-top Guideline 27a. *BJOG* 2019; **126**: e12–48.

Jauniaux E, Alfirevic Z, Bhide AG, *et al.*; Royal College of Obstetricians and Gynaecologists. Vasa praevia: diagnosis and management. Green-top Guideline 27b. *BJOG* 2019; **126**: e49–61.

Lilker SJ, Meyer RA, Downey KN, Macarthur AJ. Anesthetic considerations for placenta accreta. *Int J Obstet Anesth* 2011; **20**: 288–92.

Snegovskikh D, Clebone A, Norwitz E. Anesthetic management of patients with placenta accreta and resuscitation strategies for associated massive hemorrhage. *Curr Opin Anaesthesiol* 2011; **24**: 274–81.

Taylor NJ, Russell R. Anaesthesia for abnormally invasive placenta: a single-institution case series. *Int J Obstet Anesth* 2017; **30**: 10–15.

Viñas MT, Chandraharan E, Moneta MV, Belli AM. The role of interventional radiology in reducing haemorrhage and hysterectomy following caesarean section for morbidly adherent placenta. *Clin Radiol* 2014: **69**: e345–51.

Placental abruption

Placental abruption is defined as premature placental separation, and it occurs in around 1% of pregnancies. Major degrees of abruption have an incidence of 0.2%, with a perinatal mortality of 50%.

Risk factors for abruption are a previous history of abruption, an overdistended uterus (twins, polyhydramnios), pre-eclampsia, multiparity, greater maternal age, smoking, trauma and use of drugs such as cocaine and amphetamines.

Problems and special considerations

The diagnosis of abruption is clinical, supported by ultrasound. The usual presentation is of bleeding in the third trimester which, unlike the differential diagnosis of placenta praevia, is associated with abdominal pain due to uterine distension. The uterus commonly starts contracting, and this will exacerbate the underlying pain. Cardiotocography may show evidence of fetal compromise in the form of loss of fetal heart rate variability, decelerations or bradycardia. Minor degrees of abruption may be diagnosed retrospectively after an uneventful delivery. Abruption that is retroplacental, as opposed to at the edge of the placenta, may be concealed; if severe, these patients may present with a hard, tense abdomen, hypovolaemic shock and even disseminated intravascular coagulation.

It is easy to underestimate blood loss in abruption, especially if the membranes have not ruptured, since much of the bleeding will be concealed. Cardiovascular changes occur late, probably because of the sympathetic activity engendered by abdominal pain and because patients are generally young and fit.

Coagulopathy is an early development in placental abruption, since coagulation factors are rapidly consumed by the intrauterine clot. Where abruption is severe enough to cause fetal death, the risk is as high as 50%. The risk of amniotic fluid embolism is also thought to be increased, especially in severe cases.

Management options

Management is dependent on whether the fetus is still alive at presentation, and on the condition of the mother. If there is no evidence of placental insufficiency, then the mother may be allowed to labour, with careful fetal and maternal monitoring. Basic fluid resuscitation is essential, and platelet count, coagulation tests and fibrin degradation products should be measured on admission and at regular intervals. Regional analgesic techniques are not contraindicated, but normovolaemia and unimpaired coagulation are of paramount importance if they are used. Blood should be cross-matched and available. Early artificial rupture of the membranes may reduce the risk of coagulopathy and amniotic fluid embolism.

When the fetus has already died, then vaginal delivery is the technique of choice. Particular attention should be paid to the risk of coagulopathy.

Caesarean section

Caesarean section is indicated if there is fetal or maternal compromise. As with placenta praevia, general anaesthesia is the method of choice in the mother with cardiovascular decompensation, and should also be used in the presence of clotting disorders (see Chapter 71, *Abnormal placentation*). If an epidural catheter is already in situ, then this may be used to provide anaesthesia unless there are major contraindications. Unlike placenta praevia, where the mother may be put at risk if caesarean section is carried out before blood is available, there are benefits for both fetus and mother in operating without delay in the case of abruption: coagulopathy may be prevented and the risk of causing massive bleeding by having to cut through the placenta is not an issue.

After delivery

Postpartum haemorrhage is far more common following abruption. This may arise as a result of coagulopathy or because the uterus fills with blood and cannot contract (Couvelaire uterus).

Key points

- Blood loss may be underestimated in abruption.
- Coagulopathy is common.
- Caesarean section should not be delayed once the mother has been resuscitated.
- Regional anaesthesia may be used in the absence of hypovolaemia or impaired coagulation.

Further reading

Oyelese Y, Ananth CV. Placental abruption. *Obstet Gynecol* 2006; **108**: 1005–16.
Tikkanen M. Placental abruption: epidemiology, risk factors and consequences. *Acta Obstet Gynecol Scand* 2011; **90**: 140–9.

Cord prolapse

Cord prolapse occurs when the umbilical cord prolapses through the birth canal, either preceding or simultaneously with the presenting part, and often before the cervix is fully dilated. It is generally more common when the fetus does not fully occlude the pelvic inlet and is frequently associated with obstetric interventions, such as artificial rupture of the membranes with a high presenting part, or manoeuvres to correct fetal malposition or presentation. The incidence of cord prolapse is around 0.1–0.6%, but exceeds 1% with breech presentations. Other risk factors include polyhydramnios, multiple pregnancy, preterm labour and cord abnormalities.

Problems and special considerations

Overt prolapse occurs when the cord advances beyond the presenting part and is palpable or visible in the vagina, while occult prolapse is when the cord descends alongside the presenting part but is neither visible nor palpable in the vagina. Almost invariably, the result is compression of the cord by the presenting part of the fetus, which effectively cuts off its own blood supply, making it a true obstetric emergency with a fetal mortality rate of up to 10%. Delivery must be achieved very rapidly to prevent hypoxic–ischaemic damage to the fetus, ideally within a few minutes of prolapse.

By definition, there is usually little, if any, warning of a cord prolapse. It usually occurs during procedures such as assessment of progress or artificial rupture of membranes, when it is detected by the appearance of the cord through the introitus or the palpation of a pulsatile vaginal mass, but it may present spontaneously as acute, severe fetal distress or the mother noticing 'something coming down'. When there is high suspicion that artificial rupture of membranes may result in a prolapsed cord, a 'controlled' rupture of membranes is often done in the operating theatre.

Management options

The successful management of cord prolapse requires immediate delivery by caesarean section, although vaginal spontaneous or assisted delivery may occasionally be performed when delivery is imminent and cardiotocography is reassuring. Local guidelines should be developed, and a well-established mechanism for handling emergencies of this nature should be in place. Regular simulated drills will highlight weak points in the process and ensure that all staff are familiar with their roles. Well-recognised areas of delay include transfer of the patient to the operating theatre, gathering the theatre team, and waiting for inappropriate investigations or cross-matched blood.

The other danger of the need for rapid delivery is that important preparations may be overlooked in the rush: for example anaesthetic assessment, antacid premedication and removal of dentures. Damage to the bladder may occur if it is not emptied preoperatively.

However rapidly delivery can be achieved, every effort should be made to relieve the occlusion of the umbilical cord by manually lifting the presenting part off the cord. This can be difficult, but may be helped by maintaining a steep head-down tilt until delivery is imminent. Rapid transfer of the patient in this position, especially with a midwife supporting the fetus with her hand inside the birth canal, can be very fraught indeed. Instillation of saline into the bladder via a catheter may assist this manoeuvre, and tocolytics may be administered in the presence of fetal bradycardia or non-resolving abnormalities of the fetal heart trace.

General anaesthesia

Caesarean section in these circumstances is often best managed by induction of general anaesthesia. It is a fast and reliable technique, and the manoeuvres needed to relieve the pressure on the cord often preclude positioning the patient for a de novo regional block. If general anaesthesia is to be used, a preoperative airway assessment is mandatory. If a problem with intubation is anticipated, the anaesthetist may have to make the difficult decision – in conjunction with the obstetrician – of whether an attempt at regional anaesthesia is appropriate. It is impossible to give general guidance for individual cases of this nature, but the main precept is that the mother's life should take priority over the fetus's.

Steps should always be taken to protect against aspiration of gastric contents (see Chapter 59).

Regional anaesthesia

Cord prolapse does not necessarily rule out a regional block for caesarean section, especially if the mother already has a functioning epidural in situ. It is obviously better to avoid the risks of general anaesthesia in the unprepared patient if possible, and many mothers express a strong wish to be awake to witness the birth of their baby, if its viability is in doubt. The obvious problem with using an epidural block is the time delay while it takes effect, but various recipes for rapid top-up have been described (see Chapter 35, *Epidural anaesthesia for caesarean section*). Even if this is not fully effective by the time the operation starts, the first 2–3 minutes of surgery before the peritoneum is manipulated can be managed with a relatively low block. It is important in these circumstances for the anaesthetist to reassure the mother constantly (and often the partner as well). Good, sympathetic communication may mean the difference between failure and success.

Spinal anaesthesia is not recommended for the inexperienced, but a 'rapid-sequence' technique has been reported in such cases and may be attempted in the presence of a reassuring fetal heart trace. A strict time limit, however, should be applied and the clock watched by an independent observer. If a 3-minute cut-off point is used, and the mother is preoxygenated during the spinal attempt, then no time is lost if conversion to general anaesthesia is necessary. As with epidural anaesthesia, the mother may need support during the first few minutes before the block is fully established.

Key points

- The successful management of cord prolapse depends on good communication and well-rehearsed guidelines.
- General anaesthesia may be the best option, but the risks to the mother should be borne in mind.
- Regional anaesthesia is often possible, but should not be allowed to delay delivery.

Further reading

Holbrook BD, Phelan ST. Umbilical cord prolapse. *Obstet Gynecol Clin North Am* 2013; **40**: 1–14.
Kinsella SM, Girgirah K, Scrutton MJ. Rapid sequence spinal anaesthesia for category-1 urgency caesarean section: a case series. *Anaesthesia* 2010; **65**: 664–9.
Royal College of Obstetricians and Gynaecologists. *Umbilical Cord Prolapse*. Green-top Guideline 50. London: RCOG, 2014. www.rcog.org.uk/en/guidelines-research-services/guidelines/gtg50 (accessed December 2018).

Fetal distress

Fetal distress is a loosely defined term used to indicate that the baby is compromised and in need of delivery.

Problems and special considerations

The main problem is that the diagnosis of 'fetal distress' can be difficult and must take into account many clinical parameters, together with the woman's previous obstetric history and her age. Although cardiotocography (CTG) and the presence of meconium are most commonly used to indicate fetal distress, fetal heart rate changes and meconium do not always correlate with acidosis or hypoxia, and the sensitivity and specificity for predicting a poor neonatal outcome are relatively low. In particularly high-risk cases, these signs may be more significant; in such cases antenatal diagnosis of impending fetal distress may be possible, based on ultrasound scans, Doppler blood flow studies and CTG monitoring.

Fetal distress is often used as a label to hasten operative delivery. The difficulty of associating intrapartum signs with outcome means that the allowable time before delivery is uncertain. At one end of the spectrum is the baby that needs to be delivered as soon as possible since there is immediate threat to its life, for example from placental abruption. At the other end of the spectrum, the baby needs to be delivered soon but there is time to plan the delivery. Most units' guidelines call for a maximum of 15–30 minutes between the decision to deliver by caesarean section and delivery itself, for urgent (category-1) caesarean section. However, these times are derived largely from animal experiments over 30 years ago and their relevance is arguable, especially since most cerebral palsy is now known to be related to factors arising before labour. In addition, most units find it difficult to meet these time limits.

Delivery of babies who are diagnosed as being 'distressed' before labour (see Chapter 12, *Antenatal care*) often needs the support of the neonatal intensive care unit (NICU); thus the time and place of delivery must also take account of neonatal cot availability when the gestation of the baby meets the level of NICU care. For women in labour, transfer to another unit is usually not possible, thereby often necessitating ex-utero transfer of the baby.

For the above reasons, the term 'fetal distress' has fallen out of favour. For example, in UK national guidance on CTG monitoring, it is not used at all, and potentially abnormal CTG patterns are described as being 'non-reassuring', 'suspicious' or 'pathological'. In practice, however, the term is still often used to indicate a potentially compromised fetus.

Management options

It is crucial that there is good communication between all members of the team, the mother and her partner. In particular, obstetricians should describe the clinical situation to their anaesthetic colleagues in more detail than just saying there is 'fetal distress' – and anaesthetists must be aware of the various signs that might indicate fetal compromise, so that they can put such descriptions into context. The choice of anaesthetic technique will depend on maternal factors and the degree of urgency of the case, the onus resting with the obstetrician to indicate the latter.

The ability to improve the fetus's condition while preparing for delivery is often forgotten. Intrauterine resuscitation includes ensuring that the mother is in the left lateral position, giving her oxygen (although there is little hard evidence that this is beneficial, and some have suggested that it may be potentially harmful), giving intravenous fluids and treating any hypotension, stopping oxytocic drugs and giving tocolytic drugs such as salbutamol or terbutaline 100–250 µg intravenously, or glyceryl trinitrate 50 µg intravenously or 200–400 µg sublingually.

Fetal distress is a descriptive label for a variety of diagnoses and clinical situations, but if the anaesthetist understands that not all fetal distress is a life-threatening emergency, the care of the mother will improve. There are few situations in which there is not time to institute or extend a regional block to provide regional anaesthesia. For extreme cases, general anaesthesia is often used; although not necessarily faster than a spinal anaesthetic, it is generally more reliable, if more hazardous.

Key points

- 'Fetal distress' is an ill-defined term, and signs of 'fetal distress' are poorly correlated with poor neonatal outcome.
- Degree of urgency of delivery is a useful guide for anaesthetists to plan the anaesthetic technique, although definitions are vague.
- Anaesthetists must communicate with their obstetric and midwifery colleagues.
- Intrauterine resuscitation should always be remembered.

Further reading

Committee on Obstetric Practice, American College of Obstetricians and Gynecologists. ACOG Committee Opinion. Number 326, December 2005. Inappropriate use of the terms fetal distress and birth asphyxia. *Obstet Gynecol* 2005; **106**: 1469–70.

National Institute for Health and Care Excellence. *Intrapartum Care for Healthy Women and Babies.* Clinical Guideline 190. London: NICE, 2014 (updated 2017). www.nice.org.uk/guidance/cg190 (accessed December 2018).

Yentis SM. Whose distress is it anyway? 'Fetal distress' and the 30-minute rule. *Anaesthesia* 2003; **58**: 732–3.

Shoulder dystocia

Shoulder dystocia is an obstetric emergency caused by impaction of one or both fetal shoulders against the mother's symphysis pubis after the head has been delivered, that is not relieved by gentle traction, and requires additional obstetric manoeuvres for delivery. The incidence is variable and is quoted to be 0.6–1.4% of all vaginal deliveries. In 50% of cases it is unanticipated, and although there is a recognised association with fetal macrosomia, it may occur in fetuses with a normal birth weight. Maternal risk factors include a previous history of shoulder dystocia, diabetes (gestational and pre-existing), post-dates pregnancy and cephalopelvic disproportion. It is also associated with a prolonged second stage and assisted deliveries.

It is important for obstetric anaesthetists to understand shoulder dystocia and its management, since they may be required to provide immediate assistance, and prompt intervention may be life-saving.

Problems and special considerations

Fetal brachial plexus injury, most commonly Erb's palsy, occurs in 4–16% of cases. Most recover, usually within 6–12 months, but up to 10% of affected babies suffer some permanent damage. Humeral and clavicular fractures have also been reported.

Fetal hypoxia may occur, and if prolonged this can lead to severe fetal morbidity or even death.

Maternal soft tissue damage with extensive third- or fourth-degree tears have been reported. Uterine atony leading to massive obstetric haemorrhage, and uterine rupture, may occur.

Management options

A previous history of shoulder dystocia does not mandate induction of labour or delivery by caesarean section in subsequent pregnancies. However, measures should be taken to anticipate this obstetric emergency if the mother has any associated risk factors.

The classic sign of shoulder dystocia is described as the 'turtle sign', in which the head appears on the perineum with contractions and then retracts between contractions. Another is fetal facial swelling caused by venous obstruction. Manoeuvres to dislodge the impacted shoulder are described in shoulder dystocia guidelines and include the McRoberts manoeuvre, in which the mother's legs are flexed and abducted to enable cephalad rotation of the pelvis and augmentation of uterine contractions. Suprapubic pressure applied downwards and laterally with the McRoberts manoeuvre may enable the passage of the anterior shoulder under the symphysis pubis. Other manoeuvres include internal rotation, and placing the mother on all fours to facilitate descent of the posterior shoulder.

Rarely, extreme measures such as deliberate fracture of the fetal clavicle, maternal symphysiotomy or the Zavenelli manoeuvre (attempting to push the fetal head back in the vagina and delivering the baby by caesarean section) have been attempted, though their place has been questioned. Symphysiotomy is classically done under local anaesthesia but the Zavenelli manoeuvre (a high-risk procedure for both mother and fetus) requires general anaesthesia – which must be administered in the most difficult and fraught circumstances and therefore should not be undertaken lightly.

Key points

- Shoulder dystocia is an obstetric emergency associated with significant fetal and maternal complications.
- Anticipation and preparation are paramount in cases where risk factors exist.
- The anaesthetist may be called upon to administer general anaesthesia in a situation that is stressful for all concerned.

Further reading

Dahlke JD, Bhalwal A, Chauhan SP. Obstetric emergencies: shoulder dystocia and postpartum haemorrhage. *Obstet Gynecol Clin North Am* 2017; **44**: 231–43.

Hansen A, Chauhan SP. Shoulder dystocia: definitions and incidence. *Semin Perinatol* 2014; **38**: 184–8.

Lim MN, Gale A, Debroy B. Early resort to general anaesthesia in severe shoulder dystocia. *J Obstet Gynaecol* 2008; **28**: 436–7.

Royal College of Obstetricians and Gynaecologists. *Shoulder Dystocia*. Green-top Guideline 42. London: RCOG, 2012 (updated February 2017). www.rcog.org.uk/en/guidelines-research-services/guidelines/gtg42 (accessed December 2018).

Intrauterine death

Most pregnancy loss occurs during the first trimester, and it is estimated that after 20 weeks' gestation fewer than 1% of all pregnancies end with fetal death. Of these, approximately a third occur with no explicable fetal or maternal cause.

Problems and special considerations

Intrauterine death may cause major obstetric as well as psychological sequelae. It is unusual in the UK for intrauterine death to remain undiagnosed for several days, but if this situation arises it is potentially life-threatening, since the mother is at risk of developing disseminated intravascular coagulation (DIC) and sepsis.

Fetal death occurring during the second half of pregnancy may be suspected by the mother when she fails to feel fetal movements. The diagnosis is confirmed by an absent fetal heartbeat on ultrasonography. In the majority of cases, the pregnancy will have been progressing apparently normally until shortly before fetal death occurs, and the diagnosis is devastating for the mother and her partner. The psychological as well as the medical wellbeing of the parents must be considered.

Labour will normally be induced at the earliest possible opportunity after diagnosis of intrauterine death, and adequate analgesia must be provided. Vaginal delivery is the mode of delivery recommended by the Royal College of Obstetricians and Gynaecologists, but some women may be delivered by caesarean section in the presence of a maternal indication. Coagulation may become deranged secondary to the release of tissue thromboplastin from the fetus, which does not usually occur until 3–5 weeks after intrauterine death, or from the placenta if there has been any placental separation. Coagulopathy may also be triggered by an intrauterine infection or uterine perforation, and in some of these cases may develop without an obvious risk factor.

All the potential complications of labour and delivery may occur, including slow progress in labour, difficulty with delivery and postpartum haemorrhage. While the use of oxytocics is not limited by concerns about fetal welfare, the risk of over-stimulating uterine contractions and causing uterine rupture must be considered, especially in the multiparous woman or the woman with a uterine scar. It may, very occasionally, be necessary for the obstetrician to perform destructive procedures to the fetus to achieve vaginal delivery, or alternatively to perform hysterotomy. Intrapartum care of the mother is stressful and traumatic not only for the mother and her partner but also for midwifery and medical staff.

Management options

Analgesia for labour should be discussed with the mother and her midwife before active labour begins. Parenteral opioids (usually diamorphine) are often used, sometimes with sedatives such as benzodiazepines. If opioid analgesia is used, consideration should be given to the use of intravenous patient-controlled analgesia (PCA), although extreme care should be taken to provide adequate observation and monitoring if remifentanil PCA is used. This is because reported cases of respiratory or cardiac arrest with remifentanil PCA have often been in women with intrauterine death, presumably because these are more likely to be managed in quiet and darkened rooms with minimal disturbance.

Epidural analgesia can provide more effective pain relief without clouding maternal consciousness. Although this may appear distressing for the mother at the time, parents often appreciate memories of seeing and holding their baby. Epidural analgesia is contra-indicated if there is a coagulopathy, although DIC is rarely seen in practice. Units should have guidelines on the management of these women, including the need for coagulation studies.

The anaesthetist should be aware of the possible risks of uterine rupture and postpartum haemorrhage in multiparous women.

Following delivery, the parents are usually encouraged to see and hold their dead baby. Photographs of the baby should be taken and kept with the medical records even if the parents do not wish to see the baby. The obstetric and midwifery staff should ensure that help is available for registering the stillbirth, discussing post-mortem examination and making any funeral arrangements.

Intrauterine death of one twin is a recognised risk of monochorionic twin pregnancy. Recommended management is usually conservative, although there have been recent reports that early delivery (by hysterotomy) of the dead twin improves outcome for the remaining twin. The psychological sequelae for both the parents and the surviving twin may be particularly difficult to deal with and may persist into the surviving twin's adult life.

Key points

- Intrauterine death is devastating for the parents; it is often completely unexpected and occurs towards the end of an apparently normal pregnancy.
- Standard obstetric management is induction of labour, with the aim of achieving vaginal delivery whenever possible.
- The obstetric anaesthetist should be able to advise about suitable analgesia, and should be available to deal with any complications of vaginal delivery.
- The situation demands the highest standard of communication skills and sensitivity from all medical and midwifery staff.
- The presence of coagulopathy or sepsis may have implications for regional anaesthesia.

Further reading

Royal College of Obstetricians and Gynaecologists. *Late Intrauterine Fetal Death and Stillbirth.* Green-top Guideline 55. London: RCOG, 2010. www.rcog.org.uk/en/guidelines-research-servi ces/guidelines/gtg55 (accessed December 2018).

Uterine inversion

Uterine inversion is a rare but potentially fatal complication of pregnancy. It may be incomplete or complete, depending on whether the fundus is delivered through the cervix. Nearly all cases occur within 24 hours of birth, although subacute (up to 4 weeks) and chronic forms have also been described.

The incidence is said to be between 1 in 2000 and 1 in 50,000 deliveries; this variation is thought to relate to the management of the third stage of delivery. Uterine inversion is more likely to occur when vigorous fundal pressure or cord traction is exerted before adequate placental separation. Coughing and vomiting, fundal insertion of the placenta and uterine atony are all thought to contribute to the risk of uterine inversion.

Problems and special considerations

Uterine inversion is an obstetric emergency. The presentation of the uterus through the cervix, usually with the placenta still attached, causes pain and severe vagal shock, the most important manifestation of which is bradycardia. This is often followed by severe haemorrhage.

Management options

Initial treatment is aimed at basic resuscitation, including intravenous fluids (including blood), oxygen and atropine to treat the bradycardia when indicated.

Replacement of the uterus should take place as soon as possible, since oedema quickly develops in the extruded uterus, hampering efforts to return it to its correct position. Urgent manual replacement may be successful without general anaesthesia in the first few minutes after the patient has collapsed, but general anaesthesia is usually required and should not be delayed. In the absence of shock or haemorrhage, regional anaesthesia may be suitable. Manual replacement of the uterus may be facilitated by uterine relaxation (see Chapter 64, *Oxytocic and tocolytic drugs*). Traditionally, deep halothane anaesthesia was used but this was associated with marked hypotension and prolonged uterine atony; more recently glyceryl trinitrate, β-adrenergic agonists and magnesium have been used.

If the above method is not successful, hydrostatic pressure may be considered. In this technique, warm isotonic fluid is allowed to run into the uterus. Up to 5 litres of fluid may be required; therefore, there is a risk of systemic absorption. An open abdominal method of treatment has also been described but this is rarely required.

After the uterus has been replaced, oxytocic drugs are required straight away. It is important to remember that the relaxant effects of tocolytic drugs may persist for some time.

Key points

- Uterine inversion may present with collapse, severe bradycardia and haemorrhage.
- Anaesthesia is usually required for replacement of the uterus.
- Uterine relaxation may be required to enable its replacement.
- Good communication between anaesthetists and obstetricians is essential, with minimal delay in initiating treatment.

Chapter 78

Major obstetric haemorrhage

Successive reports of the Confidential Enquiries into Maternal Deaths have highlighted major obstetric haemorrhage (MOH) as a significant direct cause of maternal mortality, accounting for about 10% of direct maternal deaths in recent years. In many cases, care is suboptimal; women at particular risk of haemorrhage are not identified beforehand, or else management is inadequate when bleeding does occur. A similar situation exists in other countries, especially developing ones, where haemorrhage is one of the leading causes of death, often related to a lack of resources.

Obstetric haemorrhage may be antepartum or postpartum. The most common causes of antepartum bleeding are placenta praevia and placental abruption. Postpartum haemorrhage is most commonly associated with uterine atony, trauma to the genital tract, ruptured uterus and caesarean section (see Chapter 79, *Postpartum haemorrhage*). There is no consensus on a definition of MOH; suggested criteria include:

- Blood loss > 1000 ml with ongoing loss or signs of clinical shock
- Blood loss > 1500 ml
- Loss of 50% of blood volume in 3 hours
- Transfusion > 4 units of packed red cells
- Decrease in haemoglobin of > 40 g/l

Problems and special considerations

The extent of bleeding may be underestimated because it is concealed, for example in the vagina or on bedclothes, between the legs (at caesarean section) or within the abdomen, or because it is mistaken for bloodstained amniotic fluid.

Pregnant women are generally healthy and tolerate blood loss well. The patient may therefore remain cardiovascularly stable even when there has been a significant decrease in her circulating blood volume. Consequently, the presence of hypotension, tachycardia and vasoconstriction in an obstetric patient represents severe hypovolaemia. A widely used classification of haemorrhagic shock is that of the American College of Surgeons (originally devised for trauma), which is shown in Table 78.1. It is important to consider the percentage of circulating volume lost rather than absolute loss, as the weight of pregnant women and their circulating volume (approximately 100 ml/kg) may vary substantially.

Apparently moderate bleeding in obstetric patients may rapidly progress to MOH.

Coagulopathy may be an underlying cause of haemorrhage, but severe haemorrhage may also result in impaired coagulation. Previously, coagulopathy as a result of haemorrhage was thought to be largely dilutional, and although this may occur, it is thought that

Table 78.1 Classification of haemorrhagic shock

	Class I	Class II	Class III	Class IV
Blood loss (ml)	< 750	750–1500	1500–2000	> 2000
Blood loss (%)	< 15	15–30	30–40	> 40
Heart rate (beats/minute)	< 100	> 100	> 120	> 140
Blood pressure	Normal	Decreased	Decreased	Decreased
Respiratory rate (breaths/minute)	14–20	20–30	30–40	> 40
Urinary output (ml/hour)	> 30	20–30	5–15	Negligible
CNS symptoms	Normal	Anxious	Confused	Lethargic

coagulopathy develops also as a result of a rapid consumption of clotting factors, in particular fibrinogen, as occurs in trauma. In certain conditions (e.g. placental abruption), disseminated intravascular coagulation may also occur.

Management options

The anaesthetist's first priority is resuscitation of the patient, but the management of MOH must involve the whole delivery suite as a team, with strong leadership and communication a priority. An MOH protocol should be activated, thus allowing the emergency to be acknowledged, and informing all members of the team including laboratory staff and porters.

The diagnosis and treatment of the cause of bleeding should be carried out during the primary resuscitation. If intravenous access is problematic owing to peripheral vascular shutdown, intraosseous access may be used. The blood lost must be replaced urgently, and time should not be wasted placing monitoring lines. It is increasingly considered that blood products should be given early (and without blood filters, to avoid delay), as in trauma, and although baseline blood tests may be sent to the laboratory, resuscitation should not be delayed and/or based on the results of samples that have been sent 30–60 minutes previously. Equally, point-of-care tests of haemoglobin concentration (e.g. HemoCue) may give false reassurance, and anaesthetists should be guided by the acute clinical situation. Blood gas and lactate measurement may help monitor tissue perfusion and adequacy of resuscitation.

Many protocols for MOH have changed to follow those used in the armed forces, where red cells and clotting factors are given in a ratio of 1:1 or 2:1, which should be considered once product replacement reaches 50% of the estimated circulating volume. Plasma and platelets may be provided as part of an MOH 'shock pack', facilitating rapid replacement. Since there is evidence that fibrinogen levels fall rapidly early on in obstetric haemorrhage, it has been suggested that cryoprecipitate or fibrinogen concentrate be given early, bearing in mind that normal fibrinogen levels in the third trimester are raised (usually > 4 g/l); a level above 2 g/l should be maintained. All fluids given should be warmed, as hypothermia will exacerbate the situation.

Increasingly, thromboelastography- or thromboelastometry-guided protocols have been established, with specific blood products indicated according to the profiles obtained. Advantages that have been claimed include more targeted use of products, thus reducing costs and unnecessary transfusion with attendant risks, as well as earlier treatment, since initial results may be obtained from the point-of-care device within a few minutes.

If a surgical procedure is required (e.g. examination under anaesthesia, removal of retained placenta, caesarean section, hysterectomy, etc.), the presence of severe hypovolaemia combined with a possible coagulopathy usually precludes regional anaesthesia; general anaesthesia with careful administration of induction agents is usually preferable. Extubation should be delayed until resuscitation is adequate and bleeding has stopped. If an epidural catheter is already in situ, removal should be delayed until coagulation has been checked and any deficits corrected.

When major haemorrhage continues, aortic compression, uterine or internal iliac artery occlusion/ligation or hysterectomy (which may be life-saving) should be considered. Embolisation of the uterine arteries under radiological control has been used, but this requires special expertise.

Intraoperative cell salvage is well described now in obstetrics, and the risk of infusing amniotic fluid into the mother's circulation is no longer considered a major concern. However, the benefit of using the intraoperative cell saver has been questioned in the emergency situation for obstetric haemorrhage; surveys in the UK have shown that the return of salvaged blood is often minimal and that its use is limited by the lack of availability of equipment and staff trained in its use. In addition, by the time it is set up much of the potentially salvageable blood may already have been lost.

Although the use of recombinant activated factor VII (rFVIIa; usual dose 75–100 mg/kg) in intractable haemorrhage has been reported, it is no longer advocated routinely as there have been case reports of thromboembolic events and also of non-responders. If rFVIIa is given, any existing coagulopathy should be corrected first. Tranexamic acid (usual dose 1 g) has been shown to reduce deaths from postpartum haemorrhage and has the advantages of being relatively cheap and non-prothrombotic, and is now widely used early in MOH.

Major obstetric haemorrhage guidelines must be available on all delivery suites and should be rehearsed regularly by all the delivery suite staff. Guidelines are published and recommended in the Confidential Enquiries reports, although they may be adapted for local use. The guidelines should be brief, easily understood, with standard abbreviations and restricted to one A4 sheet so that they can be readily referred to in an emergency (Table 78.2).

It is good practice for a delivery suite to have all the equipment that may be needed for massive haemorrhage collected together for easy access, preferably on a mobile trolley that can be quickly wheeled to the patient's bedside. This trolley should be checked and stocked on a daily basis. Multidisciplinary clinical review of all cases of haemorrhage greater than 1500 ml and an opportunity to debrief offered to the woman and her partner are recommended by the Royal College of Obstetricians and Gynaecologists.

Table 78.2 Example of a major obstetric haemorrhage (MOH) guideline

Aims	To resuscitate the patient To treat the cause
Inform/summon (MOH call)	Obstetrician (including senior staff) Anaesthetist (including senior staff) Midwives (including midwife in charge) Anaesthetic assistants and porters Haematologist (including senior staff)
Initial blood sample	Full blood count Coagulation screen/TEG/ROTEM/fast fibrinogen Venous blood gas analysis Cross-matching for at least six units of blood (or as per 'shock pack' protocol)
Initial monitoring	Pulse rate Blood pressure Pulse oximetry
Initial fluids	Crystalloid usually recommended until blood ready In dire emergency, un-cross-matched blood (patient's own ABO and Rh group if possible; un-cross-matched O Rh negative if immediate transfusion is required)
Subsequent monitoring	Direct arterial blood pressure + arterial blood gas analysis Urine output Temperature Central venous pressure
Specific obstetric management	May require general anaesthesia
Subsequent blood samples	As above, for assessment and guidance of therapy
Subsequent fluids	Blood/blood products according to condition. Fluids must be administered through warming equipment. A pressure bag or a rapid infusion device is required
Subsequent management	Early transfer to an intensive care unit should be considered

Key points

- Obstetric haemorrhage continues to be a major contributor to maternal mortality.
- Major haemorrhage guidelines should be in place in all delivery suites and should be regularly rehearsed.

Further reading

Allam J, Cox M, Yentis SM. Cell salvage in obstetrics. *Int J Obstet Anesth* 2008; **17**: 37–45.

Bell SF, Rayment R, Collins PW, Collis RE. The use of fibrinogen concentrate to correct hypofibrinogenaemia rapidly during obstetric haemorrhage. *Int J Obstet Anesth* 2010; **19**: 218–23.

Cotton BA, Au BK, Nunez TC, *et al.* Predefined massive transfusion protocols are associated with a reduction in organ failure and postinjury complications. *J Trauma* 2009; **66**: 41–8.

Mallaiah S, Barclay P, Harrod I, Chevannes C, Bhalla A. Introduction of an algorithm for ROTEM-guided fibrinogen concentrate administration in major obstetric haemorrhage. *Anaesthesia* 2015; **70**: 166–75.

Mercier FJ, Bonnet MP. Use of clotting factors and other prohemostatic drugs for obstetric hemorrhage. *Curr Opin Anaesthesiol* 2010; **23**: 310–16.

Plaat F, Shonfeld A. Major obstetric haemorrhage. *Contin Educ Anaesth Crit Care Pain* 2015; **15**: 190–3.

WOMAN Trial Collaborators. Effect of early tranexamic acid administration on mortality, hysterectomy, and other morbidities in women with post-partum haemorrhage (WOMAN): an international, randomised, double-blind, placebo-controlled trial. *Lancet* 2017; **389**: 2105–16.

Chapter 70

Postpartum haemorrhage

Placental separation involves the sudden exposure of a vascular bed receiving up to 20% of the maternal cardiac output. Prevention of potentially massive haemorrhage requires contraction of uterine and arteriolar muscle, activation of circulating and endothelial clotting factors and platelet aggregation and deposition.

Postpartum haemorrhage (PPH) occurs in ~2% of deliveries and is defined as a blood loss of over 500 ml after delivery of the placenta. A PPH occurring within 24 hours of childbirth is termed primary PPH and is divided into minor (500–1000 ml) and major (> 1000 ml), the latter further subdivided into moderate (1001–2000 ml) and severe (> 2000 ml). (Note that lower cut-offs are appropriate in women < 60 kg.)

A secondary PPH occurs within the next 12 weeks and is usually due to retained products of conception and/or infection.

Postpartum haemorrhage can be one of the most frightening obstetric emergencies and may be associated with maternal mortality.

Problems and special considerations

There are a number of different causes of PPH (Table 79.1). These have been summarised into four descriptive groups as an aide-memoire: tone, trauma, tissue and thrombin ('the four Ts'). Although initial management is the same (i.e. resuscitation), subsequent management depends on the cause, which may be difficult to ascertain in the face of continuing haemorrhage.

After a normal delivery, attention is often focused on the baby, and thus PPH may be unnoticed initially. This is compounded by the ability of normal pregnant women to compensate until hypovolaemia is severe (see Chapter 78, *Major obstetric haemorrhage*).

There may be few medical and midwifery staff in close attendance if PPH occurs without warning, especially following a spontaneous vaginal delivery in a delivery room. The severity of blood loss may be underestimated in such circumstances, and there may be a delay in resuscitation unless staff are well versed in the emergency management of such cases.

Management options

The first priority of the anaesthetist arriving at a PPH is resuscitation, followed by urgent assessment of the cause of bleeding. Initial management is as for major obstetric haemorrhage (MOH; see Chapter 78), including activation of an MOH protocol and early evaluation of coagulation using point-of-care devices if available.

Table 79.1 Causes of postpartum haemorrhage

Obstetric	Uterine atony
	• Large placental site, e.g. multiple pregnancy
	• Long or precipitous labour
	• Prolonged oxytocic infusion
	• Grand multiparity
	• Chorioamnionitis
	• Drugs, e.g. volatile anaesthetic agents, tocolytic drugs
	• Inverted or ruptured uterus
	Retained intrauterine products (placenta or membranes)
	Trauma to the cervix, birth canal or perineum
Non-obstetric	Coagulopathy
	• Primary, e.g. von Willebrand's disease
	• Secondary, e.g. disseminated intravascular coagulation, HELLP syndrome, post-massive transfusion coagulopathy, drugs

The extent of haemorrhage is often underestimated. Any woman who has an unexplained tachycardia or a hypotensive episode in the postpartum period should be treated as having had a major blood loss until proven otherwise. If PPH does not occur immediately after delivery, the use of a modified early obstetric warning score (MEOWS) may help identify changing physiology and trigger an early response to haemorrhage (see Chapter 156, *Modified early obstetric warning scores*).

The most common cause of PPH is uterine atony. It is routine practice to administer oxytocics at the delivery of the anterior shoulder of the baby (see Chapter 64, *Oxytocic and tocolytic drugs*). This hastens placental separation and encourages uterine contraction in the third stage of labour. If the uterus fails to contract and bleeding continues, further oxytocic drugs may be given (Table 79.2), aided by manual rubbsng of the uterus to stimulate contraction. If the uterus continues to relax, the possibility of retained products of conception should be considered, which necessitates exploration of the uterus. A retained placenta may involve the whole or part of the placenta, and manual removal of the placenta is indicated.

Genital tract trauma should be sought, and this may require anaesthesia. Ideally, primary resuscitation of the patient, together with confirmation of preparation of blood for transfusion, should be established before anaesthesia is administered. It is often necessary to proceed to anaesthesia before the blood is available; general anaesthesia may be preferable in the haemodynamically unstable patient.

If there is continued uterine bleeding, the abdomen needs to be opened. Hysterectomy may sometimes be avoided by packing the uterus or using an intrauterine balloon, compression (B-Lynch) sutures, and ligation or embolisation of the uterine or internal iliac arteries or use of intravascular balloon catheters (depending on expertise and the proximity of the radiology department). Recent evidence suggests the incidence of peripartum hysterectomy in the UK is 4–5 per 10,000 births (ranging from 1 in 30,000 for a first vaginal delivery, to 1 in

Table 79.2 Prevention and drug treatment of uterine atony causing postpartum haemorrhage (PPH)

Routine prophylaxis	Oxytocin 10 U intramuscularly at delivery of the anterior shoulder
PPH occurs	Oxytocin 5–10 U given slowly, intravenously, or an infusion containing 40 U oxytocin + 500 ml saline at a rate depending on the clinical response but usually over a 4-hour period
PPH persists	Ergometrine 250–500 µg intramuscularly, repeated after an hour
PPH unresponsive to the above	Carboprost (PGF$_{2\alpha}$) 250 µg given by deep intramuscular injection, repeated at intervals of > 15 minutes, up to a total dose of 2 mg (8 doses). Direct injection into the myometrium is not recommended
Various [a]	Misoprostol 200–1000 µg depending on the route. Oral, sublingual, vaginal, rectal, and intrauterine administration have been described

[a] Use of misoprostol may vary according to local protocols, but it has been used to prevent as well as treat PPH.
N.B. Consider retained placenta, genital tract trauma and other causes of haemorrhage.
See Chapter 78, *Major obstetric haemorrhage*, for general management of haemorrhage.

220 for a third caesarean section, to 1 in 32 for placenta praevia). Tranexamic acid (1 g) has been shown to reduce the incidence of death from PPH, especially if given early.

Key points

- Any postpartum haemorrhage must be seen as a potential major obstetric haemorrhage and should be treated early and aggressively.
- Senior help should be sought at an early stage.
- Full resuscitation should not be regarded as being complete until the cause of the bleeding has been identified and treated.

Further reading

Kayem G, Kurinczuk JJ, Alfirevic Z, *et al.* Specific second-line therapies for postpartum haemorrhage: a national cohort study. *BJOG* 2011; **118**: 856–64.

Knight M; UKOSS. Peripartum hysterectomy in the UK: management and outcomes of the associated haemorrhage. *BJOG* 2007; **114**: 1380–7.

Liabsuetrakul T, Choobun T, Peeyananjarassri K, *et al.* Treatment for primary postpartum haemorrhage. *Cochrane Database Syst Rev* 2007; (1): CD003249.

Mavrides E, Allard S, Chandraharan E, *et al.*; Royal College of Obstetricians and Gynaecologists. Prevention and management of postpartum haemorrhage. Green-top Guideline 52. *BJOG* 2016; **124**: e106–49.

Royal College of Obstetricians and Gynaecologists. The role of emergency and elective interventional radiology in postpartum haemorrhage. *Good Practice* **6**. London: RCOG, 2007. www.rcog.org.uk/globalassets/documents/guidelines/goodpractice6roleemergency2007.pdf (accessed December 2018).

Weeks A. The prevention and treatment of postpartum haemorrhage: what do we know, and where do we go to next? *BJOG* 2015; **122**: 202–10.

Collapse on the labour ward

Maternal collapse is defined as an acute cardiorespiratory or neurological event resulting in impaired consciousness during pregnancy or up to 6 weeks postpartum. Although uncommon, collapse of a mother in the delivery suite may represent serious underlying pathology and demands rapid treatment; the mother may also rapidly respond to relatively simple measures, thus avoiding disaster.

Problems and special considerations

The management of a collapsed mother on the labour ward presents a challenge to all staff concerned. Typically, labour ward staff are less familiar with emergency equipment and drugs than staff in the operating theatres, so continuous support and education of staff is required; regular 'drills' have been recommended, though this may be difficult in a busy and possibly understaffed unit. In addition, the labour ward is often situated in an isolated or remote area of the hospital, so access to other key clinical areas, such as the radiology suite and intensive care unit, is not always easy. Finally, pregnant women are usually fit and healthy and often clinical deterioration may go unnoticed; the use of a modified early obstetric warning score (see Chapter 156) may help earlier detection.

Collapse on the labour ward may have several causes, some of which require specific investigation and/or management (Table 80.1).

Management options

Initial resuscitation in the undelivered patient is influenced by the risk of aortocaval compression and aspiration, and the fact that the fetus is at risk. The airway should be secured, the lungs ventilated and the circulation supported with fluids, vasoactive drugs or cardiac massage as appropriate, with measures taken to displace the uterus or deliver the fetus.

Concurrent with treatment is the need to determine the cause, with further management directed as appropriate.

All staff should be familiar with basic resuscitative techniques, and protocols should exist for the more important causes, for example eclampsia and haemorrhage. Rapid delivery of relevant information about the collapsed mother to the medical staff resuscitating her is also crucial in directing management towards a particular possible cause. This will be easier in delivery suites where there is good multi-professional communication about routine as well as problem cases.

Table 80.1 Causes of collapse on the labour ward

A:	Anaesthesia	Regional anaesthetic sympathetic block, local anaesthetic toxicity, total spinal
B:	Bleeding	Antenatal, e.g. placenta praevia, abruption; postnatal, e.g. splenic artery rupture
C:	Cardiac	Congenital heart disease, infarction/arrest, arrhythmias, vasovagal syncope, aortocaval compression
	Cerebral	Epilepsy, stroke, tumour
D:	Drugs	Magnesium, antihypertensives, opioids, sedatives, illicit drug use
E:	Embolism	Amniotic fluid, air, thrombus
F:	Fever	Sepsis
G:	General	Anaphylaxis, hypoxia, electrolyte disturbance
H:	Hypertension	Eclampsia

Key points

- Collapse on the labour ward has many causes including obstetric, anaesthetic and medical factors.
- Immediate management is as for the non-pregnant patient, but with avoidance of aortocaval compression.

Further reading

Royal College of Obstetricians and Gynaecologists. *Maternal Collapse in Pregnancy and the Puerperium*. Green-top Guideline 56. London: RCOG, 2011. www.rcog.org.uk/en/guidelines-research-services/guidelines/gtg56 (accessed December 2018).

Maternal cardiopulmonary resuscitation

Although the basic principles of cardiopulmonary resuscitation (CPR) are the same as in the non-pregnant state, the underlying causes of collapse are generally different, and the presence of the fetus has major implications for management and outcome.

Problems and special considerations

Because most mothers are healthy, cardiac arrest is rare in this group (estimated at 1 in 30,000) and thus resuscitative skills are easily forgotten, especially by those not regularly exposed to patients requiring cardiorespiratory support. There may be delay in recognising and responding to cardiorespiratory arrest. Midwives and obstetricians (and also anaesthetists) may be unfamiliar with protocols for life support and the drugs and equipment required, which may easily become faulty or out of date if not checked regularly. The maternity suite is often an unfamiliar place to the regular cardiac arrest team.

Although the pregnant population is fit and healthy generally, all causes of cardiac arrest pertaining to the non-pregnant population should be considered, as well as those specifically associated with pregnancy. Most cases of peripartum cardiorespiratory arrest or collapse will involve causes other than ischaemic heart disease (see Chapter 80, *Collapse on the labour ward*).

The effect of the gravid uterus needs to be taken into account, and left uterine displacement must be continuously applied during resuscitative measures. Although previously left lateral tilt was recommended during CPR, it is now thought to be less effective than manual uterine displacement. Similarly, current guidance states that hand placement for chest compressions should be at the lower part of the sternum as for non-pregnant patients rather than higher up as previously recommended. Effective chest compressions are important for resuscitation to be successful, and the patient can remain supine, allowing this, if manual uterine displacement is applied. However, even with manual uterine displacement, return of spontaneous circulation is unlikely in the presence of a heavily gravid uterus.

The pregnant patient has limited oxygen reserve, thus requiring prompt oxygenation/ ventilation. However, airway management may be more difficult, and the presence of a gravid uterus may hinder effective artificial ventilation and increase the risk of regurgitation by exerting pressure on the stomach. It may also increase the risk of injury to the liver, spleen and ribs because of the increased intra-abdominal pressure and altered shape of the chest.

Management options

Some cases of cardiac arrest may be prevented by general training and development of protocols in airway management and cardiovascular monitoring, identification of high-risk cases, good communication and organisation of facilities, equipment, etc.

All staff who work in the maternity suite must receive training and regular updates in CPR, including use of the defibrillator and other equipment. Drills have been shown to improve retention of skills, although they may be very disruptive to a busy unit.

Actual management of cardiac arrest is as for the non-pregnant patient, including the positioning of the hands on the sternum (previously recommended as placed higher up on the sternum). Relief of aortocaval compression is paramount, as mentioned above. Intravenous access must be secured above the diaphragm. If CPR is unsuccessful after 4 minutes, the decision to perform a perimortem caesarean section should be made, aiming for delivery of the fetus by 5 minutes; the purpose of this is to improve maternal venous return rather than for the benefit of the fetus, and fetal monitoring should not occur during resuscitative attempts. The only equipment required is a scalpel (although clamps and forceps may be useful), which should therefore be included on all cardiac arrest trolleys on the labour ward. The operator should use whichever technique he/she feels most comfortable with, but a vertical incision may allow better access and reduce blood loss. There are many reported cases of return of spontaneous cardiac output and maternal survival once delivery has been achieved, where CPR has failed initially. Neonatal outcome is usually poor, although this depends on the gestation, the cause of collapse, the delay before delivery and the effectiveness of CPR; speedier delivery is associated with improved outcome.

The risk of regurgitation and aspiration of gastric contents should be remembered, and cricoid pressure should be applied, if hands are spare, until the trachea has been intubated.

If resumption of cardiac output does occur, there is some evidence that mild induced hypothermia may improve neurological outcome in the non-pregnant population; as cardiac arrest in pregnancy is rare, data in this patient group are limited to anecdotal reports.

Key points

- For CPR, the same principles apply to the pregnant population as to the non-pregnant population.
- Regular training of staff and maintenance of equipment are required.
- Maternal cardiopulmonary resuscitation is usually impossible in late pregnancy unless aortocaval compression is relieved.

Further reading

Eldridge AJ, Ford R. Perimortem caesarean deliveries. *Int Journal Obs Anesth* 2016; **27**: 46–54.

Jeejeebhoy FM, Zelop CM, Lipman S, *et al.* Cardiac arrest in pregnancy: a scientific statement from the American Heart Association. *Circulation* 2015; **132**: 1747–73.

Kikuchi J, Deering S. Cardiac arrest in pregnancy. *Semin Perinatol* 2018; **42**: 33–8.

Lipman S, Cohen S, Einav S, *et al.* The Society for Obstetric Anesthesia and Perinatology Consensus Statement on the Management of Cardiac Arrest in Pregnancy. *Anesth Analg* 2014; **118**: 1003–16.

Truhlář A, Deakin CD, Soar J, *et al.* European Resuscitation Council Guidelines for Resuscitation 2015: Section 4. Cardiac arrest in special circumstances. *Resuscitation* 2015; **95**: 148–201.

Chapter 82

Amniotic fluid embolism

Amniotic fluid embolism (AFE) has traditionally been estimated to occur in 1 in 8000 to 1 in 80,000 deliveries, the wide range reflecting the difficulty in its accurate diagnosis. More recent evidence suggests an incidence in the UK of ~2 in 100,000 births. Despite its rarity, AFE has been implicated in 10–12% of direct maternal deaths in the UK, making it one of the major causes of mortality; it is ranked as the fifth leading cause of direct maternal death in the 2018 report of the Confidential Enquiries into Maternal Deaths.

The traditional explanation of AFE is that amniotic fluid enters the maternal circulation following forceful contractions, causing embolic obstruction similar to thromboembolism. However, the mechanism now proposed is systemic release of inflammatory mediators causing cardiovascular collapse, although the trigger for mediator release is still disputed (amniotic fluid, meconium, fetal cells or other substances all having been suggested). The role of amniotic fluid itself is uncertain, since infusion of amniotic fluid may be well tolerated experimentally. The UK Obstetric Surveillance System (UKOSS) has reported that AFE is associated with increased maternal age, induction of labour and multiparity, and is seen more in women from ethnic minorities. Although AFE is most common during labour, it may also occur during caesarean section or even after delivery.

Problems and special considerations

Features of AFE include cardiovascular collapse with left ventricular failure, respiratory failure secondary to pulmonary hypertension and ventilation–perfusion mismatch, and disseminated intravascular coagulation (DIC). Thus symptoms may include dyspnoea, cyanosis and haemodynamic collapse or non-specific complaints including sweating, shivering, convulsions and unexplained fetal compromise (in 20% of cases). Collapse is typically profound, rapid and resistant to treatment; thus the initial problem of AFE is its immediate management.

In addition, there are many causes of sudden collapse (see Chapter 80, *Collapse on the labour ward*), and it may be difficult to diagnose the underlying condition. Although the diagnosis of AFE is often based on the demonstration of fetal squames in the maternal circulation or lung, this has been shown to be neither a sensitive nor a specific test, since normal mothers may demonstrate circulating fetal squames while 'classic' cases of AFE may not. For reporting purposes to UKOSS, the diagnostic criteria include:

- The absence of an alternative clear cause, and either
    - Acute maternal collapse with one or more of the following features: acute fetal compromise; cardiac arrest; cardiac rhythm problems; coagulopathy; hypotension;

maternal haemorrhage; premonitory symptoms, e.g. restlessness, numbness, agitation, tingling; seizures; shortness of breath, or

– The finding of fetal squames or hair in the lungs of women at post-mortem.

Women with maternal haemorrhage as the first presenting feature in whom there was no evidence of early coagulopathy or cardiorespiratory compromise are excluded.

A final problem – and one that hinders development of effective methods of prevention and treatment – is the debate over the nature of AFE itself, even whether it represents a separate entity at all (the term 'sudden obstetric collapse syndrome' has been suggested as being more appropriate). Since the mechanism is so poorly understood, the condition remains an enigma.

AFE is a theoretical risk of intraoperative cell salvage. However, leucocyte depletion filters have been shown to reduce amniotic fluid contamination significantly, and no cases of AFE associated with cell salvage use in obstetrics have been reported as yet.

Management options

Management is supportive, with basic resuscitative manoeuvres (remembering uterine displacement), management of bleeding and correction of DIC. If cardiac arrest occurs, perimortem caesarean section should occur within 5 minutes. Concurrent triggering of the major obstetric haemorrhage protocol is advised (see Chapter 78, *Major obstetric haemorrhage*). There have been limited case reports of novel techniques being used successfully in the treatment of AFE, including intravenous steroids, prostacyclin, plasma exchange, inhaled nitric oxide, cardiopulmonary bypass and extracorporeal membrane oxygenation. A mortality rate of 60–80% was traditionally reported, but the lower mortality rate in more recent reports (~20%) suggests that recognition and management of the syndrome has improved.

Key points

- Amniotic fluid embolism is probably a misnomer, but represents a catastrophic event on the labour ward.
- Features include convulsions, respiratory and cardiovascular collapse, disseminated intravascular coagulation and fetal compromise.
- There is no specific treatment, but with prompt recognition and supportive therapy the prognosis is improved.

Further reading

Knight, M, Berg C, Brocklehurst P, *et al.* Amniotic fluid embolism incidence, risk factors and outcomes: a review and recommendations. *BMC Pregnancy Childbirth* 2012; **12**: 7.

Knight M, Nair M, Tuffnell D, *et al.*; MBRRACE-UK. *Saving Lives, Improving Mothers' Care: Lessons learned to inform maternity care from the UK and Ireland Confidential Enquiries into Maternal Deaths and Morbidity 2013–15*. Oxford: National Perinatal Epidemiology Unit, University of Oxford, 2017.

McDonnell NJ, Percival V, Paech MJ. Amniotic fluid embolism: a leading cause of maternal death yet still a medical conundrum. *Int J Obstet Anesth* 2013; **22**: 329–36.

Pacheco LD, Saade G, Hankins GD, Clark SL; Society for Maternal–Fetal Medicine. Amniotic fluid embolism: diagnosis and management. *Am J Obstet Gynecol* 2016; **215**: B16–24.

Cholestasis of pregnancy (obstetric cholestasis)

Cholestasis of pregnancy (intrahepatic cholestasis of pregnancy) is thought to result from an exaggerated cholestatic effect of oestrogens. It occurs in approximately 0.2% of pregnancies (except in Scandinavia and South America, where incidences of up to 10% have been reported) and is associated with multiple pregnancy. Its presenting symptom is localised (usually to the hands and feet) or generalised pruritus, occurring particularly at night. This is caused by the deposition of bile acids in the skin. Symptoms usually occur during the third trimester and may be sufficiently distressing to necessitate induction of labour. The condition is specific to pregnancy, and patients are invariably asymptomatic within 6 weeks after delivery. The condition tends to recur in subsequent pregnancies.

Problems and special considerations

Although symptoms usually occur in the third trimester, the condition may present at any stage of pregnancy. There is a personal or family history of jaundice while using the oral contraceptive pill, or during a previous pregnancy, in about 50% of cases.

Jaundice occurs in up to 50% of cases if untreated or undelivered. Clinical examination is otherwise normal except for scratch marks because of the severe itching. Fat malabsorption occurs, and the mother may complain of steatorrhoea. Malabsorption may result in vitamin K deficiency. Symptoms tend to precede changes in liver function tests, which reveal predominantly conjugated bilirubinaemia, with markedly increased alkaline phosphatase and mildly increased transaminases. Liver ultrasound is usually normal.

While the prognosis is favourable for mothers, the condition is not as benign for babies. There is an increased risk of premature delivery (spontaneous and iatrogenic), fetal distress and intrauterine death, presumed to be secondary to reduced placental blood flow or a direct effect of bile salts. Risk of fetal morbidity and mortality increases with gestational age, and early delivery is often recommended.

Management options

Treatment with cholestyramine, antihistamines or topical preparations has variable success. Corticosteroids have also been used, but most women are now treated with ursodeoxycholic acid, which has been shown to improve symptoms and reduce serum bile acid levels. Both the mother and the neonate should receive vitamin K therapy.

The mother's coagulation should be checked during the antenatal period and before considering insertion of an epidural or spinal needle, although coagulopathy is rare. While it is acknowledged that changes in coagulation are not rapid, guidance issued by the Association of Anaesthetists of Great Britain and Ireland (AAGBI) recommends that clotting studies be checked in the 24 hours preceding neuraxial intervention. If coagulation studies are within normal limits, the mother should be encouraged to have epidural analgesia for labour, since there is an increased incidence of caesarean section.

Key points

- Cholestasis of pregnancy is a benign and self-limiting condition for the mother but is associated with an increased incidence of preterm labour, fetal distress and caesarean delivery.
- Coagulopathy may occur secondary to vitamin K malabsorption.
- The only definitive treatment is delivery.
- Epidural analgesia should be encouraged unless contraindicated by coagulopathy.

Further reading

Joshi D, James A, Quaglia A, Westbrook RH, Heneghan MA. Liver disease in pregnancy. *Lancet* 2010; **375**: 594–605.

Royal College of Obstetricians and Gynaecologists. *Obstetric Cholestasis*. Green-top Guideline 43. London: RCOG, 2011 (updated 2014). www.rcog.org.uk/en/guidelines-research-services/guide lines/gtg43 (accessed December 2018).

Westbrook RH, Dusheiko G, Williamson C. Pregnancy and liver disease. *J Hepatol* 2016; **64**: 933–45.

Acute fatty liver of pregnancy

Acute fatty liver of pregnancy is an uncommon (estimated 1 in 22,000 births in the UK) but serious complication of predominantly primiparous women, especially those with multiple pregnancy and possibly low body mass index (BMI). The condition was first reported in the literature in 1934, and traditionally the mortality for both mother and fetus has been reported to be as high as 85%, secondary to multi-organ failure. Current figures estimate maternal mortality to be about 10–20%, the improvement being attributed to earlier diagnosis and delivery. The median gestation at diagnosis is 36 weeks.

In some cases, the condition may be associated with long-chain-3-hydroxyacyl-CoA dehydrogenase (LCHAD) deficiency; this is an enzyme that catalyses a reaction in the oxidation of fatty acids, and its deficiency allows a build-up of fatty acids. Both parents have 50% of normal LCHAD activity and the fetus has no LCHAD activity, with the fetal liver dysfunction apparently causing fatty liver disease in the mother. Other enzyme deficiencies have also been correlated with acute fatty liver, so deficiency of LCHAD does not account for all the cases.

Symptoms usually present in the third trimester and tend to be non-specific: malaise, nausea and vomiting (which may be severe), headache and diffuse right upper quadrant or epigastric pain. Liver function may deteriorate rapidly, leading to acute liver failure. There is overlap between acute fatty liver and pre-eclampsia, and it has been suggested that acute fatty liver is a manifestation of pre-eclampsia, as is the HELLP (haemolysis, elevated liver enzymes and low platelet count) syndrome (see Chapter 85). It is often difficult to differentiate between HELLP and acute fatty liver.

The only treatment for acute fatty liver of pregnancy is delivery of the fetus regardless of gestational age; expectant management is not appropriate. As with pre-eclampsia, there may be a time lag of several days between delivery and clinical improvement.

Recovery is usually complete, with no evidence of chronic liver disease. Recurrence in subsequent pregnancies is said to be uncommon, although there have not been a large number of documented pregnancies in survivors of acute fatty liver. In cases associated with LCHAD deficiency, the risk of acute fatty liver is 25% in each pregnancy.

Problems and special considerations

The differential diagnoses at initial presentation include pre-eclampsia, acute viral hepatitis, drug-induced hepatitis, cholestasis of pregnancy and biliary tract disease. Pruritus is uncommon in acute fatty liver and is highly suggestive of cholestasis (see Chapter 83).

The mother is usually, but not invariably, jaundiced. Although she may complain of abdominal pain, it is unusual to find marked liver tenderness on examination, and this finding is suggestive of viral hepatitis or HELLP syndrome. If presentation occurs late, all the stigmata of acute liver failure may be present, including hepatic encephalopathy, disseminated intravascular coagulation (DIC) and renal failure. The prognosis is poor if the disease presents in this advanced state.

The Swansea criteria may be used to diagnose acute fatty liver, in which six or more of the following are present in the absence of another cause: vomiting; abdominal pain; polydipsia/polyuria; encephalopathy; elevated bilirubin; elevated transaminases; elevated ammonia; hypoglycaemia; renal impairment; coagulopathy; elevated urate; leucocytosis; ascites or bright liver echo texture on ultrasound; and microvesicular steatosis on liver biopsy.

Management options

Acute fatty liver of pregnancy is uncommon but has a high maternal and fetal mortality if the diagnosis is delayed. A high index of clinical suspicion is needed for the non-specifically unwell mother with pre-eclampsia, especially if there is any indication that she may be jaundiced.

Once the diagnosis is confirmed, the mother should be stabilised as necessary and the baby delivered. Medical support is likely to include administration of glucose, blood, clotting factors and platelets. Hypertension associated with pre-eclampsia should be controlled. Careful fluid balance is required, as acute kidney injury and propensity towards pulmonary oedema may be present. Increased likelihood of postpartum haemorrhage should be anticipated.

Regional analgesia and anaesthesia are contraindicated in the presence of any coagulopathy. If regional analgesia is contraindicated, analgesia for labour can be provided by using cautious doses of opioid drugs, preferably by using intravenous patient-controlled analgesia (PCA). Elimination of opioid drugs is likely to be prolonged, and remifentanil PCA may be advantageous. Adjuvant sedative drugs such as promazine and promethazine should not be given. General anaesthesia may adversely affect hepatic encephalopathy. Because of impaired metabolism, atracurium is the preferred neuromuscular blocking drug for general anaesthesia.

Operative delivery is not indicated unless the obstetrician considers that successful vaginal delivery is unlikely to be achieved. If operative delivery is needed, persistent bleeding from surgical sites should be anticipated and prophylactic wound drains are advisable. Close observation is essential following delivery, and intensive care management including multi-organ support may be required. Transfer to a specialist liver unit may be necessary. Mildly affected mothers should have a low-protein diet and scrupulous fluid and electrolyte management until clinical and laboratory findings return to normal.

Key points

- Acute fatty liver of pregnancy potentially has a very high mortality unless diagnosed and treated promptly.
- Some cases are caused by long-chain-3-hydroxyacyl-CoA dehydrogenase (LCHAD) deficiency and have an increased risk of recurrence.
- Delivery of the fetus is the only definitive treatment.

- Acute liver failure and multi-organ derangement can occur rapidly. Regional analgesia and anaesthesia are usually contraindicated because of abnormal clotting studies.
- Pre-eclampsia frequently coexists with acute fatty liver, and it is possible that acute fatty liver is a variant of pre-eclampsia.

Further reading

Kia L, Rinella ME. Interpretation and management of hepatic abnormalities in pregnancy. *Clin Gastroenterol Hepatol* 2013; **11**: 1392–8.

Knight M, Nelson-Piercy C, Kurinczuk JJ, Spark P, Brocklehurst P; UK Obstetric Surveillance System. A prospective national study of acute fatty liver of pregnancy in the UK. *Gut* 2008; **57**: 951–6.

Rajasri AG, Srestha R, Mitchell J. Acute fatty liver of pregnancy: an overview. *J Obstet Gynaecol* 2007; **27**: 237–40.

Tran TT, Ahn J, Reau NS. ACG clinical guideline: liver disease and pregnancy. *Am J Gastroenterol* 2016; **111**: 176–94.

Chapter 85

HELLP syndrome

HELLP (haemolysis, elevated liver enzymes and low platelet count) syndrome is one of the presentations of pre-eclampsia and may occur before or soon after delivery (usually within 48 hours). Severe HELLP syndrome is associated with disseminated intravascular coagulation (DIC) and placental abruption, and may progress to multi-organ failure. It is associated with a high fetal and maternal morbidity and mortality.

Problems and special considerations

The mother with HELLP syndrome may not necessarily have presented with other symptoms or signs of pre-eclampsia. The main presenting feature may be abdominal pain, perhaps with nausea and vomiting, so a high index of suspicion is needed. The first presentation may be a seizure.

Mild changes in liver function tests have been reported in up to 50% of women with pre-eclampsia, but more serious dysfunction may occur, including periportal haemorrhage and hepatic infarction. There have also been several reported cases of liver rupture associated with severe HELLP syndrome. Acute fatty liver of pregnancy is also considered by many authorities to be part of the spectrum of pre-eclampsia/eclampsia.

Other complications of HELLP syndrome include renal failure, DIC, pulmonary oedema, pleural effusions, acute respiratory distress syndrome, retinal detachment and cerebral oedema. About 16% of women who are undelivered and who develop HELLP syndrome present with placental abruption.

Management options

The treatment of HELLP syndrome is supportive; delivery of the placenta is the definitive treatment.

Women should be delivered as soon as the maternal condition has been optimised, usually by caesarean section. Recommendations vary regarding pre- or perioperative platelet transfusion, with some centres suggesting platelet transfusion if the platelet count is below $50 \times 10^9/l$ and others not giving platelets until the count falls below $20 \times 10^9/l$.

The benefits of invasive pressure monitoring must be balanced against the potential hazards. Careful fluid balance is important, and may be guided with central venous pressure monitoring and urine output. However, many anaesthetists believe that the hazards of central venous lines and their use on the labour ward for fluid balance outweigh the benefits, and there is little evidence in the literature supporting an improved outcome.

Regional anaesthesia is relatively contraindicated in the presence of thrombocytopenia, but ultimately the anaesthetist must choose the anaesthetic technique that he or she judges to be the safest in the circumstances. The choice of regional anaesthesia in a woman with a platelet count of less than 75×10^9/l should only be made by an experienced consultant obstetric anaesthetist. In women with progressive thrombocytopenia, a platelet count should be checked immediately before performing neuraxial anaesthesia. Thromboelastography/thromboelastometry has been used to aid management.

If general anaesthesia is used, attempts must be made to attenuate the hypertensive response to intubation, usually by use of an intravenous opioid as part of the induction sequence (see Chapter 86, *Hypertension, pre-eclampsia and eclampsia*). Tracheal intubation should be carried out as atraumatically as possible, and difficult intubation secondary to airway oedema should be anticipated.

There is no specific treatment for HELLP syndrome other than symptomatic treatment of the associated complications, although there is some evidence to support steroid therapy, e.g. two doses of dexamethasone 10 mg 12 hours apart followed by 5 mg at 24 and 36 hours. Plasma exchange has been anecdotally reported to be useful, although the evidence for it is weak. Magnesium sulfate is indicated for seizure prophylaxis. Women with HELLP syndrome should be managed in a high-dependency or intensive care environment. Postnatal management is entirely supportive.

Key points

- HELLP syndrome is part of the spectrum of pre-eclampsia/eclampsia and may present without prodromal symptoms and signs of pre-eclampsia.
- It may present before or after delivery, and is associated with significant maternal and fetal morbidity and mortality.
- Epigastric pain, nausea and vomiting are common presenting features, and a high index of suspicion is essential in every pregnant woman presenting with abdominal pain.
- Treatment consists of delivery and supportive management of the associated complications.

Further reading

del-Rio-Vellosillo M, Garcia-Medina JJ. Anesthetic considerations in HELLP syndrome. *Acta Anesthesiol Scand* 2016; **60**: 144–57.
Fitzpatrick KE, Hinshaw K, Kurinczuk JJ, Knight M. Risk factors, management, and outcomes of hemolysis, elevated liver enzymes, and low platelets syndrome and elevated liver enzymes, low platelets syndrome. *Obstet Gynecol* 2014; **123**: 618–27.
Haram K, Svendsen E, Abildgaard U. The HELLP syndrome: clinical issues and management. A review. *BMC Pregnancy Childbirth* 2009; **9**: 8.

Hypertension, pre-eclampsia and eclampsia

Hypertension in pregnancy is diagnosed either by raised absolute values of systolic or diastolic pressure (> 140 mmHg and > 90 mmHg respectively) or by increases in systolic or diastolic pressures above those at booking (> 30 mmHg and > 15 mmHg respectively). Pressures should be raised on two separate occasions using appropriate methods of measurement (see below).

Hypertensive disorders of pregnancy are divided into chronic hypertension, gestational hypertension and pre-eclampsia.

Chronic hypertension and gestational hypertension

Chronic hypertension occurs in 3–5% of pregnancies, though the incidence is increasing in the UK as maternal age increases. It is diagnosed by pre-existing hypertension, hypertension that occurs before 20 weeks' gestation (although the diagnosis may be masked by the normal slight fall in blood pressure that occurs in early pregnancy, and pre-eclampsia may rarely present earlier than 20 weeks), or hypertension that develops in pregnancy and persists postpartum. The risk of pre-eclampsia is approximately doubled, and there is also a greater risk of abruption and fetal growth restriction, but if the blood pressure is controlled, women with chronic hypertension would be expected to have good outcomes.

Gestational hypertension describes hypertension after 20 weeks' gestation without any features of pre-eclampsia, and occurs in 6–7% of pregnancies. The risk of pre-eclampsia is increased slightly, this risk increasing the earlier the hypertension develops. Blood pressure usually returns to normal within 1–2 months of delivery.

Pre-eclampsia

Pre-eclampsia is now defined as hypertension that develops after 20 weeks' gestation in a previously normotensive woman, that is associated with proteinuria or impairment of one or more organ system. This may include renal, hepatic, respiratory, neurological, haematological or uteroplacental disease. Because of practical difficulties in quantifying 24-hour proteinuria, measurement of a random urine protein/creatinine ratio (PCR) is often done instead, a PCR above 30 mg/mmol correlating with a 24-hour protein excretion greater than 300 mg. It is possible to develop non-proteinuric pre-eclampsia, and also to have eclamptic seizures with minimal or even no hypertension. Pre-eclampsia occurs in 5–6% of pregnancies overall (up to 25% in patients with pre-existing hypertension).

Pre-eclampsia/eclampsia is a major cause of direct maternal death worldwide. The pathophysiology of pre-eclampsia is still only partially understood, but it is known that failure of placentation occurs early in pregnancy and this leads to vascular endothelial cell damage and dysfunction. The endothelial cell damage is thought to lead to release of vasoactive substances, which promote generalised vasoconstriction and reduced organ perfusion. This is exacerbated by an increased sensitivity to circulating catecholamines. Pre-eclamptic women demonstrate an imbalance of the normal thromboxane/prostacyclin ratio and increased free radical activity.

Pre-eclampsia encompasses HELLP (haemolysis, elevated liver enzymes and low platelet count) syndrome, eclampsia and possibly acute fatty liver of pregnancy. Although the disease is progressive, a mother may be asymptomatic until she presents with an eclamptic fit, and although pre-eclampsia is a disease of pregnancy, terminated only by delivery, pre-eclampsia, HELLP syndrome and eclampsia may all present for the first time after delivery.

There have been many attempts to prevent development of pre-eclampsia, for example with dietary vitamins, antioxidants and minerals, with no clear benefit found. There is evidence that low-dose aspirin may be beneficial in selected high-risk women.

Problems and special considerations

Blood pressure measurements should be made with the mother sitting (or on her side in late pregnancy) to avoid aortocaval compression. Most automated blood pressure measuring devices have not been validated in pregnancy, and many tend to under-read blood pressure, especially in pre-eclampsia, giving a false sense of security (though they can be used to monitor trends, so long as manual measurements are taken at intervals). If manual methods of measurement are used, it is now recommended that Korotkoff phase V sounds should be used to measure diastolic pressure, not phase IV, since the former are more reproducible and better correlated with true diastolic pressure in pregnancy.

Pre-eclampsia is frequently asymptomatic despite significant disease. Symptoms are often non-specific and include headache (commonly frontal), visual disturbance and epigastric or right upper quadrant pain. The most commonly occurring signs are hypertension, oedema and hyperreflexia, although the last of these is subjective and unreliable as a prognostic indicator (though sustained clonus is pathological). Severe pre-eclampsia is characterised by features of significant end-organ dysfunction that may include pulmonary oedema, cerebral haemorrhage, elevated transaminases (doubling of the normal level or ALT > 70 IU/L), renal dysfunction (proteinuria > 5 g/24 h, 3+ protein dipstick or doubling of serum creatinine in the absence of other pathology) or coagulopathy, e.g. thrombocytopenia, haemolytic anaemia or DIC. Oedema may also affect the airway, and pleural and pericardial effusions may occur. Occasionally the clinical presentation may be dramatic – ruptured liver has been reported.

Chronic impairment of uteroplacental blood flow causes fetal growth restriction, and this may be one of the first signs of pre-eclampsia. There is an increased risk of prematurity. Placental abruption may occur in severe disease.

The normal expansion of blood volume that takes place in early pregnancy fails to occur in pre-eclamptic women, and there is therefore a relatively hypovolaemic state. This is exacerbated by leaky capillaries, which allow inappropriate fluid shifts between compartments. Colloid osmotic pressure is low in women with pre-eclampsia, and any increased hydrostatic pressure due to iatrogenic fluid overload, impaired left ventricular function or postpartum fluid shifts may therefore readily precipitate pulmonary oedema.

Results of the numerous studies (both invasive and non-invasive) of the haemodynamic changes occurring in pre-eclampsia are confusing. There is generalised vasoconstriction and therefore systemic vascular resistance is usually increased. Cardiac index and cardiac output may be high, low or normal but this is frequently a reflection of drug therapy. In severe pre-eclampsia, especially if there is pulmonary oedema, right atrial pressure may not accurately reflect pulmonary artery pressure, and central venous pressure monitoring may therefore be an unreliable guide to treatment.

In the UK, approximately 1–2% of pre-eclamptic women develop eclampsia (~2–3 per 10,000 births), though the incidence is higher in the developing countries. Forty per cent of eclamptic fits occur after delivery, most commonly within the first 3 days and rarely more than 1 week postpartum. In approximately a third of cases, there are minimal prodromal signs or symptoms, and only ~40% have proteinuria or hypertension in the preceding week. Recurrent seizures are associated with increased maternal morbidity and mortality. Twenty per cent of eclamptic patients experience pre-eclampsia in the next pregnancy, and 2% have eclampsia.

Posterior reversible encephalopathy syndrome (PRES) is a particular complication that is not specific to pregnancy or to pre-eclampsia, but is increasingly described in association with the latter. Clinical features include headache, convulsions, confusion and visual loss. Several mechanisms for PRES have been hypothesised; it is thought to be a manifestation of cerebral oedema caused either by impaired cerebral autoregulation with accelerated hypertension, or by cerebral vasospasm that results in reduced cerebral blood flow and cytotoxicity. Magnetic resonance imaging (MRI) is the gold standard for diagnosis and follow-up and should be obtained ideally 1–2 days after the initial event. T2-weighted imaging typically reveals bilateral hyperintensities, predominantly in the parieto-occipital region. Magnesium sulfate is the first line of treatment and may be used concomitantly with antihypertensive therapy. Recovery usually takes several days, though neurological deficits may persist.

Management options

The management of chronic and gestational hypertension consists of antihypertensive drugs and close monitoring for development of pre-eclampsia or fetal growth restriction.

The reports of the Confidential Enquiries into Maternal Deaths (CEMD) strongly recommend that every obstetric unit should have written guidelines for the management of pre-eclampsia and eclampsia. There have also been recommendations that every obstetric unit should have an 'eclampsia pack' containing everything necessary to treat eclamptic women with magnesium.

Women who do not present with severe features or major fetal compromise are usually offered a trial of vaginal delivery, while those with severe pre-eclampsia (especially < 37 weeks' gestation) are likely to be delivered by caesarean section (although some evidence exists to support expectant care). The anaesthetist should assess the mother, paying particular attention to any symptoms of pre-eclampsia, drug treatment, the airway, the level of hypertension, the results of haematological and biochemical investigations, and the proposed mode of delivery.

Hypertension

Treatment of hypertension does not modify the course of the underlying disease process but may reduce the morbidity and mortality attributable to uncontrolled hypertension. Whether treatment of mild hypertension during pregnancy is worthwhile is unclear, but because of the risk of haemorrhagic stroke most guidelines suggest treating a systolic blood pressure of 160 mmHg or more. The first-line treatment of hypertension includes methyldopa, which has a long safety record for the fetus, labetalol, nifedipine and other β-adrenoreceptor blockers such as metoprolol and propranolol. Patients already receiving angiotensin-converting enzyme inhibitors or anti-angiotensin receptor agents should have them withdrawn because of their fetotoxic effects.

Hydralazine is the most commonly used agent for management of acute hypertension. Administration of small repeated intravenous boluses (e.g. 5 mg) is preferable to continuous infusion. Hydralazine acts primarily as a vasodilator and should therefore be used with caution and preferably in conjunction with gentle volume replacement, since acute vasodilatation may cause an uncontrolled fall in blood pressure and thus provoke fetal distress. (Reduction in maternal blood pressure is associated with a significantly greater percentage reduction in uteroplacental perfusion.)

Labetalol (10 mg boluses) may be used parenterally in the acute situation, and oral nifedipine (5–10 mg) has also been used, acting within 15–30 minutes. Although there have been concerns over sublingual nifedipine and the risk of uncontrolled hypotension, particularly in combination with magnesium sulfate, this is not thought to be a common problem, especially with slow-release preparations.

Nitroprusside and glyceryl trinitrate may be used for acute control of hypertension but are not commonly used in the UK.

Angiotensin-converting enzyme inhibitors are contraindicated in pre-eclampsia, as their use is associated with unacceptably high fetal morbidity and mortality.

Convulsions

Magnesium sulfate has been shown to reduce the incidence of eclampsia in pre-eclampsia by approximately half, although whether it should be offered routinely to women with pre-eclampsia is controversial, since only 1–2% of them go on to develop eclampsia in the UK, and a significant proportion of eclamptics cannot be identified beforehand (see Chapter 87, *Magnesium sulfate*).

In women who have had a convulsion, magnesium sulfate reduces the incidence of recurrent convulsions by about half compared with phenytoin and diazepam, and 'magnesium packs' should be available on every labour ward.

The optimum treatment of convulsions themselves is less clear. Both magnesium sulfate and diazepam have been used, though some authorities claim that eclamptic fits are self-limiting and that no treatment other than initiation of the magnesium sulfate regimen is needed.

Analgesia for labour

Regional analgesia is the method of choice, since it prevents hypertensive episodes associated with contraction pain and may be beneficial to the compromised fetus by improving uteroplacental perfusion. Although epidural analgesia may lower blood pressure, it should not be considered a treatment for hypertension. A combination of low-dose local anaesthetic and opioid may be given by continuous epidural infusion or intermittent boluses, and this can be supplemented as necessary should instrumental or operative delivery be required.

The platelet count should be measured before insertion of the epidural (if trends suggest that platelet numbers are decreasing significantly, a platelet count should be repeated immediately before epidural insertion; otherwise, a platelet count within the last ~4 hours is usually considered adequate). Current opinion suggests that a platelet count of at least 75 × 10^9/l is advisable before instituting central neural blockade, although any stated lower safe limit is entirely arbitrary, and the relative risks and benefits of regional analgesia and anaesthesia must be considered for each patient. Several studies have confirmed that if the platelet count is at least $100 × 10^9$/l there is no need to perform further coagulation studies. In some centres, thromboelastography/thromboelastometry or similar techniques are used to assist decision making concerning epidural insertion.

If epidural analgesia is contraindicated, it is important to control the blood pressure by using appropriate agents (hydralazine, nifedipine, labetalol) and to provide alternative analgesia. Patient-controlled intravenous opioids offer the mother the psychological benefit of being in control of her analgesia and are more predictable than intramuscular opioids.

Anaesthesia for caesarean section

Regional anaesthesia

Regional is preferable to general anaesthesia, both for the mother and for the fetus. Although the use of spinal anaesthesia in pre-eclampsia was traditionally avoided because of the fear of causing severe hypotension, there is now evidence that so long as there is no hypovolaemia, cardiovascular stability is maintained better in pre-eclamptic patients than in non-pre-eclamptic ones. Furthermore, there is evidence that uterine artery velocity and neonatal condition are unaffected by spinal anaesthesia if systolic arterial pressure remains at least 80% of baseline.

Combined spinal–epidural anaesthesia confers the benefits of dense anaesthesia (especially of the sacral nerve roots) with the flexibility of epidural anaesthesia and postoperative analgesia.

The untreated pre-eclamptic mother may exhibit greater sensitivity to vasoconstrictors than the normotensive mother. Adrenaline-containing epidural solutions are sometimes avoided in severe cases, although their use appears to be safe.

General anaesthesia

General anaesthesia may be necessary if there is great urgency to deliver the mother or if regional anaesthesia is contraindicated by coagulopathy or major haemorrhage. Extreme prematurity does not contraindicate regional anaesthesia, and nor does eclampsia.

The additional risks of general anaesthesia for caesarean section (see Chapter 36) are compounded in the pre-eclamptic woman by the potential for a significantly compromised airway and the hypertensive response to intubation and extubation. There may also be potential drug interactions, especially between magnesium sulfate and neuromuscular blocking agents.

Laryngeal oedema is uncommon but may be sufficient to obscure all normal anatomy at laryngoscopy. Each obstetric theatre should include small-sized tracheal tubes on the intubation trolley for this eventuality.

Uncontrolled hypertension in response to tracheal intubation may provoke cardiac arrhythmias, myocardial ischaemia or cerebrovascular catastrophe. Numerous agents have been used to attenuate this response, but the most commonly used agents in the UK are fentanyl 1–4 μg/kg or alfentanil 7–10 μg/kg and labetalol 10–20 mg. Other opioids, β-blockers and lidocaine may be used; magnesium sulfate 30 mg/kg also appears to be effective.

Monitoring and fluid therapy

All women with moderate or severe pre-eclampsia should have continuous electronic fetal monitoring. Direct arterial pressure monitoring is more accurate than non-invasive methods, because of the inaccuracy of most non-invasive monitors. The relative benefits of intra-arterial monitoring must be balanced against the familiarity of midwifery staff with its use. Central venous pressure catheters may provide guidance for fluid administration during regional anaesthesia, although their use is uncommon in the UK. Access via the antecubital fossa rather than via neck veins is sometimes recommended, especially in the undelivered mother. Pulmonary artery catheterisation is rarely used. Transthoracic echocardiography has an increasing role in the assessment of volume status and ventricular function in patients with severe disease.

All pre-eclamptic women should have a urinary catheter inserted and an accurate hourly fluid balance recorded. Fluid management is controversial. The risks of volume overload and iatrogenic pulmonary oedema must be balanced against the risk of hypotension if vasodilators are given without concomitant volume replacement. In general, the emphasis has shifted away from liberal use of fluids in order to encourage urine output, towards careful restriction, since long-term problems from renal failure are rare, whereas deaths from pulmonary oedema are well reported.

Postoperative management

In both HELLP syndrome and eclampsia, the risks of deterioration in blood pressure control do not end immediately with delivery of the placenta. Women with pre-eclampsia with severe features should be monitored in a high-dependency environment for at least 24–48 hours after delivery. Invasive monitoring and antihypertensive treatment should be continued during this time.

Key points

- Hypertensive disorders of pregnancy are divided into chronic hypertension, gestational hypertension and pre-eclampsia.
- Pre-eclampsia and eclampsia are major causes of maternal death.
- Although the classic presentation of the disease is hypertension and proteinuria occurring after 20 weeks of pregnancy, pre-eclampsia is a multisystem disease and may present atypically.
- HELLP syndrome is part of the spectrum of pre-eclampsia and may not be preceded by significant pre-eclampsia.
- Pre-eclampsia can only be effectively treated by delivery of the placenta, although symptomatic treatment attenuates maternal morbidity.
- Effective control of hypertension in pre-eclampsia reduces cardiovascular and cerebrovascular morbidity and mortality.
- Eclampsia may occur without premonitory symptoms or signs, and 40% of eclamptic fits occur after delivery.

Further reading

Dennis AT, Castro JM. Hypertension and haemodynamics in pregnant women: is a unified theory for pre-eclampsia possible? *Anaesthesia* 2014; **69**: 1183–9.

Hofmeyr R, Matjila M, Dyer R. Preeclampsia in 2017: obstetric and anaesthesia management. *Best Pract Res Clin Anaesthesiol* 2017; **31**: 125–38.

Leffert LR. What's new in obstetric anesthesia? Focus on preeclampsia. *Int J Obstet Anesth* 2015; **24**: 264–71.

Mol BWJ, Roberts CT, Thangaratinam S, *et al*. Pre-eclampsia. *Lancet* 2016; **387**: 999–1011.

National Institute for Health and Care Excellence. *Hypertension in Pregnancy: Diagnosis and Management*. Clinical Guideline 107. London: NICE, 2010. www.nice.org.uk/guidance/CG107 (accessed December 2018).

Stocks G. Preeclampsia: pathophysiology, old and new strategies for management. *Eur J Anaesthesiol* 2014; **31**: 183–9.

Chapter 87

Magnesium sulfate

Magnesium was first reported to be effective in preventing further convulsions in eclamptic women in 1925. The Collaborative Eclampsia Trial, reporting in 1995, confirmed that magnesium sulfate is significantly more effective than either diazepam or phenytoin in preventing recurrence of convulsions in eclamptic women.

The MAGPIE Trial, reporting in 2002, showed that magnesium sulfate was also effective in reducing (by about half) the incidence of eclampsia when given to pre-eclamptic women. However, since the incidence of eclampsia in the UK is low (~1–2% of pre-eclamptic cases), the number needed to treat (NNT) in order to prevent a single woman having a convulsion is ~110 in the UK. This has led to controversy about whether magnesium should be routinely given to all pre-eclamptics, especially since there was no overall effect on maternal and neonatal morbidity and mortality in the trial. In populations in which the incidence is higher, as in some African countries, or in those with severe pre-eclampsia, the NNT is lower, so administration to such cases is less controversial. However, it is impossible to predict which women will go on to develop eclampsia; as a result magnesium is now used frequently in cases of severe pre-eclampsia across the world, including in the UK, as a result of these two trials. These two studies have changed clinical practice around the world but especially in the UK, where magnesium used to be infrequently used for pre-eclampsia/eclampsia.

Magnesium sulfate is widely used in the USA as a tocolytic agent in preterm labour, but randomised trials have failed to confirm its efficacy for this purpose. Its beneficial effect as a neuroprotective agent in the premature fetus has, however, been established, and it has been shown to reduce the incidence of cerebral palsy in preterm neonates, although there is no evidence of a significant reduction in fetal mortality with its use.

Site of action

Magnesium is essential for potassium and calcium metabolism. It acts as a calcium antagonist, probably reducing systemic and cerebral vasospasm via action at calcium channels and intracellular sites. It is a cofactor in the sodium–potassium–ATPase system and is also an N-methyl-D-aspartate (NMDA) receptor antagonist; it is thought that its anticonvulsant action is mediated through these systems. Production of endothelial prostacyclin is increased by magnesium, and this may help to restore the thromboxane–prostacyclin imbalance that occurs in pre-eclampsia. Magnesium is also thought to reduce levels of circulating angiotensin-converting enzyme (ACE), which may contribute to its antihypertensive action.

Magnesium sulfate relieves the cerebral vasospasm associated with pre-eclampsia and eclampsia; transcranial Doppler studies have demonstrated an increase in cerebral blood flow.

Side effects

Magnesium sulfate has widespread effects, not all of which are beneficial. Its use has been associated with increased obstetric haemorrhage (presumably due to generalised vasodilatation and uterine atony), increased length of labour and increased rate of caesarean section. Prophylactic use of magnesium sulfate before induction of general anaesthesia for caesarean section (e.g. in severe pre-eclampsia) can prolong the effects of neuromuscular blocking agents; use of a peripheral nerve stimulator is mandatory.

Toxicity is possible during infusion, although this is unlikely at the usual dosage unless there is concomitant renal impairment. Symptoms and signs of toxicity occur as blood levels increase (Table 87.1). Magnesium toxicity is reversed by intravenous calcium gluconate (10 ml of 10% solution, given by slow intravenous injection), and calcium should always be available when magnesium therapy is given.

Dose

The Collaborative Eclampsia and MAGPIE trials used an intravenous loading dose of 4–5 g magnesium sulfate (given over 5–15 minutes) followed by either 5 g intramuscularly into each buttock and a further 5 g intramuscularly every 4 hours for 24 hours, or an intravenous infusion of 1–2 g/h after the intravenous loading dose.

There is controversy about whether an intravenous maintenance infusion of 1 g/h produces adequate plasma levels, with some studies suggesting that 3 g/h is required to guarantee therapeutic levels (4–8 mg/dl). The Collaborative Eclampsia group has stated that use of higher doses would increase the risk of toxicity without conferring proven benefit, and in the MAGPIE Trial side effects occurred in a quarter of cases.

Monitoring

If the regimen used in the two above trials is used, clinical monitoring is considered to be adequate. Assessment of respiratory rate and patellar tendon reflexes every 15 minutes, and monitoring of hourly urine output, should be performed. Monitoring of plasma levels is

Table 87.1 Signs and symptoms of magnesium toxicity at various blood levels

Symptoms	Magnesium level	
	mg/dl	mmol/l
Normal adult levels	1.7–2.4	0.7–1.1
Therapeutic range	4–8	2–4
Loss of patellar reflexes, warmth, flushing, somnolence	9.5–12	4.2–5
Respiratory depression	12–16	5–6.5
Muscle paralysis	15–17	6.2–7
Cardiac conduction defects	> 18	> 7.5
Cardiac arrest	30–35	12.5–14.5

advisable if larger doses of magnesium sulfate are used, if there is impaired renal function, if symptoms/signs of toxicity occur or a convulsion occurs despite therapy.

Key points

- Magnesium sulfate is the only drug proven to be effective in preventing recurrence of convulsions in eclampsia.
- In pre-eclampsia, magnesium sulfate reduces the incidence of eclamptic convulsions, but its use for this purpose is controversial because there is no reliable method of predicting eclampsia.
- Both intramuscular and intravenous regimens are effective, and clinical monitoring is adequate.
- Calcium gluconate should be available at the bedside of every woman receiving magnesium sulfate.

Further reading

Dean C, Douglas J. Magnesium and the obstetric anaesthetist. *Int J Obstet Anesth* 2013; **22**: 52–63.
Duley L, Gülmezoglu AM, Henderson-Smart DJ, Chou D. Magnesium sulphate and other anticonvulsants for women with pre-eclampsia. *Cochrane Database Syst Rev* 2010; (11): CD000025.
Duley L, Henderson-Smart DJ, Chou D. Magnesium sulphate versus phenytoin for eclampsia. *Cochrane Database Syst Rev* 2010; (10): CD000128.
Duley L, Henderson-Smart DJ, Walker GJ, Chou D. Magnesium sulphate versus diazepam for eclampsia. *Cochrane Database Syst Rev* 2010; (12): CD000127.
Duley L, Matar HE, Almerie MQ, Hall DR. Alternative magnesium sulphate regimens for women with pre-eclampsia and eclampsia. *Cochrane Database Syst Rev* 2010; (8): CD007388.

Chapter

88

Hyperemesis gravidarum

Nausea and vomiting during early pregnancy occurs in about 70–90% of women, although in most cases it is not severe and has diminished by the mid-second trimester. Rarely, severe vomiting continues throughout pregnancy, and it may require hospitalisation in about 3–10 per 1000 women. It is referred to as hyperemesis gravidarum when there has been 5% of pre-pregnancy weight loss, dehydration and electrolyte imbalance, and other causes of vomiting have been excluded. It is more common in first pregnancies and with younger maternal age, obesity, multiple pregnancy, previous history of hyperemesis, metabolic disorders and eating disorders. The aetiology is unknown but hormonal (particularly oestrogen and human chorionic gonadotrophin), metabolic and psychological factors have been implicated.

Anaesthetists may be asked to advise on antiemetic therapy or to assist in establishing peripheral or central venous access for fluid replacement and/or nutrition. They may also be involved in providing analgesia or anaesthesia for delivery or, rarely, for termination of pregnancy if hyperemesis is very severe.

Problems and special considerations

Clinical symptoms are non-specific, and it is important to consider other causes of nausea and vomiting (Table 88.1). There may be evidence of malnutrition and/or dehydration, with associated biochemical and metabolic derangement including ketonuria, renal and particularly hepatic impairment and mineral/vitamin deficiency, for example Wernicke's encephalopathy. The muscle bulk is virtually always reduced in severe cases, and there may be fetal growth restriction. Because of the importance of psychological factors, these patients may need psychological or psychiatric support, which may be difficult in the maternity suite; in early pregnancy they are often managed on general gynaecological wards.

Management options

Initially, non-pharmacological methods of management are usually proffered, such as frequent small snacks (e.g. dry crackers), ginger root tea, hypnosis and use of acupressure bands or acupuncture to stimulate an area on the ventral surface of the wrist between the long flexor tendons. Electrolyte replacement drinks and oral nutritional supplements, if tolerated, are advocated. The evidence for the more esoteric treatments is somewhat mixed, although is probably strongest for acupressure or acupuncture for its general (as opposed to obstetric) antiemetic effect. Psychological support is generally advocated.

Standard antiemetics such as prochlorperazine and cyclizine are usually tried first; promazine has traditionally been used. Second-line drugs include metoclopramide (because

Table 88.1 Causes of vomiting in pregnancy

Infective	Gastroenteritis
	Urinary tract infection
	Hepatitis
Surgical	Intra-abdominal pathology
	Primary gastrointestinal
	Severe reflux oesophagitis
Neurological	Increased intracranial pressure
	Migraine
Metabolic	Diabetes
	Hypercalcaemia
	Uraemia
	Acute fatty liver of pregnancy
Drug-related	Antibiotics
	Analgesics
	Alcohol
Psychogenic	

of the increased incidence of extrapyramidal side effects in young women), domperidone and ondansetron. It should be remembered that the effects of these drugs on the fetus are unclear and that few are licensed for use in pregnancy.

There is some evidence to support the use of steroids as treatment (e.g. intravenous hydrocortisone 100 mg, twice daily, then prednisolone 45–50 mg/day, reduced to the lowest possible dose). The use of diazepam has been studied in randomised trials, and its success is thought to be a result of its sedative properties. However, sedative drugs are not recommended because of their addictive properties and because of possible adverse effects on the fetus.

In cases where dehydration is apparent, hospitalisation and intravenous rehydration (and occasionally resuscitation) is required; use of glucose-containing solutions (after administration of thiamine) may provide a small amount of calorific intake, but excessive administration may result in hyponatraemia, so crystalloids containing sodium and potassium are recommended. Vitamin and mineral supplementation is advisable, and enteral nasogastric nutrition has been used. In very severe cases, parenteral nutrition may be required; use of parenteral nutrition has even been advocated as a treatment in its own right, and there are several reports of its apparent success, occasionally on repeated occasions throughout the same pregnancy. Oesophagitis may be severe and is treated by using standard methods. Thromboprophylaxis may be indicated for hospital admission with reduced mobility.

Key points

- Nausea and vomiting occurs in about 75% of pregnancies.
- Hospitalisation is required in about 3–10 per 1000 women.
- Urea and electrolyte disturbances and hepatic impairment may occur.

- There are few randomised controlled trials of therapy but many different non-pharmacological and pharmacological therapies have been used.

Further reading

Boelig RC, Barton SJ, Saccone G, *et al.* Interventions for treating hyperemesis gravidarum. *Cochrane Database of Syst Rev* 2016; (5): CD010607.

Royal College of Obstetricians and Gynaecologists. *The Management of Nausea and Vomiting of Pregnancy and Hyperemesis Gravidarum.* Green-top Guideline 69. London: RCOG, 2016. www.rcog.org.uk/en/guidelines-research-services/guidelines/gtg69 (accessed December 2018).

Chapter 89

Maternal mortality

There has been continuous audit of maternal deaths in England and Wales since 1952 (and the whole of the UK since 1984), the results of which have been published regularly as reports of the Confidential Enquiries into Maternal Deaths (CEMD). Other countries have established reviews of maternal deaths but none is as well established or complete as the CEMD.

The organisation of the Enquiry has changed in recent years, being administered previously by various bodies including the Confidential Enquiry into Maternal and Child Health (CEMACH) until 2009 and then the Centre for Maternal and Child Enquiries (CMACE). In 2012 a new consortium, MBRRACE-UK (Mothers and Babies – Reducing Risk through Audits and Confidential Enquiries across the UK), was appointed by the Healthcare Quality Improvement Partnership (HQIP) to run the maternal and perinatal death enquiries. The CEMD reports now consist of an annual report into deaths, with a rolling three-year analysis, and chapters focusing on selected topics that rotate over a three-year cycle (e.g. sepsis, psychiatric causes, cardiac disease, anaesthesia); previously a single comprehensive report was produced annually. The 2014 report examined anaesthetic mortality in detail, and this was further reviewed in the 2017 report, which covered the years 2013–15 (see below).

The 2018 CEMD report (covering the years 2014–16) found the following:

- The UK maternal mortality rate (equals number of indirect + direct deaths per 100,000 maternities; see below) was 9.8, which was similar to 2011–13 data, but a 37% decrease since 2003–05.
- The maternal mortality ratio (MMR, the international definition: equals number of indirect + direct deaths (from birth certificates only) per 100,000 live births) was 4.65 (2012–14 data), down from 5.57 (comparable with other northern European countries; in the USA, MMR was 14 in 2015; in sub-Saharan Africa it is around 1000).
- Cardiac disease was the overall leading cause of maternal death, followed by thromboembolism, neurological disease, psychiatric disease and sepsis (Figure 89.1).

Definitions and data collection

A maternal death is any death occurring during or within 42 days of the pregnancy ending. The enquiry into any maternal death is initiated by local reporters in each unit and organised by regional offices. Each death is assessed by obstetric anaesthetic, midwifery and pathology assessors as appropriate.

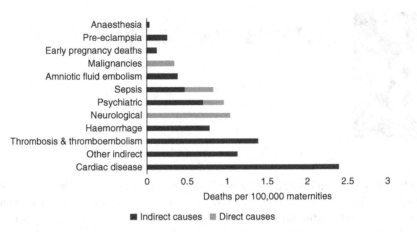

Figure 89.1 Major causes of death in the 2018 CEMD report (data from 2014–16). Original source: Knight M, Bunch K, Tuffnell D, *et al.*; MBRRACE-UK. *Saving Lives, Improving Mothers' Care: Lessons learned to inform maternity care from the UK and Ireland Confidential Enquiries into Maternal Deaths and Morbidity 2014–16.* Oxford: National Perinatal Epidemiology Unit, University of Oxford, 2018

Maternal deaths are classified as:

- Direct (resulting from obstetric complications of pregnancy) – 98 cases in 2014–16.
- Indirect (deaths resulting from previous existing disease or disease that developed during pregnancy and that was not due to direct obstetric causes but was aggravated by the physiological effects of pregnancy) – 127 cases in 2014–16.
- Late (occurring after 42 days and within one year of the pregnancy ending) – 286 cases in 2014–16.
- Coincidental (from unrelated causes, such as road traffic accident) – 34 cases in 2014–16.

Since 1994–96 the number of indirect deaths has outnumbered that of direct deaths. Deaths were previously categorised also according to whether they were associated with substandard care, a term used not only to denote failure of clinical care, but also to indicate failure of the woman to take responsibility for her own health (such as refusal of blood transfusion or refusal to be admitted) and inadequate resources for staffing, intensive care and back-up services. More recent reports have moved away from such pejorative terms and focus instead on areas where care could be improved and lessons learned. The reports continue to make recommendations for improved care, and these tend to include similar themes over the years – for example:

- The importance of early recognition of critically unwell parturients
- The importance of early involvement of senior clinicians and referral to other relevant specialists
- The need for local provision of intensive care (not necessarily on the intensive care unit)
- The need for protocols for common, potentially serious conditions, e.g. pre-eclampsia, major haemorrhage
- The need for regular drills and training in life-threatening emergencies and human factors
- The need for better record keeping and communication generally

Anaesthetic deaths

Although anaesthesia is no longer one of the three leading causes of maternal death, as it was in the 1980s, there are still lessons to be learned from the deaths associated with anaesthesia and the cases in which anaesthesia was felt to have contributed to the death. In the 2017 report (2013–15 data), there were two direct anaesthetic deaths as a result of anaphylaxis and pulmonary aspiration (Table 89.1). Recurrent anaesthetic themes in the reports highlighted as learning points include adequate resuscitation before extubation, management of hypotension secondary to aortocaval compression or regional anaesthesia, and appropriate care planning for women with complex needs. Other issues include follow-up of postdural puncture headache and effective communication between team members. Difficulties in airway management including tracheal intubation are regularly highlighted, even though the number of failed intubations is now low.

Table 89.1 Anaesthetic deaths since 1985 in the CEMD reports

Triennium	Direct anaesthetic deaths	Proportion of direct deaths	Rate per 100,000 maternities
1985–87	6	4.3%	0.26
1988–90	4	2.8%	0.17
1991–93	8	6.3%	0.35
1994–96	1	0.7%	0.05
1997–99	3	2.8%	0.14
2000–02	6	5.7%	0.30
2003–05	6	4.5%	0.28
2006–08	7	6.5%	0.31
2009–11	3	3.6%	0.12
2012–14	2	3.0%	0.09
2013–15	2	2.3%	0.08
2014–16	1	1.0%	0.04

Key points

- Obstetric anaesthesia is high-risk anaesthesia.
- The severity of coexisting medical disease is easily underestimated.
- Adequate monitoring equipment and trained anaesthetic assistance are required for obstetric anaesthesia.
- Intensive care facilities may be required.
- The anaesthetic record is a legal document and is essential for adequate evaluation of morbidity and mortality.

Further reading

Knight M, Bunch K, Tuffnell D, *et al.*; MBRRACE-UK. *Saving Lives, Improving Mothers' Care: Lessons learned to inform maternity care from the UK and Ireland Confidential Enquiries into Maternal Deaths and Morbidity 2014–16.* Oxford: National Perinatal Epidemiology Unit, University of Oxford, 2018.

Knight M, Nair M, Tuffnell D, *et al.*; MBRRACE-UK. *Saving Lives, Improving Mothers' Care: Lessons learned to inform maternity care from the UK and Ireland Confidential Enquiries into Maternal Deaths and Morbidity 2013–15.* Oxford: National Perinatal Epidemiology Unit, University of Oxford, 2017.

Lucas DN, Bamber JH. UK Confidential Enquiry into Maternal Deaths: still learning to save mothers' lives. *Anaesthesia* 2018; **73**: 416–20.

Yentis SM. From CEMD to CEMACH to CMACE to … ? Where now for the confidential enquiries into maternal deaths? *Anaesthesia* 2011; **66**: 859–60.

Chapter

Allergic reactions

Patients may be mildly allergic to many substances, and this may become better or worse during pregnancy. Severe reactions, however, are rare on the labour ward, with anaphylaxis thought to complicate up to 3.4 in 100,000 deliveries. Although these reactions are divided into anaphylactic (release of histamine and other inflammatory mediators from mast cells via cross-linkage of IgE molecules on the cell surface by the antigen, after prior exposure), anaphylactoid (direct release of mediators from mast cells via interaction of molecules – e.g. drugs – with the cell surface) and others (e.g. direct complement activation), the distinction is largely academic since the clinical presentation is identical.

Most severe reactions on the labour ward are caused by drugs, especially antibiotics, intravenous anaesthetic drugs (particularly suxamethonium) and oxytocin; in the recent 6th National Audit Project (NAP6), all cases of severe obstetric anaphylaxis occurred in the operating theatre.

Traditionally, up to 10% of individuals with true penicillin allergy have been thought to be allergic to cephalosporins; more recent estimations put this figure at 1% for cross-reactivity with first-generation cephalosporins, and a negligible risk with third- and fourth-generation cephalosporins. Allergy to amide local anaesthetic drugs is rare but has been reported, as has allergy to preservatives used in local anaesthetic and other drug preparations. Symptoms related to local anaesthetic injection are more often due to a vasovagal episode, accidental intravascular injection or toxicity.

Non-steroidal anti-inflammatory drugs and paracetamol often cause rashes, but these are usually mild following brief oral or rectal courses, although severe reactions have been reported following intravenous administration. Reactions may also follow administration of gelatine intravenous fluids and blood. Latex allergy is more common in subjects with multiple exposures to latex such as medical or nursing staff, cleaners, those with neurological disease requiring repeated bladder catheterisation (e.g. spina bifida), and those with allergy to certain foodstuffs including avocados, bananas, kiwi fruit and chestnuts. Finally, other conditions not primarily allergic may also present in a similar way, for example amniotic fluid embolism.

Patients may have a history of previous allergic reactions to drugs or other substances, although many patients who give only a vague history are not truly allergic.

Problems and special considerations

Features range from mild skin rashes to severe urticaria, hypotension, bronchospasm, mouth/laryngeal swelling, abdominal pain, diarrhoea, a 'feeling of impending doom' and cardiovascular collapse. Initial hypotension is largely related to profound vasodilatation,

271

which is followed by leakage of intravascular fluid into the interstitium. Cardiac depression (thought to be caused by circulating inflammatory mediators) may also contribute to hypotension. The cardiovascular effects are exacerbated by aortocaval compression. Maternal anaphylaxis can lead to compromised uterine blood flow and maternal hypoxia, and subsequent fetal compromise.

Features usually occur within a few seconds or minutes of exposure to the allergen. During caesarean section in latex-allergic subjects, anaphylaxis typically occurs 10–15 minutes after induction of anaesthesia and once surgery has started, since the most provocative stimulus is exposure via mucous membranes.

In NAP6, diagnosis and specific treatment of anaphylaxis were more likely to be delayed in obstetric than in non-obstetric cases. Since clinical features may develop at a time of great physiological change, e.g. during caesarean section or during/after delivery, it may be difficult to assess the situation and determine what has happened. Differential diagnoses include pulmonary embolism, amniotic fluid embolus, cardiac disease, complications of anaesthesia (including high neuraxial block and local anaesthetic toxicity), sepsis and haemorrhage. Administration of many different drugs together or within a short time is common, and this may further hinder the diagnosis (and is suspected of increasing the risk of a reaction).

Management options

Immediate management of severe reactions consists of intravenous adrenaline 50 μg boluses (or 0.5 mg intramuscularly if not experienced at giving intravenous vasopressors) with prompt assessment and management of the airway and administration of 100% oxygen. Intravenous fluid resuscitation is required to correct the deficit caused by decreased systemic vascular resistance and extravasation secondary to increased vessel permeability; the patient should always be monitored for signs of volume overload that may be precipitated by the physiological changes that ensue after delivery. An adrenaline infusion may be required if several boluses are required. Aortocaval compression must be avoided at all times, and fetal monitoring should be instituted. Adrenaline may cause uteroplacental vasoconstriction and uterine hypotony, which may contribute to fetal hypoxia and postpartum haemorrhage respectively; however it remains first-line treatment and should not be withheld when indicated. Intravenous chlorpheniramine 10 mg and hydrocortisone 200 mg may be given to reduce the effects of subsequent inflammatory mediator release. Urgent caesarean delivery may be considered in cases of fetal compromise or to reduce maternal hypotension secondary to aortocaval compression, but this may be challenging in the presence of maternal hypoxia and cardiovascular instability. For less severe reactions (e.g. urticaria only), chlorpheniramine alone may suffice.

In an acute reaction, blood should be taken for tryptase levels as soon as possible and at 1–2 and 24 hours. The enzyme is normally present in mast cells and in minuscule amounts in the plasma; an increase in plasma concentration therefore represents mast cell degranulation (but does not distinguish between anaphylactic and anaphylactoid reactions). Immunoglobulin and complement levels may be suggestive, but not diagnostic, of an allergic response. If a severe reaction is suspected, the anaesthetist involved should refer the patient for testing; a suggested referral form and a list of allergy centres can be found on the Association of Anaesthetists of Great Britain and Ireland (AAGBI) website. Normally investigation will involve skin tests (prick testing ± intradermal testing). Further tests may be performed on plasma (e.g. radioallergoabsorbent test (RAST) looking for concentrations of a specific antibody, e.g. to latex) or occasionally basophils or other cellular components, if skin testing is not diagnostic. The patient should be advised to obtain a 'MedicAlert' bracelet and given written details of all the drugs tested and the results, in case she should require a subsequent anaesthetic. A copy of the letter should also be sent to her general practitioner.

It is important that mothers with a previous history of severe allergic reactions are identified antenatally and on arrival to the labour ward. Wherever possible, the previous anaesthetic record should be obtained and a plan for the woman's care documented. Management of the known allergic case includes a general state of readiness (emergency preparedness) and awareness as well as the obvious avoidance of any known allergens. Latex-allergic patients may be identified from the history in most cases by asking about food allergies and skin reactions after exposure to rubber gloves, condoms, etc. If patients have had a previous severe reaction where the allergen is unknown, pre-treatment with H_1- and H_2-antagonists ± steroids should be considered, although whether this should be routinely done if the allergen is known and can be avoided is controversial. Routine screening of all women by using skin or blood testing is generally not indicated, since precautions should be taken on the basis of a strong history even if testing produces negative results.

Key points

- In severe allergic reactions, immediate management is with oxygen, adrenaline and intravenous fluids.
- Hydrocortisone and chlorpheniramine are second-line drugs.
- Blood should be taken for mast cell tryptase levels as early as possible and at 1–2 and 24 hours.
- Subsequent testing should include skin testing.

Further reading

Adriaensens I, Vercauteren M, Soetens F, et al. Allergic reactions during labour analgesia and caesarean section anaesthesia. *Int J Obstet Anesth* 2013; **22**: 231–42.

Association of Anaesthetists of Great Britain and Ireland. Management of a patient with suspected anaphylaxis during anaesthesia. London: AAGBI, 2009. www.aagbi.org/sites/default/files/ana_we b_laminate_final.pdf (accessed December 2018).

Cook TM, Harper N. *Anaesthesia, Surgery and Life-Threatening Allergic Reactions. Report and Findings of the Royal College of Anaesthetists' 6th National Audit Project: Perioperative Anaphylaxis.* London: RCoA, 2018. www.nationalauditprojects.org.uk/NAP6Report (accessed December 2018).

Hepner DL, Castells M, Mouton-Faivre C, Dewachter P. Anaphylaxis in the clinical setting of obstetric anesthesia: a literature review. *Anesth Analg* 2013; **117**: 1357–67.

Soar J, Perkins GD, Abbas G, et al. European Resuscitation Council Guidelines for Resuscitation 2010, Section 8. Cardiac arrest in special circumstances: electrolyte abnormalities, poisoning, drowning, accidental hypothermia, hyperthermia, asthma, anaphylaxis, cardiac surgery, trauma, pregnancy, electrocution. *Resuscitation* 2010; **81**: 1400–33.

Cardiovascular disease

In the 2018 Confidential Enquiries into Maternal Deaths (CEMD), cardiac disease remained the leading overall cause of maternal death in the UK between 2014 and 2016, accounting for nearly a quarter of maternal deaths. Over three-quarters of these women were not known to have pre-existing cardiac disease, so the possibility of undiagnosed cardiac disease must be remembered. The spectrum of pre-existing cardiac disease affecting pregnant women has changed in the UK as rheumatic heart disease has become less common (though it is still a major problem in other parts of the world) and congenital heart disease more common, partly related to the improved survival of girls with congenital heart disease who undergo surgery during infancy and childhood.

The most common acquired cardiac disease in the UK is ischaemic heart disease. Possible epidemiological factors include an increased prevalence of risk factors such as smoking among younger women, increased age and obesity.

Problems and special considerations

Although different sorts of cardiac disease require different management, there are general principles that are applicable to this heterogeneous group. Many of these have been high-lighted in recent CEMD reports, which have found the following:

- There is a general failure fully to understand the impact of the normal physiological changes of pregnancy on pre-existing cardiovascular pathology (see Chapter 11, *Physiology of pregnancy*).
- Symptoms such as a raised respiratory rate, chest pain, persistent tachycardia or breathlessness, or orthopnoea may indicate exacerbation of known or undiagnosed cardiac disease.
- Management of women with cardiac disease is often undertaken by inappropriately experienced medical staff. Consultants from all relevant specialties should be involved in management from early pregnancy onward, with review in a joint obstetric cardiac clinic. If necessary, patients should be referred onwards to specialist cardiological units.
- There may be failure to carry out essential investigations such as chest radiography, where the radiation risks to the fetus are minimal but the information gained from the investigation may be life-saving. Equally, necessary medications such as angiotensin-converting enzyme inhibitors should not be withheld because of breastfeeding.
- There may be failure to communicate with other specialties involved in a woman's care and failure to organise clear written plans for management of labour and delivery. Anaesthetic review should occur in the second or third trimester (bearing in mind that

many cardiac patients will have a preterm delivery), and critical care staff consulted and/ or involved early as appropriate.

* The severity of the mother's condition may be underestimated, either because of the above or because symptoms are mild or absent, or because they are mistaken for those of pregnancy.

Management options

The pregnant woman with cardiac disease, whether congenital or acquired, should be seen as early as possible in her pregnancy. Ideally, she should be seen for pre-conception counselling when her risks (Table 91.1) and those of her baby can be fully discussed.

A full history and examination should be performed during the first trimester of pregnancy, and baseline cardiological investigations should be arranged. These may include electrocardiography, chest x-ray, echocardiography and possibly cardiac catheterisation. Severity of cardiac disease is frequently assessed by using the New York Heart Association (NYHA) classification, which although originally described for heart failure is a useful overall measure of severity (Table 91.2)

Women with cardiovascular disease graded NYHA I and II usually tolerate the physiological changes of pregnancy well, though it should be remembered that certain conditions (e.g. mitral and aortic stenosis, pulmonary hypertension and complex lesions) may be dangerous even in the absence of symptoms.

Studies suggest that cardiac complications (pulmonary oedema, arrhythmia, stroke or cardiac death) are more likely in women who have the following predictors: a history of previous cardiac events or arrhythmia; NYHA class IV or cyanosis; left heart obstruction; or left ventricular systolic dysfunction – with complications occurring in around a quarter of women with one predictor and three-quarters of women with more than one predictor.

Table 91.1 Risk of death or severe morbidity resulting from certain cardiac lesions in pregnancy

Low risk (mortality 0.1–1%)	Most repaired lesions
	Uncomplicated left-to-right shunts
	Mitral valve prolapse; bicuspid aortic valve; aortic regurgitation; mitral regurgitation; pulmonary stenosis; pulmonary regurgitation
Intermediate risk (mortality 1–5%)	Metal valves
	Single ventricle
	Systemic right ventricle; switch procedure
	Unrepaired cyanotic lesions
	Mitral stenosis; aortic stenosis; severe pulmonary stenosis
High risk (mortality 5–30%)	NYHA III or IV
	Severe systemic ventricular dysfunction
	Severe aortic stenosis
	Marfan's syndrome with aortic valve lesion or aortic dilatation
	Pulmonary hypertension (mortality 30–50%)

Table 91.2 New York Heart Association (NYHA) classification of cardiovascular disease, adapted version

NYHA I	No limitation of physical activity and no objective evidence of cardiovascular disease
NYHA II	Slight limitation of normal physical activity and objective evidence of minimal disease
NYHA III	Marked limitation of physical activity and objective evidence of moderately severe disease
NYHA IV	Severe limitation of activity including symptoms at rest and objective evidence of severe disease

Further risk stratification tools may be used, such as the CARPREG risk score which looks at pre-pregnancy symptoms and signs, or the modified WHO classification of maternal cardiovascular risk which looks at cardiac lesions and their surgical repair. Such stratification may help plan antenatal follow-up and labour care.

Consideration should be given to the appropriate place for both subsequent antenatal management and delivery. Referral to a local teaching hospital with facilities for cardiac surgery may be indicated, and in some cases it may be in the woman's best interests to be referred to a supra-regional unit.

Routine antenatal care is not adequate for women with cardiac disease. Antenatal appointments need to be more frequent; there must be clear communication with the general practitioner and the community midwife and also with the woman herself, who should receive instructions about symptoms that demand immediate medical attention. Serial investigations and careful documentation of symptoms should alert medical staff to any deterioration in cardiac health, and it may be useful to admit women with cardiac disease for 24–48 hours towards the end of the second trimester of pregnancy in order to repeat investigations and arrange multidisciplinary review. These women require careful monitoring for development of pre-eclampsia, since it may be poorly tolerated in the presence of cardiac disease.

Elective admission to hospital in the third or even second trimester may be useful to ensure the mother can rest, with due attention to antithrombotic prophylaxis and regular assessments. Continuous oxygen therapy may also be given if required.

As a general rule, operative delivery should only be carried out if indicated for obstetric reasons or deteriorating maternal condition, and not just because the mother has cardiac disease; caesarean delivery has not been shown to confer benefit to women with cardiac disease if they are stable. Regional analgesia and anaesthesia can be safely provided for the majority of women with cardiac disease, even in those with fixed cardiac output (though this is more controversial), although this may be precluded by anticoagulation in certain cases. Epidural anaesthesia may be advisable to reduce the pain-related cardiovascular stresses of labour, or to facilitate delivery with minimal active pushing with the associated Valsalva manoeuvre, which may be detrimental to cardiac output. Analgesia and anaesthesia should only be carried out in units familiar with the management of such high-risk patients.

Cardiac monitoring for arrhythmias/ischaemia and invasive blood pressure monitoring may be useful during labour and delivery, so long as there are appropriate personnel to manage and interpret these monitors. The risk of endocarditis should be remembered;

although recent UK guidance suggests that prophylactic antibiotics may not be indicated, many clinicians with experience of managing such patients still elect to give them, because the consequences of endocarditis can be so devastating. Cardiovascular side effects of oxytocics should be considered and weighed against the risk of postpartum haemorrhage and decreased venous return. Depending on cardiac pathology, reduced bolus doses or infusions alone may be given. Non-pharmacological methods of haemostasis should be considered early if the consequences of haemorrhage are a particular risk.

The puerperium is a time of high risk for many women with cardiac disease, and vigilance should be maintained. The mother with cardiac disease should be nursed on the delivery suite or high-dependency unit until all medical staff involved in her care agree that she can be safely returned to the general postnatal ward. Haemodynamic parameters have usually returned to normal within 3–5 days but may take longer in severe cases, and rarely may never return to pre-pregnancy values.

Key points

- Women with cardiovascular disease should be identified and assessed early in pregnancy, and referred to specialist units when necessary. Coordinated multi-professional care should occur during and after the pregnancy.
- Good communication between specialties is mandatory.
- Clear management plans should be written.
- Vigilance should be maintained into the puerperium.

Further reading

Curry R, Swan L, Steer PJ. Cardiac disease in pregnancy. *Curr Opin Obstet Gynecol* 2009; **21**: 508–13.

European Society of Cardiology. ESC guidelines on the management of cardiovascular diseases during pregnancy: the Task Force on the Management of Cardiovascular Diseases during Pregnancy of the European Society of Cardiology (ESC). *Eur Heart J* 2011; **32**: 3147–97.

Royal College of Obstetricians and Gynaecologists. Cardiac disease and pregnancy. *Good Practice* 13. London: RCOG, 2011. www.rcog.org.uk/en/guidelines-research-services/guidelines/good-prac tice-13 (accessed December 2018).

Ruys TPE, Roos-Hesselink JW, Hall R, *et al*. Heart failure in pregnant women with cardiac disease: data from the ROPAC. *Heart* 2014; **100**: 231–8.

Turnbull J, Bell R. Obstetric anaesthesia and peripartum management. *Best Pract Res Clin Obstet Gynaecol* 2014; **28**: 593–605.

Vause S, Clarke B, Thorne S, James R, on behalf of the MBRRACE-UK cardiovascular chapter writing group. Lessons on cardiovascular disease. In Knight M, Nair M, Tuffnell D, *et al*.; MBRRACE-UK. *Saving Lives, Improving Mothers' Care: Surveillance of maternal deaths in the UK 2012–14 and lessons learned to inform maternity care from the UK and Ireland Confidential Enquiries into Maternal Deaths and Morbidity 2009–14*. Oxford: National Perinatal Epidemiology Unit, University of Oxford, 2016, pp. 33–68.

Chapter 92

Arrhythmias

Pregnancy-induced hormonal, haemodynamic and autonomic changes cause an increase in the incidence of both benign arrhythmias and arrhythmias associated with cardiac disease (see Chapter 11, *Physiology of pregnancy*).

If the abnormal rhythm causes haemodynamic instability, there is potential for fetal compromise.

Problems and special considerations

Sinus tachycardia is normal during pregnancy. Superimposed supraventricular or ventricular ectopic beats occur commonly and may cause palpitations and anxiety. Underlying organic disease is extremely unlikely in healthy women, who should be reassured and advised about avoiding likely precipitators such as caffeine.

Paroxysmal supraventricular tachycardia is more common in pregnancy, and rarely indicates underlying organic disease. Palpitations, dizziness and syncope may occur, and although attacks may terminate spontaneously with rest, persistent tachycardia that does not respond to vagal manoeuvres should be treated acutely with either suitable antiarrhythmic agents (adenosine or verapamil) or with DC cardioversion. In refractory cases, His bundle studies and subsequent ablation of abnormal conduction pathways may be indicated, although it is usual to wait until after delivery for such management.

Atrial fibrillation is usually associated with mitral valve disease and less commonly with cardiomyopathy. The major risks from atrial fibrillation in pregnancy are thromboembolic disease and pulmonary oedema. Prophylactic anticoagulants are indicated, and full anticoagulation may be necessary in some situations, such as during and immediately following DC cardioversion. Pregnancy does not alter medical management of atrial fibrillation. It is essential to confirm that therapeutic plasma levels of antiarrhythmic agents are achieved throughout the pregnancy.

Ventricular tachycardia or fibrillation may occur in association with severe organic cardiac disease, such as myocardial infarction. In such potentially life-threatening situations, pregnancy is of secondary concern, and the primary goal of treatment is termination of the arrhythmia by whatever means is effective.

Symptomatic bradyarrhythmias are uncommon in pregnancy. Transient sinus bradycardia may occur in the early postpartum period and does not require treatment in an asymptomatic woman with a structurally normal heart.

Conduction disorders require referral for cardiological opinion, since some cardiologists recommend aggressive management (permanent pacing) of even first-degree heart block during pregnancy, although this is disputed.

Management options

In general, pregnant women with cardiac arrhythmias should be assessed and treated in the same way as those who are not pregnant. Underlying causes such as cardiorespiratory conditions, anaemia, thyrotoxicosis or electrolyte imbalance should not be forgotten, and women should be investigated appropriately. Women with known predisposing cardiac conditions, for example Wolff–Parkinson–White or long QT syndromes, should be referred early for cardiological advice, and plans made both for management during delivery and for the occurrence of an acute arrhythmia.

All commonly used antiarrhythmics cross the placenta (and indeed may be administered to the mother to treat a fetal arrhythmia). Consensus opinion recommends using the lowest effective dose of the most well-established drug. Maternal β-blockade may cause fetal bradycardia and make interpretation of the fetal heart rate trace difficult, and there are reports of fetal growth restriction with their use in pregnant women with heart disease.

DC cardioversion in a pregnant woman requires general anaesthesia and tracheal intubation using rapid-sequence induction. Women in the second half of pregnancy are at risk of aortocaval compression in the supine position, and adequate uterine displacement must be performed to avoid compromise to uteroplacental perfusion. Fetal heart rate monitoring should be instituted before and immediately after the procedure. Prophylactic anticoagulation should be considered during and after DC cardioversion because of the increased risk of thromboembolic disease during pregnancy.

Agents that are associated with increased heart rate (e.g. oxytocin, ephedrine, terbutaline, salbutamol) should be avoided or used very cautiously if needed, in women at risk of tachyarrhythmias.

Cardiac implantable electronic devices in pregnancy

Pregnant women with underlying structural cardiac disease or a significant arrhythmogenic disorder may occasionally present with a cardiac implantable electronic device such as a permanent pacemaker (PPM) or implantable cardioverter defibrillator (ICD) in situ, or may rarely require the insertion of one during pregnancy. These women should be managed by a team that includes an obstetrician, anaesthetist, cardiologist and cardiac electrophysiologist. A well-communicated peripartum management plan should be put in place. Information on the nature of the device, the indication for its insertion, current programmed settings, date of last check and battery status should be elicited. Anaesthetists must be familiar with the mode of operation and the specific characteristics of these devices, particularly their susceptibility to electromagnetic interference.

Electromagnetic waves generated by the use of diathermy, nerve stimulators, magnetic resonance imaging (MRI) or transcutaneous electrical nerve stimulation (TENS) machines and other medical equipment may disrupt the device's ability to sense an arrhythmia, trigger unwarranted therapy or damage its components. Strategies to minimise these risks include reprogramming the device or the application of a clinical magnet to inactivate the anti-tachyarrhythmia function of an ICD or revert a PPM to an asynchronous pacing mode; this is typically performed in an operative setting when the use of diathermy is anticipated. The decision to alter device settings must be individualised and should be based on the potential for adverse interactions with electromagnetic interference, taking into account factors such as the distance between the device and the path of electric current (15 cm is the minimum recommended distance), and patient pacemaker dependency. Bipolar diathermy poses a lower risk and should be employed whenever possible. If monopolar diathermy is used, the ground plate should be placed close to the operative site and as far away from the device as possible. Short, intermittent bursts of current at the minimum effective power levels should be used. Equipment for transcutaneous/transvenous pacing or external defibrillation must be readily available in the perioperative period.

Neuraxial blocks for labour analgesia and anaesthesia reduce the adrenergic stimulation associated with pain and anxiety and have been used successfully in this patient group. Continuous maternal heart rate monitoring is advised during labour and delivery, and invasive monitoring should be considered in women with a high-risk profile. If general anaesthesia is required, rocuronium may be preferable to suxamethonium, as the muscle fasciculations associated with use of the latter may trigger shock release by an ICD or cause inhibition of PPM function and have been reported to cause device failure on induction of anaesthesia.

The patient should remain monitored in a high-dependency environment for the initial postpartum period. After delivery, the original programmed settings must be restored and the device checked.

Device implantation during pregnancy is uncommon, but carries the risk of fetal exposure to ionising radiation, which is more hazardous during the period of organogenesis. If there is an urgent clinical need for the insertion of a cardiac electronic device, protective measures such as shielding of the mother's abdomen and limiting the dose and duration of x-ray screening must be undertaken (pulsed fluoroscopy).

Key points

- No antiarrhythmic drug is considered completely safe for use in pregnancy.
- Older, well-established agents are generally recommended for first-line management, but newer drugs should not be withheld if other means are unsuccessful.
- Relief of aortocaval compression must not be forgotten during an acute arrhythmia.
- Carefully titrated central neuraxial blocks can be used for intrapartum analgesia/anaesthesia in women with cardiac implantable electronic devices.
- Precautions are required to minimise the effect of electromagnetic interference on device function in the peripartum period.

Further reading

Laksman Z, Harris L, Silversides C. Cardiac arrhythmias during pregnancy: a clinical approach. *Fetal Maternal Med Rev* 2011; **22**: 123–43.

Metz T, Khanna A. Evaluation and management of maternal cardiac arrhythmias. *Obstet Gynecol Clin North Am* 2016; **43**: 729–45.

Salman MM, Kemp HI, Cauldwell MR, Dob DP, Sutton R. Anaesthetic management of pregnant patients with cardiac implantable electronic devices: case reports and review. *Int J Obstet Anesth* 2018; **33**: 57–66.

Stone ME, Salter B, Fischer A. Perioperative management of patients with cardiac implantable electronic devices. *Br J Anaesth* 2011; **107** (Suppl 1): i16–26.

Pulmonary oedema

The pregnant mother may be at increased risk of developing pulmonary oedema, because her cardiac output and blood volume are increased considerably compared with pre-pregnancy values. This increase is greater in the mother with multiple pregnancy. Colloid osmotic pressure is also reduced in pregnancy.

Problems and special considerations

Acute pulmonary oedema in the pregnant woman may mimic an acute asthmatic attack. Attempts to treat the latter will tend to exacerbate the former.

There are multiple aetiologies of pulmonary oedema in pregnancy, but a careful history will usually provide a diagnosis of the underlying cause. Pulmonary oedema may occur:

1. As a complication of coexisting cardiac disease
2. Secondary to complications of pregnancy, e.g. pre-eclampsia, major obstetric haemorrhage, intrauterine fetal death, amniotic fluid embolism, peripartum cardiomyopathy
3. Secondary to aspiration of gastric contents
4. Secondary to major sepsis
5. Following therapeutic or recreational drug administration, e.g. β-adrenergic agonists, glucocorticoids, oxytocics, dexamethasone, cocaine
6. Following excessive administration of intravenous fluid

Hypoxaemia caused by oedema is exacerbated by the increased oxygen demand of pregnancy and the reduced functional residual capacity and oxygen reserve.

Management options

Women who are known to be at increased risk of developing cardiac failure should receive antenatal and intrapartum care in an obstetric unit with high-dependency and intensive care facilities on site. Pulse oximetry is particularly useful, since a fall in saturation may be an early sign of pulmonary oedema.

Women receiving β-adrenergic agonists must have fluid balance and electrolytes monitored rigorously, and supplementary oxygen therapy should be considered. Invasive monitoring of central venous pressure should be considered if regional analgesia or anaesthesia is used in a woman who has been receiving β-agonists, because of the risk of fluid overloading.

Appropriate investigations should be performed, including chest radiography, since this carries negligible risk to the fetus.

In the absence of any obvious cause for cardiac failure, it is important to consider the use of illicit drugs.

Invasive cardiovascular monitoring will guide diagnosis and treatment, and the mother should be transferred to a high-dependency or intensive care unit at the earliest possible opportunity.

Oxygen therapy is invariably beneficial. Delivery of the fetus reduces oxygen demand and relieves the physical effect of the gravid uterus on the diaphragm and lungs. Further therapeutic strategies depend on the underlying cause of pulmonary oedema, but it can be helpful to differentiate between pulmonary oedema associated with pre-eclampsia and pulmonary oedema of other causes. The latter is managed in a similar fashion to pulmonary oedema in the non-pregnant adult, with diuresis and ventilatory support as required. In addition to this, pulmonary oedema associated with pre-eclampsia requires acute control of blood pressure. Intravenous glyceryl trinitrate is usually the drug of choice. Nifedipine and hydralazine may also be considered. The most appropriate place for monitoring and management is often the high-dependency or intensive care unit.

Key points

- Pulmonary oedema is uncommon in pregnancy but may be fatal.
- Chest radiography should not be withheld.
- Delivery of the fetus may be indicated.
- The mother should be managed in a high-dependency or intensive care unit.

Further reading

Dennis AT, Solnordal CB. Acute pulmonary oedema in pregnant women. *Anaesthesia* 2012; **67**: 646–59.

Sciscione AC, Ivester T, Largoza M, *et al.* Acute pulmonary edema in pregnancy. *Obstet Gynecol* 2003; **101**: 511–15.

Cardiomyopathy

Pregnant women may have a pre-existing cardiomyopathy or may develop cardiomyopathy of pregnancy (peripartum cardiomyopathy, PPCM).

The causes of pre-existing cardiomyopathy are diverse and include infection, systemic disease such as sarcoidosis, infiltrative disease such as amyloid, toxins such as alcohol and cocaine, ischaemic heart disease, obesity-related and congenital cardiomyopathies. Of this group, the most commonly encountered in the antenatal clinic is hypertrophic cardiomyopathy (HCM), with a prevalence of about 1 in 500, though restrictive and dilated cardiomyopathies may also be seen.

The aetiology of PPCM is unknown, but viral or autoimmune myocarditis, or an exaggerated response to the haemodynamic stresses of pregnancy, have been suggested. Predisposing factors seem to be multiple pregnancy, smoking, family history, prolonged use of β-agonists, diabetes and hypertension. The classic criteria for diagnosis of PPCM are:

1. Development of cardiac failure in the last month of pregnancy or within 5 months of delivery.
2. Absence of other aetiology for cardiac failure.
3. Absence of cardiac disease prior to the last month of pregnancy.
4. Echocardiography criteria have subsequently been added: ejection fraction < 45% and/or fractional shortening < 30%, and end-diastolic dimension > 2.7 cm/m^2 body surface area.

It has been suggested that the definition should be extended to include cardiac failure developing within the third trimester of pregnancy for which no other cause can be found. The incidence of PPCM is estimated to be 1 in 3000 pregnancies.

Functionally, patients with HCM have thickened myocardium and may have outflow obstruction, while those with PPCM have a dilated cardiomyopathy.

Problems and special considerations

Patients with HCM have a hypertrophied left ventricle and interventricular septum which may cause outflow obstruction and myocardial ischemia due to a mismatch between oxygen supply and demand. Mitral regurgitation is often present. Any factors that increase myocardial contractility (β-agonists, circulating catecholamines) or decrease preload or afterload (vasodilatation, hypovolaemia) will cause an increase in left ventricular outflow obstruction. Tachycardias reduce the time for diastolic filling, and atrial arrhythmias are particularly poorly tolerated.

The obstructive component of HCM varies considerably. Women with minimal obstruction usually tolerate pregnancy well, although the more severe the degree of left ventricular hypertrophy the greater the risk of myocardial ischaemia, particularly in response to the stress of pregnancy and delivery.

Patients with dilated cardiomyopathy have reduced myocardial contractility. The left ventricle is hypokinetic, ejection fraction is reduced and there is usually mitral and/or tricuspid regurgitation. Pressures in the right side of the heart are raised, and cardiac or pulmonary artery catheterisation usually confirms pulmonary hypertension. Any factors that depress myocardial contractility or increase afterload will further compromise cardio-vascular stability.

Women with PPCM usually present with the classic signs of left ventricular or congestive cardiac failure. There is a high associated risk of embolic phenomena.

Management options

Hypertrophic cardiomyopathy

Women with HCM have usually been diagnosed before pregnancy, and baseline cardiological investigations should be available. If β-blocking drugs are being used they should be continued during pregnancy.

Serial cardiological investigations (electrocardiography (ECG), echocardiography) should be performed during pregnancy. Tachycardias should be treated with suitable β-blockers, and esmolol has been recommended for use in the acute situation. Cardioversion may be required to terminate supraventricular tachycardia; amiodarone is recommended for ventricular tachycardias. Nitrates should not be used to treat angina because the consequent vasodilatation and afterload reduction further aggravates left ventricular outflow obstruction.

There is no indication to deliver women by caesarean section unless there are obstetric reasons to do so or unless the maternal condition deteriorates. Continuous ECG and arterial blood pressure monitoring should be used throughout labour and delivery and continued into the early postnatal period.

Traditionally, regional analgesia has been considered contraindicated because of the risk of acute reduction in afterload. However, provision of high-quality analgesia is beneficial, particularly for preventing pain-induced tachycardia. Intrathecal opioid analgesia is not accompanied by sympathetic blockade but is of limited efficacy in advanced labour. Epidural or combined spinal–epidural analgesia, using low-dose (< 0.1% bupivacaine) epidural local anaesthetic with fentanyl, offers good analgesia with minimum haemodynamic disturbance.

Maintenance of adequate hydration – intravenously if necessary – is important. Phenylephrine is preferable to ephedrine for treatment of hypotension because the α effects of phenylephrine on myocardial contractility and heart rate are less than those of the mixed α and β effects of ephedrine.

Dilated cardiomyopathy/PPCM

The majority of cases of PPCM present in the peripartum or immediate postpartum period. Treatment includes use of positive inotropes such as digoxin (and parenteral inotropes such as dopamine and dobutamine in the acute situation), oxygen and diuretics, vasodilators to reduce afterload (but not angiotensin-converting enzyme inhibitors before delivery), bed rest and anticoagulants (because of the risk of thromboembolic disease). Intra-aortic balloon pumps, left ventricular assist devices and heart or heart–lung transplantation may be required in severe cases that fail to respond to maximal medical therapy.

If PPCM presents antenatally, delivery is indicated as soon as the woman's condition has been optimised. Caesarean section may be necessary unless conditions are favourable for induction of labour.

Regional analgesia and anaesthesia are thought to be beneficial for the patient with dilated cardiomyopathy, since the cardiodepressant effects of most general anaesthetic drugs are avoided, and afterload is beneficially reduced. Hypotension should be treated with drugs with predominantly β activity, which stimulate myocardial contractility (ephedrine) rather than pure α-agonists (phenylephrine), which increase systemic vascular resistance. The immediate postpartum period is a particularly risky time owing to auto-transfusion and the risk of fluid overload.

PPCM is thought to have a mortality rate approaching 10% at 2 years and has a high recurrence rate, and some authorities consider further pregnancies to be contraindicated following PPCM. Others suggest that another pregnancy can be considered if there is no residual cardiomegaly by 6 months postpartum. Case series suggest that if left ventricular function is still impaired 1 year after delivery, there is a ~20% risk of death in the next pregnancy.

Key points

- Hypertrophic cardiomyopathy is usually inherited, and presents with variable left ventricular outflow obstruction.
- Treatment is directed at reduction of myocardial contractility and increasing preload and afterload.
- Tachyarrhythmias and myocardial ischaemia are particular hazards.
- Peripartum cardiomyopathy usually presents in the peripartum or early postpartum period.
- Treatment is symptomatic and is directed at maintaining myocardial contractility and reducing afterload.

Further reading

Blauwet LA, Cooper LT. Diagnosis and management of peripartum cardiomyopathy. *Heart* 2011; **97**: 1970–81.

Herrey AS. Pregnancy in inherited and acquired cardiomyopathies. *Best Pract Res Clin Obstet Gynaecol* 2014; **28**: 563–77.

Hilfiker-Kleiner D, Haghikia A, Nonhoff J, *et al.* Peripartum cardiomyopathy: current management and future perspectives. *Eur Heart J* 2015; **36**: 1090–7.

Lewey J, Haythe J. Cardiomyopathy in pregnancy. *Semin Perinatol* 2014; **38**: 309–17.

Coarctation of the aorta

Coarctation of the aorta occurs in approximately 5% of patients with congenital heart disease, and may occur as an isolated lesion or in association with other cardiovascular defects. Preductal coarctation is associated with patent ductus arteriosus, ventricular septal defect, bicuspid aortic valve and (in about 10% of cases) transposition of the great vessels. The majority of cases of preductal coarctation present with congestive cardiac failure in the neonatal period and are diagnosed and corrected surgically in infancy.

Postductal coarctation of the aorta may not be diagnosed until adolescence or adult life. There are associated berry aneurysms of the circle of Willis in approximately 10% of cases, and bicuspid aortic valve in 50% of patients.

Problems and special considerations

Corrected coarctation is considered a relatively low-risk lesion in pregnancy, unless there are associated abnormalities such as those described above. However, pregnancy in women with an uncorrected aortic coarctation or with residual hypertension, coarctation or aortic aneurysm is associated with a maternal mortality of 3–9%, and a fetal mortality of up to 20%.

Undiagnosed coarctation may present for the first time in pregnancy. There is invariably hypertension, and this may be accompanied by congestive cardiac failure, caused by inability to compensate for the increased blood volume and cardiac output of pregnancy. The generalised peripheral vasodilatation and consequent reduction in systemic vascular resistance that occur in pregnancy may also precipitate cardiac failure.

In uncorrected or undiagnosed aortic coarctation, there is a risk of aortic rupture or dissection or rupture of a cerebral aneurysm if blood pressure increases acutely, for example because of severe pain or following use of certain drugs (e.g. ergometrine, vasopressors). Increased shearing forces associated with swings in blood pressure may also be dangerous. Fetal mortality is increased because of decreased uteroplacental flow.

Hypertension is limited to the arms, and blood pressure may be reduced in the legs; palpation of the peripheral pulses frequently reveals absent foot pulses and radiofemoral delay. An aortic systolic murmur is heard on auscultation of the chest, and there may also be audible bruits over the intercostal and internal mammary vessels, which carry collateral flow to the lower limbs. A chest x-ray may show rib notching caused by the collateral vessels, and left ventricular hypertrophy.

Management options

Women with corrected coarctation should be assessed both before and early in pregnancy, and any associated abnormalities noted. Changes to usual obstetric and anaesthetic management are not generally indicated in the absence of complications or other pathology, although epidural analgesia will often be advised, particularly in the presence of hypertension.

In uncorrected coarctation, blood pressure should be controlled throughout pregnancy, even though this may further hinder uteroplacental flow, and regular monitoring of the fetus is required. There is no proven benefit of operative delivery for women with uncorrected coarctation, although anxiety about undiagnosed aneurysms of the circle of Willis may lead to recommendations for epidural analgesia and elective instrumental delivery. There is also no evidence that allowing the woman to labour increases her risks of aortic dissection or rupture, but again, epidural analgesia is usually recommended. Minimising haemodynamic disturbance is the main aim of management of delivery. Cardiac output is relatively fixed; tachycardia secondary to uncontrolled pain may precipitate cardiac failure, but bradycardia and acute reduction in systemic vascular resistance are also hazardous. Hypovolaemia leads to compromised left ventricular filling.

Invasive systemic arterial pressure monitoring allows close attention to changes in blood pressure and facilitates analgesic and anaesthetic management, although this may not be necessary in repaired coarctation with no residual obstruction or other problems. Postductal pressures (left radial) give the best indication of uteroplacental blood flow. Central venous pressure monitoring may also be useful. Epidural or combined epidural–spinal techniques can provide safe and effective pain relief in labour. Although the main risk is from hypertension, it is also important to avoid hypotension.

For caesarean section, both regional and general anaesthesia may be suitable, although many practitioners would avoid single-shot spinal anaesthesia because of the risk of uncontrolled hypotension. Combined spinal–epidural, continuous spinal or epidural techniques allow gradual extension of the anaesthetic level cephalad and minimise the risks of rapid onset of profound hypotension. If general anaesthesia is used, steps should be taken to prevent the hypertensive response to tracheal intubation.

Postoperative management in a high-dependency environment is essential; invasive monitoring should be continued postoperatively, and adequate analgesia should be ensured by using either the epidural route or patient-controlled intravenous analgesia.

Key points

- Women with corrected coarctation do not usually pose any particular problem in pregnancy, although there may be other associated cardiovascular abnormalities.
- Uncorrected coarctation may be associated with aortic dissection or rupture.
- Both general and regional anaesthesia are acceptable options but both may be hazardous in uncorrected or unstable cases.
- Invasive arterial ± central venous pressure monitoring is recommended in uncorrected coarctation or corrected cases with complications.

Further reading

European Society of Cardiology. ESC guidelines on the management of cardiovascular diseases during pregnancy: the Task Force on the Management of Cardiovascular Diseases during Pregnancy of the European Society of Cardiology (ESC). *Eur Heart J* 2011; **32**: 3147–97.

van Hagen IM, Roos-Hesselink JW. Aorta pathology and pregnancy. *Best Pract Res Clin Obstet Gynaecol* 2014; **28**: 537–50.

Aortic dissection

Aortic dissection in a pregnant woman is a rare event that carries an increased risk of maternofetal morbidity and mortality, with a risk of maternal death in the first month from presentation of over 80%. The estimated incidence of aortic dissection in the UK is around 1 per 100,000 maternities. In pregnancy, aortic dissection is more commonly associated with connective tissue disorders, particularly Marfan's syndrome and others such as Turner's, Ehlers–Danlos type IV and related syndromes. Other risk factors include structural disease such as coarctation of the aorta and bicuspid aortic valve, inflammatory vasculitides, chronic hypertension and cocaine abuse.

Approximately half of the acute dissections in women under 40 years old occur during pregnancy or after delivery. The increased risk of dissection in the obstetric population is attributed to pregnancy-induced haemodynamic stress caused by volume overload and increased downstream resistance secondary to compression by the gravid uterus. In addition, hormonal effects may alter the structural elements of the aortic wall. The haemodynamic changes become more marked in the last trimester of pregnancy and the immediate postpartum period, when the risk of dissection peaks. Stanford type A aortic dissection (DeBakey types I and II) involves the ascending aorta and is the more common type in pregnancy. Stanford type B (DeBakey type III) does not involve the ascending aorta.

Problems and special considerations

The initial presentation may include a myriad of clinical symptoms that overlap with other conditions and can cause a diagnostic dilemma. Early diagnosis is crucial, as mortality increases by 1% per hour for the first 48 hours after presentation.

Acute dissection typically presents with severe chest or interscapular pain of abrupt onset that is described as tearing, stabbing or sharp and may radiate to the jaw, arm or epigastrium. The pain may be migratory in nature and may manifest in the abdomen or legs with type B dissections. Other associated features may include systolic hypertension, tachycardia, dyspnoea, syncope or neurological symptoms. Pulse deficits, asymmetric blood pressure or focal neurology may be elicited on examination. Cardiac auscultation may reveal a diastolic murmur of acute aortic regurgitation. Cardiovascular decompensation may indicate heart failure, myocardial infarction, aortic rupture or cardiac tamponade.

Women who present with severe unexplained pain requiring opioid analgesia must be reviewed by a senior clinician and be fully investigated. Electrocardiography may reveal ST segment changes, and a plain chest x-ray may show a widened mediastinum, but both tests may be normal or inconclusive. Imaging must be expedited, and transthoracic echocardiography is recommended as an initial investigation. Magnetic resonance imaging, computerised tomography and transoesophageal echocardiography have comparable accuracy in confirming or ruling out the diagnosis of aortic dissection, but the latter two may be more appropriate in the haemodynamically compromised patient.

Management

Pre-pregnancy counselling and inter-specialty management is essential in women with known aortic disease. Prophylactic surgical repair may be considered in some patients. Pregnant women with a dilated aortic root should have adequate blood pressure control and regular echocardiographic monitoring. Women with a history of aortic dissection should be delivered in a hospital equipped with facilities for cardiothoracic surgery.

Conservative management may be appropriate in small uncomplicated type B dissection, with strict blood pressure control and close surveillance. Other cases may require open surgery (with or without caesarean section depending on gestational age and severity) or endovascular repair. Anaesthesia for aortic root repair is as for cardiac surgery of any kind in pregnancy, taking particular care to avoid hypertension.

Key points

- Aortic dissection is an uncommon disease that carries an over 80% risk of death in the first month from presentation.
- Pregnant women presenting with abrupt-onset severe chest or back pain must be thoroughly investigated.
- Timely diagnosis allows the initiation of life-saving treatment and an improved chance of survival.

Further reading

Erbel R, Aboyans V, Boileau C, et al.; ESC Committee for Practice Guidelines. 2014 ESC Guidelines on the diagnosis and treatment of aortic diseases: Document covering acute and chronic aortic diseases of the thoracic and abdominal aorta of the adult. The Task Force for the Diagnosis and Treatment of Aortic Diseases of the European Society of Cardiology (ESC). *Eur Heart J* 2014; **35**: 2873–926.

European Society of Cardiology. ESC guidelines on the management of cardiovascular diseases during pregnancy: the Task Force on the Management of Cardiovascular Diseases during Pregnancy of the European Society of Cardiology (ESC). *Eur Heart J* 2011; **32**: 3147–97.

Rajagopalan S, Nwazota N, Chandrasekhar S. Outcomes in pregnant women with acute aortic dissections: a review of the literature from 2003 to 2013. *Int J Obs Anes* 2014; **23**: 348–56.

Smok D. Aortopathy in pregnancy. *Semin Perinatol* 2014; **38**: 295–303.

Chapter 97

Valvular heart disease

Most women presenting to a UK antenatal clinic with valvular lesions will have congenital heart disease, although immigrants from the Indian subcontinent and some parts of eastern Europe still have a high incidence of acquired valve disease. As with most types of heart disease, pregnancy presents a challenge to women with valvular disease due to the altered cardiovascular physiology seen. Specific concerns and management depend on how the valvular lesion functions and how the haemodynamic changes of pregnancy will be tolerated.

Women with a prosthetic heart valve present an additional challenge owing to the need for anticoagulation, and the potential catastrophic consequences of inadequate anticoagulation. Prosthetic valves may also not function optimally before or during pregnancy. Women with corrected valvular heart disease and a prosthetic valve have increased morbidity in pregnancy, especially if they are anticoagulated.

Problems and special considerations

Morbidity is related to the severity of the underlying valvular lesion and cardiac function. Regurgitant and right-sided lesions tend to be better tolerated than stenotic and left-sided lesions in pregnancy, due to the reduction in systemic vascular resistance which encourages right-to-left flow.

Mitral stenosis is a particularly high-risk lesion, and those with moderate to severe disease should be counselled against pregnancy until treated. Even if a woman is asymptomatic to start with, the increase in blood volume and heart rate in pregnancy will often lead to decompensation. Those with a mitral valve replacement have a relatively fixed cardiac output and are also at risk of developing cardiac failure during pregnancy. They have an increased risk of thromboembolism and atrial fibrillation; most will be anticoagulated throughout pregnancy, and if arrhythmia occurs it should be treated promptly, by cardioversion if necessary.

A bicuspid aortic valve is one of the most common congenital heart defects seen, affecting up to 2% of the population; it is more likely to affect women than men and results in accelerated aortic stenosis, usually presenting from the third decade. Women with aortic valve lesions or replacement tend to tolerate the physiological changes of pregnancy relatively well, unless they have severe aortic stenosis (valve area < 1.0 cm^2 and mean gradient > 40 mmHg) or are symptomatic before pregnancy.

Prosthetic heart valves

The relative risk of pregnancy in women with prosthetic heart valves depends not only on the underlying cardiac abnormality and residual impairment of cardiac function, but also on the type of valve replacement used. Observational data from the UK Obstetric Surveillance System (UKOSS) suggest that maternal complications in women with prosthetic valves are more common than previously thought, with a mortality of 9% and morbidity of 41%; these figures are higher than in recent reports from a multinational registry of pregnancy and cardiac disease (ROPAC; mortality 1.5%), which may reflect differences in outcomes in specialist versus non-specialist centres. Prosthetic heart valves may be mechanical, xenograft (usually porcine) or human allograft (homograft). While mechanical valves provide superior durability and haemodynamic performance to biological valves, the need for long-term anticoagulation increases maternal and fetal morbidity and mortality, so they are usually second choice for women of reproductive age.

Mechanical valves

The most important risks for women with mechanical valves are those associated with the increased thrombotic risk during pregnancy (estimated to be as high as 29%), the need for anticoagulation and the risk of endocarditis. Both warfarin and heparin therapy are associated with significant maternal morbidity and fetal morbidity and mortality. Warfarin is better for maternal health and the risk of thrombosis but worse for the fetus, while heparin is better for the fetus and worse for the mother.

Warfarin is teratogenic, causing mental retardation, short stature and multiple facial abnormalities. Its use in the second trimester of pregnancy is associated with fetal blindness, microcephaly and mental retardation. There is also an increased risk of fetal internal haemorrhage and maternal haemorrhage in women taking warfarin. The ROPAC group has reported an association between miscarriage and late fetal death and use of vitamin K antagonists.

Administration of heparin during pregnancy is also associated with increased rates of spontaneous abortion, fetal and maternal haemorrhage and stillbirth. Prolonged use of heparin may cause maternal osteoporosis and heparin-induced thrombocytopenia, though these are less common with low-molecular-weight heparins. However, the main risk with heparin is thromboembolism involving the heart valves, increasing maternal morbidity and mortality. Optimal dose of heparins can be difficult with the altered pharmacokinetics of pregnancy. Dose adjustment according to anti-Xa levels can reduce the risk of thrombosis.

Traditionally, British practice has been to convert women to heparin for the first trimester of pregnancy and then maintain them on warfarin before reverting to heparin for the last few weeks of pregnancy and for delivery, while practice in the USA has been to heparinise women throughout pregnancy. In particular high-risk cases, low-dose aspirin may be added to heparin therapy in an attempt to improve maternal outcome. It has been suggested that as there is no clear-cut optimal anticoagulation regimen, women should be informed of the risks and benefits of all options and encouraged to help choose their own therapy.

Xenograft valves

The major risks of xenograft valves are thromboembolic events and valve failure. The rate of valve degeneration at 10 years is estimated at 50–60%. There is some evidence that pregnancy accelerates the degeneration of xenograft valves, and it is therefore imperative to follow these women closely during pregnancy and to investigate immediately any possibility of deteriorating cardiac function.

Although an advantage of xenograft compared with mechanical valves is that anti-coagulation is not needed routinely, women with atrial fibrillation or a history of thromboembolic events are likely to require full anticoagulation, with its attendant risks.

Homograft valves

These valves are used primarily for aortic valve replacement, and the available evidence suggests that they are associated with a significantly lower morbidity in pregnancy than either xenograft or mechanical valves. There is no need for anticoagulant therapy and there do not appear to be the same risks of degenerative change as with xenograft valves.

Management options

Pre-pregnancy counselling should be offered to women with valvular heart disease, firstly to advise those with congenital heart disease of the increased risks of congenital heart disease in their offspring, and secondly to advise those who are dependent on anticoagulants of the risks of such therapy in pregnancy. Valve function and cardiac status should also be assessed before pregnancy if possible.

All women with valvular heart disease, and in particular those with prosthetic heart valves, should be regarded as having high-risk pregnancies and should be delivered in large maternity units, preferably in or near to centres with facilities for cardiac surgery. Multidisciplinary management should involve the obstetric, cardiology, haematology and anaesthetic teams, with input from midwifery and critical care staff as appropriate. Cardiac function should be assessed early in the first trimester of pregnancy and at regular intervals throughout the pregnancy. It is particularly important for women with prosthetic valves to receive regular dental care during pregnancy, and any dental treatment should be preceded by prophylactic antibiotics. Similarly, any intercurrent infection during pregnancy should be aggressively treated. Most units continue to give prophylactic antibiotics to cover delivery in women with prosthetic heart valves, despite recent guidelines suggesting this is unnecessary.

In general, management and monitoring will depend on the severity of residual cardiac disease and the underlying lesion, and the requirements of each woman must be determined on an individual basis. Aortocaval compression and the consequent reduction in preload must be avoided in all types of valvular heart disease. An arterial line may be useful to monitor changes in blood pressure and allow a rapid response.

In the presence of a stenotic valvular lesion, tachycardia, hypovolaemia and a reduction in afterload are poorly tolerated and should be avoided. If anaesthesia is required, general anaesthesia is often chosen over spinal anaesthesia. However, pain-mediated tachycardia may increase flow across the valve and precipitate cardiac failure; carefully titrated regional analgesia may be beneficial, and neuraxial anaesthesia is not contraindicated.

In the presence of a regurgitant lesion, forward flow increases with a drop in systemic vascular resistance, so regional analgesia/anaesthesia is usually advised. Normal blood pressure and a high-normal heart rate should be maintained. Most anaesthetists would avoid spinal anaesthesia in favour of a more gradual epidural or combined spinal–epidural technique.

Sinus rhythm should be maintained if possible. Particular attention to fluid balance is necessary in the postpartum period.

Prosthetic heart valves

The presence of a prosthetic heart valve is not in itself an indication for operative delivery. There are obvious advantages in planned induction of labour in anticoagulated women to allow appropriate management of anticoagulation over the period of induction and delivery; an individualised plan for labour and delivery should be agreed in advance by the multidisciplinary team. This would usually involve stopping low-molecular-weight heparin 24 hours before planned induction and converting to unfractionated heparin, which can then be stopped at an appropriate time before delivery. This enables regional analgesic and anaesthetic techniques to be used (following laboratory assessment of coagulation status) if appropriate. If regional analgesia is contraindicated, patient-controlled intravenous opioid analgesia is the most appropriate alternative for labour, and also for provision of post-operative analgesia if general anaesthesia has been used for caesarean section.

Key points

- Women with prosthetic heart valves and valvular heart disease are not a homogeneous group. They differ in their underlying cardiac disease, degree of impairment of cardiac function and type of prosthetic valve.
- Pre-pregnancy counselling is recommended whenever possible.
- Antenatal care and delivery should be undertaken in a hospital with facilities for high-dependency care.
- Regular assessment of cardiac function during pregnancy is important.
- Anaesthetic goals include maintaining normal cardiovascular parameters, sinus rhythm and fluid status.

Further reading

Dennis AT. Valvular heart disease in pregnancy. *Int J Obstet Anesth* 2016; **25**: 4–8.

European Society of Cardiology. ESC guidelines on the management of cardiovascular diseases during pregnancy: the Task Force on the Management of Cardiovascular Diseases during Pregnancy of the European Society of Cardiology (ESC). *Eur Heart J* 2011; **32**: 3147–97.

Lawley CM, Lain SJ, Algert CS, *et al.* Prosthetic heart valves in pregnancy, outcomes for women and their babies: a systematic review and meta-analysis. *BJOG* 2015; **122**: 1446–55.

McLintock C. Thromboembolism in pregnancy: challenges and controversies in the prevention of pregnancy-associated venous thromboembolism and management of anticoagulation in women with mechanical prosthetic heart valves. *Best Pract Res Clin Obstet Gynaecol* 2014; **28**: 519–36.

Thorne S. Pregnancy and native heart valve disease. *Heart* 2016; **102**: 1410–17.

van Hagen IM, Roos-Hesselink JW, Ruys TP, *et al.*; ROPAC investigators. Pregnancy in women with a mechanical heart valve: data of the European Society of Cardiology Registry of Pregnancy and Cardiac Disease (ROPAC). *Circulation* 2015; **132**: 132–42.

Vause S, Clarke B, Tower CL, Hay C, Knight M; UKOSS. Pregnancy outcomes in women with mechanical prosthetic heart valves: a prospective descriptive population based study using the United Kingdom Obstetric Surveillance System (UKOSS) data collection system. *BJOG* 2017; **124**: 1411–19.

Windram JD, Colman JM, Wald RM, *et al.* Valvular heart disease in pregnancy. *Best Pract Res Clin Obstet Gynaecol* 2014; **28**: 507–18.

Congenital heart disease

About 70–80% of children with congenital heart disease (CHD) now reach adult life (16 years and over) and thus reproductive age. Unfortunately, there is still a significant mortality rate among young adults with corrected CHD. In the pregnant population, cyanotic CHD is associated with a higher maternal and fetal morbidity and mortality than non-cyanotic disease, but both groups of women should be regarded as high-risk patients.

Problems and special considerations

Patients primarily with disorders of cardiac output may experience cardiac failure as pregnancy progresses, because of the increased demands placed on the cardiovascular system and the increased oxygen demand. Patients with cyanotic (or potentially cyanotic) disorders may experience worsening cyanosis as the decreasing systemic vascular resistance encourages shunting of blood across the heart; this is compounded by increased oxygen demand. Both types of patients are prone to arrhythmias and venous thromboembolism, and tolerate hypovolaemia poorly.

A maternal haematocrit of greater than 60%, arterial oxygen saturation of less than 80%, right ventricular hypertrophy and episodes of syncope are all considered poor prognostic factors. Women with cyanotic disease have higher rates of spontaneous abortion, and these are said to correlate with haematocrit.

The World Health Organization (WHO) classification of pregnancy risk depending on cardiac condition is given in Table 98.1.

Regardless of the maternal cardiac condition, the fetus of the mother with CHD has an increased risk of CHD (Table 98.2). Other fetal risks include prematurity, fetal growth restriction and perinatal death.

Bolus doses of oxytocin cause a transient but sometimes profound fall in arterial blood pressure; the drug should be given by intravenous infusion if at all. Ergometrine causes a sharp rise in arterial, central venous and intracranial pressures and should generally be avoided in women with CHD, although it may be preferable to oxytocin in certain fixed-output states without pulmonary hypertension. If caesarean section is performed, the need for oxytocics may be avoided by performing a brace suture through the uterus to provide mechanical, rather than pharmacological, uterine compression.

Women may be receiving therapeutic doses of anticoagulants and this may preclude regional analgesia and anaesthesia, though the latter is still possible if timed appropriately.

Table 98.1 Modified WHO classification of maternal risk by cardiac condition

WHO pregnancy risk		
1: Risk no higher than general population	**2 or 3: Increased risk of maternal mortality and morbidity**	**4: Pregnancy contraindicated: very high risk of maternal mortality or severe morbidity**
Uncomplicated, small or mild: • pulmonary stenosis • ventricular septal defect • patent ductus arteriosus • mitral valve prolapse Successfully repaired simple lesions, e.g.: • ostium secundum atrial septal defect • ventricular septal defect • patent ductus arteriosus • total anomalous pulmonary venous drainage Isolated ventricular extrasystoles and atrial ectopic beats	*WHO 2 if well:* • unoperated atrial septal defect • repaired tetralogy of Fallot • most arrhythmias *WHO 2/3 depending on patient:* • mild left ventricular impairment • hypertrophic cardiomyopathy • native or tissue valvular heart disease • Marfan's syndrome without aortic dilatation • heart transplantation *WHO 3:* • mechanical valve • systemic right ventricle • Fontan circulation • cyanotic heart disease	Previous peripartum cardiomyopathy with any residual impairment of left ventricular function Severe systemic ventricular dysfunction (NYHA III–IV or LVEF < 30%) Pulmonary arterial hypertension Severe left heart obstruction Marfan's syndrome with aorta dilated > 40 mm

LVEF, left ventricular ejection fraction; NYHA, New York Heart Association.
Adapted from: Thorne S, MacGregor A, Nelson-Piercy C. Risks of contraception and pregnancy in heart disease. *Heart* 2006; **92:** 1520–5.

Management options

Women with CHD must be identified early in pregnancy (preferably seen for pre-conception counselling) and managed jointly by the obstetrician, cardiologist and obstetric anaesthetist. Appropriate investigations and plans should be instituted (see Chapter 91, *Cardiovascular disease*) and placed clearly in the patient's notes. Some units have a register in which high-risk patients approaching term delivery can be entered. The anaesthetists involved should have a clear understanding of the underlying cardiac lesion and/or correction, and its implications for cardiac output and likely complications that may be encountered.

Table 98.2 Risk of neonatal cardiac lesions when at least one parent has congenital heart disease

Tetralogy of Fallot	2–3%
Persistent ductus arteriosus; aortic coarctation	4%
Atrial septal defect	5–11%
Pulmonary stenosis	6–7%
Ventricular or atrioventricular septal defect	10–16%
Aortic stenosis	15–18%
Marfan's/Di George's syndrome	50%

Caesarean section is not indicated for women with CHD unless there are obstetric indications or worsening maternal condition. Concerns regarding caesarean delivery include the haemodynamic response to anaesthesia, the risk of increased blood loss, and the increased risk of postoperative complications such as bleeding and infection. Planned induction of labour may appear to have obvious benefits, but carries the risk of an increased likelihood of obstetric intervention. Elective instrumental delivery avoids the fall in cardiac output that accompanies pushing, and should be recommended for most cases, although a maximum of 15–30 minutes' pushing can be allowed for mild cases. The left lateral position is often advised for examinations and labour to avoid aortocaval compression.

Invasive arterial and/or central venous pressure monitoring is generally recommended except for mild conditions; the use of pulmonary artery catheters is controversial and is usually impractical outside the intensive care unit.

Depending on the lesion and repair, there may be increased risk of a paradoxical embolism; all intravenous injections must be administered with care, and a loss-of-resistance to saline technique is advisable if epidural anaesthesia is employed.

Cautious use of low-dose epidural bupivacaine (0.1% or less) in combination with an opioid (usually 2.0–2.5 µg/ml fentanyl) provides optimal analgesia for women with CHD. Intrathecal opioids and continuous spinal analgesia have also been used. The use of high concentrations of bupivacaine (0.25%) in labour is contraindicated because of the risk of rapid and uncontrolled decrease in cardiac output.

Anaesthesia for caesarean delivery in women with CHD carries high risks. The options are for slow induction of regional anaesthesia (e.g. epidural, continuous spinal or combined spinal–epidural with a very small spinal component) or a 'cardiac' general anaesthetic (which may necessitate prompt neonatal resuscitation and some hours of maternal and neonatal postoperative ventilatory support). There are no absolute rules; the relative risks and benefits in each individual case must be considered. A consultant anaesthetist with expertise in the management of high-risk pregnancy should be involved in the decision making.

Management of intrapartum anticoagulation should be discussed with both the haematologist and the cardiologist. Recent guidelines have not recommended routine prophylactic antibiotic cover for labour but many centres continue to give this, and it is recommended that this should be discussed with the patient. All drug therapy should be discussed with a cardiologist with expertise in the management of CHD.

Key points

- Cyanotic congenital heart disease is associated with high maternal and fetal morbidity and mortality.
- Multidisciplinary antenatal and intrapartum care is essential, and an individualised plan for delivery should be made.
- Regional analgesia for labour is usually beneficial; choice of anaesthetic technique for caesarean section is controversial.

Further reading

Connolly HM. Managing congenital heart disease in the obstetric patient. *Semin Perinatol* 2018; **42**: 39–48.

European Society of Cardiology. ESC guidelines on the management of cardiovascular diseases during pregnancy: the Task Force on the Management of Cardiovascular Diseases during Pregnancy of the European Society of Cardiology (ESC). *Eur Heart J* 2011; **32**: 3147–97.

Stout K. Pregnancy in women with congenital heart disease: the importance of evaluation and counselling. *Heart* 2005; **91**: 713–14.

Swan L. Congenital heart disease in pregnancy. *Best Pract Res Clin Obstet Gynaecol* 2014; **28**: 495–506.

Pulmonary hypertension and Eisenmenger's syndrome

Primary pulmonary hypertension is associated with an extremely high maternal mortality (40–60%) and is one of the few remaining maternal conditions in which pregnancy is considered absolutely contraindicated.

Secondary pulmonary hypertension may occur as a result of chronic pulmonary disease (e.g. connective tissue disease) or congenital heart disease such as severe aortic or mitral stenosis, or, more usually, chronic left-to-right shunt, and tends to have a lower mortality rate. These conditions are also associated with high maternal mortality, particularly left-to-right shunt leading to Eisenmenger's syndrome (reversal of the shunt when pulmonary pressures exceed systemic pressures).

Although women are advised against pregnancy and termination is offered, many do not heed this advice.

Problems and special considerations

Pulmonary artery pressures may be close to systemic arterial pressures and are associated with a high pulmonary vascular resistance. There is right ventricular hypertrophy and a relatively fixed low cardiac output. Increases in pulmonary vascular resistance, decreases in systemic vascular resistance or falls in cardiac output can all have catastrophic and potentially fatal consequences. In Eisenmenger's syndrome, peripheral vasodilatation increases shunt across the heart and thus worsens hypoxaemia and leads to a low cardiac output state.

The increased cardiac output that occurs during pregnancy is poorly tolerated, since it causes further increase in pulmonary artery and right ventricular pressures, and volume overload. Right ventricular dilatation and tricuspid regurgitation may occur, and left ventricular function and cardiac output may become increasingly impaired. The major haemodynamic changes occurring during parturition and the puerperium can prove fatal. Major haemorrhage causing hypovolaemia, or autotransfusion with the third stage of labour causing volume overload, are both poorly tolerated.

Preterm delivery and fetal growth restriction are both likely and perinatal mortality is increased, particularly in the presence of cyanosis.

Management options

Close antenatal monitoring is essential, and women with pulmonary hypertension are frequently admitted for inpatient care in the third trimester of pregnancy or even earlier – most women resting more in hospital than is possible at home. Beta-blockers, diuretics and pulmonary vasodilators may be used for symptom relief. Prophylactic anticoagulation is controversial, but prophylactic heparin is often given in addition to simple antithromboembolism measures such as graduated compression stockings. Care must be taken to avoid prolonged immobility in hospital. The risks of aortocaval compression if women adopt supine or semi-supine positions are not confined to labour, and the lateral position should be adopted for any antenatal examinations of mother or fetus.

Pulmonary hypertension itself is not considered an indication for caesarean section, though it may be required should maternal condition deteriorate or if there is fetal compromise. Recent data from a large European registry of pregnancies and cardiac disease reported that nearly two-thirds of deliveries in women with pulmonary hypertension were by caesarean section, although a third of these were unplanned. The advantages of choosing to deliver by caesarean section include avoiding a prolonged second stage and the adverse effects of bearing down, and also avoiding uncontrolled vaginal haemorrhage. Continuous oxygen therapy may be beneficial for both mother and fetus. The mother may describe 'funny spells', and these should be taken seriously as potential indicators of episodes of severe pulmonary hypertension. Induction of labour is an option if the cervix is favourable, but is associated with a higher rate of operative delivery than spontaneous labour.

For delivery, maternal monitoring should include electrocardiography and invasive right atrial and arterial blood pressure measurement. Use of a pulmonary artery catheter is more controversial and has been associated with an increased risk of thrombosis; other methods of cardiac output monitoring have been used intraoperatively. Scrupulous care must be taken to avoid accidental injection of air, because of the risk of systemic embolism in women with shunts. Episodes of hypotension should be treated promptly with fluids or vasopressors to stop an increase in right-to-left flow.

Oxygen is a readily available and easily administered pulmonary vasodilator and should be given continuously throughout labour and delivery. Hypoxia, hypercarbia and acidosis all tend to increase pulmonary artery pressure and pulmonary vascular resistance. Prolonged labour, use of systemic opioids and inadequate hydration are all, therefore, risk factors for these women.

Regional analgesia has been used successfully. Epidural infusions or intermittent boluses of low concentrations of local anaesthetic and opioid (0.0625–0.1% bupivacaine with fentanyl 2.0–2.5 µg/ml; alternatively opioid alone) provide good analgesia without compromising haemodynamic stability. Combined spinal–epidural analgesia is a suitable alternative but offers little advantage over low-dose epidural analgesia, except possibly more profound analgesia if opioids alone are used. Use of air to identify the epidural space should be avoided because of the risk of air embolism.

Although general anaesthesia has traditionally been recommended for women with pulmonary hypertension, regional anaesthesia has been successfully used for both Eisenmenger's syndrome and primary pulmonary hypertension. It is imperative to use a slow titration technique and invasive central monitoring if regional anaesthesia is chosen.

General anaesthesia offers potentially greater haemodynamic stability, and the opportunity to minimise oxygen consumption by eliminating the work of breathing and maximising arterial oxygen saturation. It also facilitates transoesophageal echocardiography and the administration of inhaled pulmonary vasodilators such as 100% oxygen, nebulised prostacyclin or nitric oxide; use of the latter two has been described, although their place in improving oxygenation is still uncertain. However, the cardiodepressant effects of general anaesthesia with associated reduction in cardiac output are still hazards for these women, as is the potentially increased risk of thromboembolism. A high-dose opioid 'cardiac' general anaesthetic provides maximal haemodynamic stability. There is no particular advantage in elective ventilation postoperatively, but high-dependency or intensive care nursing is mandatory.

Postoperative and post-delivery analgesia can be provided by patient-controlled intravenous opioids or by epidural or intrathecal opioids. Intensive care admission should be planned, and invasive monitoring must be continued for several days; women with pulmonary hypertension are frequently successfully delivered, only to die during the first 2 weeks after delivery because of acute increases in pulmonary vascular resistance coupled with volume overload. Mortality is associated with pulmonary hypertensive crises, thromboembolism or refractory right heart failure.

Key points

- Pregnancy is extremely hazardous for women with pulmonary hypertension.
- Maternal mortality may be as high as 60%.
- The physiological changes of normal pregnancy are poorly tolerated by women with pulmonary hypertension.
- Hypovolaemia and any increase in pulmonary vascular resistance must be avoided.
- Cautious use of regional analgesia for vaginal delivery, with full invasive cardiovascular monitoring, is recommended.
- Both general and epidural anaesthesia have been used for operative delivery; both have significant risks.

Further reading

Curry R, Swan L, Steer PJ. Cardiac disease in pregnancy. *Curr Opin Obstet Gynecol* 2009; **21**: 508–13.

Lane CR, Trow TK. Pregnancy and pulmonary hypertension. *Clin Chest Med* 2011; **32**: 165–74.

Rex S, Devroe S. Anesthesia for pregnant women with pulmonary hypertension. *Curr Opin Anaesthesiol* 2016; **29**: 273–81.

Sliwa K, van Hagen IM, Budts W, *et al.*; ROPAC investigators. Pulmonary hypertension and pregnancy outcomes: data from the Registry Of Pregnancy and Cardiac Disease (ROPAC) of the European Society of Cardiology. *Eur J Heart Fail* 2016; **18**: 1119–28.

Chapter 100

Ischaemic heart disease

Myocardial infarction (MI) during pregnancy is uncommon, with a reported incidence of ~2–6 per 100,000 deliveries; these figures do not, however, include unstable angina. In the 2016 report of the Confidential Enquiries into Maternal Deaths (CEMD), ischaemic heart disease accounted for over a fifth of all cardiac deaths. The risk of coronary syndromes is increased fourfold in pregnancy, owing to altered physiology such as hypercoagulability, increased myocardial demand and vascular dysfunction.

Ischaemic heart disease in the antenatal population may result from atherosclerotic coronary artery disease or acute coronary artery dissection. Risk factors include smoking, obesity, hypertension, older maternal age and the use of illegal drugs, particularly crack cocaine, which can cause hypertension, left ventricular hypertrophy and coronary artery vasospasm. Postpartum MI has been reported as a complication of pre-eclampsia. Women who have had previous MI, with or without previous coronary artery bypass grafting, may also present to the obstetrician and obstetric anaesthetist.

Problems and special considerations

A high index of suspicion is necessary. Myocardial ischaemia may not be considered in the differential diagnoses of a pregnant woman presenting with chest pain, and the presentation may be atypical. The woman who has been using cocaine is frequently an unreliable historian, and may conceal or deny her drug abuse. Clinical examination and investigations may be difficult to interpret; a systolic murmur is common during pregnancy, and it should be remembered that left axis deviation with non-specific ST and T wave changes is commonly seen in the healthy pregnant patient. Serial ECGs to detect dynamic changes are useful, as is cardiac troponin I since it is unaffected by pregnancy, labour and delivery.

Maternal mortality of acute MI during pregnancy has been reported to be as high as 30–50%, with the highest mortality associated with MI during the third trimester and also delivery within two weeks of an MI. Recent studies suggest a lower mortality rate, of under 10%.

Myocardial ischaemia and infarction caused by cocaine are associated with a high incidence of cardiac arrhythmias.

Antenatal considerations include: the use of antiplatelets and anticoagulants; planning of place, time and mode of delivery; use of intrapartum invasive monitoring; and choice of analgesia and anaesthesia for delivery.

Management options

These women should be managed by a multidisciplinary team. Reported treatments include drug therapy, percutaneous coronary intervention, the use of intra-aortic balloon counter-pulsation and coronary artery bypass grafting.

Mode of delivery

There is no consensus of opinion in the literature about the preferred mode of delivery of a woman who has had an antenatal MI, nor about the method of anaesthesia. Vaginal delivery eliminates the stress of surgery and the need to provide anaesthesia. The risk of peripartum thromboembolism is also reduced, as is the potential for obstetric haemorrhage. However, induction of labour carries an increased risk of further obstetric intervention, whereas allowing spontaneous onset of labour is unpredictable. Pushing in the second stage should be limited. Caesarean delivery can be optimally timed to permit senior staff from all concerned specialties to be involved. There is adequate time to institute full invasive monitoring and to organise cardiovascular support, but surgical intervention increases the risks of complications. Blood loss may precipitate cardiac ischaemia in women with pre-existing coronary artery disease.

Monitoring

Most authorities suggest using intra-arterial pressure monitoring, pulse oximetry and continuous electrocardiographic monitoring. The use of pulmonary artery pressure monitoring is now not advised as it is associated with significant risks that may outweigh potential benefits. Central venous catheterisation allows infusion of cardioactive drugs as well as an additional mode of monitoring, albeit of right-sided pressures only.

Analgesia and anaesthesia

For analgesia in labour, epidural analgesia minimises haemodynamic instability caused by the pain and stress of labour. Use of low-dose local anaesthetic and opioid infusions or boluses avoids the risk of hypotension. Combined spinal–epidural analgesia would also be a suitable alternative.

Both 'cardiac' (high-dose opioid) general anaesthesia and epidural anaesthesia have been used successfully for caesarean section. The major concerns with general anaesthesia are the uncontrolled hypertensive response to tracheal intubation, the risks of potentially life-threatening arrhythmias (particularly in cocaine users) and the need for postoperative ventilatory support because of the high doses of opioids used.

The major concern with regional anaesthesia is haemodynamic instability caused by rapid onset of sympathetic blockade. For this reason, if a regional technique is chosen, a slow incremental technique is preferred to single-shot spinal anaesthesia; epidural, continuous spinal, and combined spinal–epidural anaesthesia have been used successfully.

Oxytocic drugs

Ergometrine causes acute hypertension and is contraindicated in women with ischaemic heart disease; its use has been implicated in maternal deaths in recent CEMD reports. Large intravenous boluses (> 5 U) of oxytocin cause transient hypotension and may compromise coronary filling; it is therefore preferable to use an intravenous infusion of oxytocin during management of the third stage of labour. Carboprost can cause significant haemodynamic effects and is often avoided in patients with known cardiac disease. Non-pharmacological methods of haemostasis should be considered early, to avoid major blood loss and reduce the use of drugs that may cause haemodynamic compromise.

Puerperium

The fluid shifts that occur during the early postpartum period contribute to potential haemodynamic instability at this time. High-dependency nursing and medical care is mandatory; intensive cardiovascular monitoring should be maintained for at least 24–48 hours after delivery. Epidural opioids are recommended for provision of postoperative analgesia. The use of prophylactic anticoagulants should be considered for 3–6 months post-delivery.

Key points

- Myocardial infarction during pregnancy has a high maternal mortality.
- The association between myocardial infarction and cocaine consumption should be considered.
- Management of labour and delivery is based on maintaining haemodynamic stability and minimising myocardial oxygen consumption.

Further reading

Bush N, Nelson-Piercy C, Spark P, *et al.* Myocardial infarction in pregnancy and postpartum in the UK. *Eur J Prev Cardiol* 2013; **20**: 12–20.

Fryearson J, Adamson DL. Heart disease in pregnancy: ischaemic heart disease. *Best Pract Res Clin Obstet Gynaecol* 2014; **28**: 551–62.

Kealey A. Coronary artery disease and myocardial infarction in pregnancy: a review of epidemiology, diagnosis, and medical and surgical management. *Can J Cardiol* 2010; **26**: 185–9.

Knight M, Nair M, Tuffnell D, *et al.*; MBRRACE-UK. *Saving Lives, Improving Mothers' Care: Surveillance of maternal deaths in the UK 2012–14 and lessons learned to inform maternity care from the UK and Ireland Confidential Enquiries into Maternal Deaths and Morbidity 2009–14.* Oxford: National Perinatal Epidemiology Unit, University of Oxford, 2016.

Roth A, Elkayam U. Acute myocardial infarction associated with pregnancy. *J Am Coll Cardiol* 2008; **52**: 171–80.

Chapter 101

Endocrine disease

The most common endocrine disorder affecting pregnancy is diabetes mellitus, which is considered separately (see Chapter 102). Although there are several other conditions that may have obstetric implications, most have little specific obstetric anaesthetic relevance over and above considerations applicable to the non-pregnant state.

Special considerations and management options

Thyroid disease

Anaesthetic implications are as for non-pregnant patients. Goitre may increase in size in pregnancy. Fetal morbidity includes neonatal encephalopathy and goitre with maternal antithyroid treatment in rare cases. Acute hyperthyroidism ('thyroid storm') is an obstetric emergency that may cause premature labour, fetal loss or, rarely, fetal hyperthyroidism, or potentially life-threatening cardiac dysfunction.

Parathyroid disease

Primary hyperparathyroidism is associated with increased maternofetal morbidity with an increased incidence of pancreatitis, pre-eclampsia and fetal loss secondary to severe hypercalcaemia. Medical management includes hydration and oral phosphates, and parathyroidectomy may be required.

Adrenal disease

Hypoadrenalism is a rare cause of collapse on the labour ward. Patients receiving steroid therapy may require extra dosage peripartum (see Chapter 150, *Steroid therapy*). Cushing's syndrome is rare in pregnancy. Treatment strategies include surgical resection and medical therapy; in advanced pregnancy, treatment may be limited to the management of clinical manifestations such as hypertension.

Phaeochromocytoma is a rare but well-recognised cause of hypertension in pregnancy and may present as part of the multiple endocrine neoplasia syndrome. The condition may initially be misdiagnosed as pregnancy-related hypertensive disease, causing a delay in treatment and a peripartum maternal mortality of up to 50%. Unlike gestational hypertension or pre-eclampsia, hypertension associated with phaeochromocytoma is of paroxysmal nature and may develop before 20 weeks' gestation. Medical management is classically with α-blockade first and then β-blockade, ensuring adequate fluid replacement. Magnesium therapy has also been used to control pre- and intraoperative hypertension. Regional anaesthesia has been safely used for labour and vaginal delivery. Combined caesarean section and excision of the tumour has been reported using both regional and general anaesthesia, with appropriate monitoring. More recently there have been reports of an elective two-step procedure, whereby patients are treated medically first, followed by caesarean section and then excision of the tumour.

Neuroendocrine disease

Most of the anaesthetic implications relate to the effects of any intracranial space-occupying lesion. Specific hormonal conditions are managed as for non-pregnant patients. Sheehan's syndrome is pituitary infarction caused by severe hypotension ('pituitary apoplexy'), originally described in association with placental abruption. Pregnant women are thought to be particularly susceptible to this phenomenon because the pituitary gland enlarges during pregnancy by about one-third and its blood supply is consequently more critical.

Other conditions

These are managed as for non-pregnant patients.

Key points

- Diabetes mellitus is the most common and important endocrine disease in pregnancy.
- General management of endocrine disease is as for non-pregnant patients.
- The clinical features of some endocrine disorders may overlap with pregnancy-related changes or conditions; a high index of suspicion is required for timely diagnosis.

Further reading

Biggar MA, Lennard TW. Systematic review of phaeochromocytoma in pregnancy. *Br J Surg* 2013; **100**: 182–90.
Frise CJ, Williamson C. Endocrine disease in pregnancy. *Clin Med (Lond)* 2013; **13**: 176–81.
Kennedy RL, Malabu UH, Jarrod G, *et al.* Thyroid function and pregnancy: before, during and beyond. *J Obstet Gynaecol* 2010; **30**: 774–83.

Chapter 102

Diabetes mellitus

In the general population, diabetes mellitus is present in about 2% of individuals, about half of them undiagnosed. In pregnancy, insulin requirements increase as peripheral sensitivity to insulin decreases (thought to be caused by the opposing action of placental hormones). Thus patients known to have diabetes may become unstable, and otherwise normal subjects may reveal themselves as having gestational diabetes if they cannot meet the increased demands (the latter occurs in up to 2–5% of pregnancies). Most women who develop gestational diabetes recover after pregnancy, although most relapse in subsequent pregnancies at an earlier gestational age, and there is a 50% risk of developing type 2 diabetes in later life.

Current UK guidelines recommend screening for gestational diabetes using the oral glucose tolerance test (OGTT) in pregnant women with risk factors, which include a history or family history of gestational diabetes, raised body mass index (BMI), or previous macrosomic baby. The OGTT includes the administration of 75 g glucose orally, followed by blood glucose measurement after 2 hours. The test is offered at 24–28 weeks' gestation but should be performed earlier in women with a history of gestational diabetes and repeated if the initial results are normal.

Problems and special considerations

Effect of diabetes on the mother

Diabetes has many effects on most organ systems, the most immediately important being renal impairment, cardiovascular disease and central and peripheral neurological disease. Women with long-standing type 1 diabetes, depending on their overall glycaemic control, may already manifest these complications, whereas those women with gestational or type 2 diabetes are usually younger than 40–45 years and systemic effects tend to be less common.

Control of blood sugar

This is important during pregnancy, since poor control is associated with an increased incidence of fetal abnormalities (see below). In pregnancy, insulin requirements increase by up to 50% at term. During labour, it is important to avoid hyper- or hypoglycaemia, the former because it results in maternal and fetal acidosis and the latter because of the risk of impaired neurological function. Insulin requirements may decrease in the first stage but increase in the second stage of labour, although this may depend on other factors such as length of labour, prelabour state, etc.

Effect of diabetes on pregnancy

Women with diabetes have an increased incidence of miscarriage, pregnancy-induced hypertension, polyhydramnios, fetal macrosomia, obstructed labour, caesarean section and preterm labour (the last may not hold for gestational diabetes). There is also an increased incidence of neonatal hypoglycaemia and hyperbilirubinaemia. In type 1 diabetes, there is a 5- to 10-fold incidence of congenital malformation if glycaemic control during pregnancy is poor, with a 5-fold increase in stillbirth rate and 4- to 5-fold increase in perinatal death rate. Good glycaemic control reduces the incidence of congenital malformation to 2%, about twice the normal.

Management options

Before conception, women known to have diabetes should be counselled and their care optimised (ideally, glycosylated haemoglobin concentration < 6.5%).

During pregnancy, careful dietary advice, and possibly also pharmacological intervention, aims to maintain normal blood glucose concentrations. Ideal glucose levels are below 5.3 mmol/l fasting, 7.8 mmol/l 1 hour postprandial and 6.4 mmol/L 2 hours postprandial. Close follow-up of diabetic pregnant women is required, with monitoring of glycaemic control as well as screening for infections, since diabetic ketoacidosis may be precipitated by infection, as in the non-pregnant state. It has been recommended that diabetic pregnant women with comorbidities such as obesity or autonomic neuropathy be reviewed by an anaesthetist in the third trimester of their pregnancy.

Increasing insulin requirements in pregnancy may reflect reduced placental function and may be an indication for induction of labour. Women with absent warning signs of hypoglycaemia should be advised against driving (pregnancy may alter awareness of hypoglycaemia, which occurs particularly in the first trimester). With regard to the fetus, women with diabetes should be offered a detailed fetal cardiac scan at 20 weeks' gestation.

During labour, most authorities advocate continuous glucose/insulin infusions; a suitable regimen comprises a 5% glucose infusion plus 20 mmol/l potassium chloride with a continuous insulin infusion using a sliding scale, according to regular (30–60-minute) blood glucose concentration monitoring (Table 102.1). The aim is to maintain blood glucose concentrations at 4–7 mmol/l; if this cannot be achieved the entire insulin infusion scale is increased by 1 U/h. If blood glucose concentration repeatedly falls below 4 mmol/l, the 5% dextrose may be changed for 10% glucose. Urine should be tested, e.g. 4-hourly, for glucose and ketones. Avoidance of glucose during labour has been popular previously, but leads to maternal and fetal acidosis. Most authorities advise continuous fetal monitoring

Table 102.1 Sample sliding scale for insulin during labour in diabetic women

Blood glucose concentration (mmol/l)	≤ 3.9	4.0–5.9	6.0–8.9	9.0–11.9	12.0–14.9	15.0–17.9	≥ 18.0
Insulin infusion rate (U soluble insulin/h)	0.5	1	2	3	4	5	6

throughout labour, and a paediatrician should attend all deliveries, with neonatal unit admission prepared. For elective caesarean section, the same intravenous regimen is started in the morning, the patient having been nil-by-mouth since midnight and having omitted her usual morning insulin.

Insulin requirements fall rapidly once delivery has occurred, and the insulin infusion rate should be halved once the baby has been born. Most women with gestational diabetes do not need insulin postpartum; insulin-dependent diabetic patients may be given a subcutaneous dose of soluble insulin (e.g. 5 U) when ready to eat and drink, and the infusion stopped 60 minutes later.

Management as far as regional or general anaesthesia is concerned is along standard lines, although the former is especially desirable. In labour, regional analgesia is thought to be beneficial by reducing catecholamine levels and thus avoiding anti-insulin effects and the propensity for acidosis. Care should be taken to assess the mother for the complications of diabetes, as above. In addition, of especial relevance to general anaesthesia, autonomic neuropathy may be associated with reduced gastric emptying, and a syndrome of stiff joints has been described in which difficult tracheal intubation has featured. The syndrome is suggested by the 'prayer sign' in which the patient is unable to lay the palmar surfaces of her index fingers fully flat against one another when pressing her palms together as if praying; when viewed from the side there is a space between the proximal phalangeal joints. The syndrome has also been implicated in causing reduced compliance of the epidural space, with the risk of spinal cord ischaemia when large volumes are injected epidurally.

Fluid therapy should be separate from intravenous dextrose/insulin; thus two intravenous cannulae are usually required if anaesthetic intervention is needed. Hartmann's solution may result in a small increase in blood glucose concentration caused by gluconeogenesis from lactate metabolism, although this is rarely a problem in practice. Patients should receive adequate diabetic follow-up postpartum. Patients who have presented with gestational diabetes in particular should be followed up with a 6-week fasting plasma glucose check, and this should be checked annually thereafter.

Diabetic ketoacidosis in pregnancy is a rare but potentially life-threatening complication that may occur in up to 3% of pregnant women with diabetes. Principles of management are as for non-pregnant patients, namely removal of the trigger, fluid resuscitation, and the correction of hyperglycaemia and metabolic derangements such as acidosis and hyperkalaemia. Particular attention must be paid to the optimisation of fetal oxygenation and the stabilisation of maternal condition before proceeding with a caesarean section for fetal indications.

Key points

- Diabetes mellitus is associated with increased incidence of fetal malformations, macrosomia and death, especially if diabetic control is poor.
- Regional analgesia and anaesthesia are especially desirable.
- Insulin and glucose infusions are used in labour.
- Insulin requirements fall rapidly after delivery.
- Diabetic ketoacidosis is rare in pregnancy but can carry significant maternal and fetal morbidity.

Further reading

Association of Anaesthetists of Great Britain and Ireland. Peri-operative management of the surgical patient with diabetes 2015. *Anaesthesia* 2015; **70**: 1427–40.

de Veciana M. Diabetes ketoacidosis in pregnancy. *Semin Perinatol* 2013; **37**: 267–73.

McCance DR. Diabetes in pregnancy. *Best Pract Res Clin Obstet Gynaecol* 2015; **29**: 685–99.

National Institute for Health and Care Excellence. *Diabetes in Pregnancy: Management from Preconception to the Postnatal Period*. NICE Guideline NG 3. London: NICE, 2015. www.nice.org.uk/guidance/ng3 (accessed December 2018).

Anaemia and polycythaemia

Anaemia in pregnancy is seen in around 40% of pregnant women worldwide (around 20% in the UK). Several definitions exist; the British Committee for Standards in Haematology defines it as a haemoglobin level < 110 g/l in the first trimester, < 105 g/l in the second and third trimesters and < 100 g/l in the postnatal period.

Pregnancy is associated with a 20–30% increase in red cell mass. Circulating plasma volume can increase by 30–50% in single pregnancies but may double in multiple pregnancies. There is therefore a physiological dilutional 'anaemia'. This increase in red cell mass and the needs of the developing fetus increase requirement for iron and folate, which often need to be supplemented. Normal iron absorption is around 1–2 mg a day; however, requirements may be as high as 7.5 mg a day in late pregnancy. Many women start pregnancy with depleted iron stores and a low haemoglobin concentration, and the likelihood of this increases with subsequent pregnancies.

Polycythaemia in pregnancy is rare and is usually secondary to other disease processes such as cyanotic heart disease. The underlying problem is usually more significant than the haemoglobin concentration itself. Primary polycythaemia (rubra vera) is a neoplastic disease more often seen in older patients than in the childbearing population.

Problems and special considerations

Anaemia

Normal vaginal delivery of a single fetus is associated with a blood loss of around 500 ml, but this may double with twin deliveries. Caesarean section is associated with a blood loss of 500–1000 ml. Following delivery, there is a fall in plasma volume caused by diuresis; this partially compensates for the drop in haemoglobin concentration resulting from blood loss.

Mothers who are already anaemic have less reserve than normal and may thus be more susceptible to the effects of haemorrhage. Since they rely on an even greater increase in cardiac output than normal to maintain oxygen delivery, cardiac depression (e.g. caused by general anaesthesia) may have profound effects on maternal and fetal oxygenation. Maternal myocardial ischaemia is also more common. Haemorrhage in Jehovah's Witnesses is a particular problem and an important cause of maternal death.

Pernicious anaemia is extremely rare in pregnancy, but the presence of a macrocytic anaemia may prompt investigation. Folate and B_{12} deficiency may cause congenital malformations in the neonate, abruption and haemorrhage. Maternal complications include neurological complications such as subacute combined degeneration of the cord. Aplastic anaemia has been reported in pregnancy and in some cases has resolved following delivery.

Polycythaemia

There have been few published cases of polycythaemia complicating pregnancy. There may be associated thrombocytopenia or thrombocythaemia. Thrombocytopenia may be dilutional and may not reflect function. Thrombotic events (arterial and venous) do occur, and prophylactic aspirin and heparin have been given to prevent them.

In cyanotic heart disease, a haemoglobin concentration greater than 160 g/l is associated with poor fetal outcome. This probably represents both a marker of severity of the underlying disease and impairment of uteroplacental oxygenation resulting from increased blood viscosity.

Coagulation times may be artefactually prolonged in severe polycythaemia.

Management options

Antenatally, treatment with iron and vitamin B_{12} supplements is routine in pregnancy to treat and prevent anaemia. In some cases of extreme iron deficiency, parenteral iron and erythropoietin have been used.

As long as the above potential problems are considered, anaesthetic management in general is routine. Simple measures such as maintenance of normothermia and normocalcaemia may help support normal coagulation mechanisms and minimise blood loss in the intra- and postpartum periods. In anaemia, the threshold for transfusion should be lower than normal. Parenteral iron and erythropoietin have also been used postpartum, especially in Jehovah's Witnesses – management of whom must include senior staff.

In polycythaemia, regional analgesia and anaesthesia may be precluded by recent administration of heparin, although the benefits usually outweigh the risk of epidural haematoma.

Key points

- A drop in haemoglobin concentration during pregnancy is normal.
- Postpartum diuresis partially compensates for peripartum blood loss.
- Polycythaemia in pregnancy is usually secondary to underlying disease.

Further reading

Achebe MM, Gafter-Gvili A. How I treat anemia in pregnancy: iron, cobalamin, and folate. *Blood* 2017; **129**: 940–9.
Annamraju H, Pavord S. Anaemia in pregnancy. *Br J Hosp Med* 2016; **77**: 584–8.
Goonewardene M, Shehata M, Hamad A. Anaemia in pregnancy. *Best Pract Res Clin Obstet Gynaecol* 2012; **26**: 3–24.
Muñoz M, Acheson AG, Auerbach M, *et al.* International consensus statement on the peri-operative management of anaemia and iron deficiency. *Anaesthesia* 2017; **72**: 233–47.

Chapter 104

Deep-vein thrombosis and pulmonary embolism

After an initial fall in the number of maternal deaths caused by thrombotic disease following the issuance of national guidelines on thromboprophylaxis in pregnancy and the puerperium in 2004, thrombosis and thromboembolism feature again in recent Confidential Enquiries into Maternal Deaths (CEMD) reports as the leading cause of direct maternal deaths during pregnancy and in the first 6 weeks postpartum. There has been no significant change in mortality due to venous thromboembolism (VTE) since 2009. The condition is associated with a high morbidity and mortality rate; the latter is around 15% with untreated calf vein thrombosis and is even higher with iliofemoral thrombosis, which is more common in pregnancy. Untreated pulmonary embolus (PE) in pregnancy may recur and is associated with a mortality of 25%.

Problems and special considerations

Physiological changes in pregnancy favour coagulation, making pregnant women far more likely to develop VTE than non-pregnant women. In addition, obesity and the gravid uterus may cause venous stasis while lying down and encourage thrombus formation. Other risk factors include bed rest, dehydration, coincident thrombophilia, pre-eclampsia, greater maternal age, higher parity, patient/family history, smoking, and caesarean section (the last by up to eight times).

Diagnosis of deep-vein thrombosis (DVT) in pregnancy may be difficult; however, a high index of suspicion is required since mortality audits have identified patients with classic symptoms and signs who were not treated effectively. Not only is the diagnosis often not considered in pregnancy, but women may be denied appropriate investigation because of their pregnant state.

Management options

Treatment of thromboembolism in pregnancy

Suspected DVT in pregnancy should be investigated with duplex ultrasonography and venography if necessary. A raised concentration of D-dimers or other fibrin degradation products may not be helpful, as both may be raised in normal pregnancy; however, low levels make the diagnosis unlikely. Suspected PE in pregnancy should be investigated with chest radiography, arterial blood gas analysis and electrocardiography, followed by a ventilation–perfusion scan or computerised tomography pulmonary angiogram depending on local protocols and availability. Magnetic resonance imaging and specialised echocardiography have also been used to diagnose PE. Bilateral duplex lower limb ultrasonography should be performed if necessary.

Treatment of VTE is with heparin, which is preferred to warfarin because of the latter's fetal effects. Intravenous unfractionated heparin has now largely been replaced by subcutaneous low-molecular-weight heparin, and this should not be delayed while awaiting investigation. Unfractionated heparin may be considered in patients with renal dysfunction, in situations where rapid reversibility of the anticoagulant action is required, and in the treatment of massive PE. Full anticoagulation precludes regional analgesia and anaesthesia (see Chapter 106, *Coagulopathy*) and can be a problem when pregnancy is complicated by ante- or postpartum bleeding.

In severe cases with cardiovascular instability, thrombolytic therapy may be required. The administration of potent intravenous fibrinolytic drugs in these women may result in massive obstetric haemorrhage or fetal bleeding. Some patients may require dispersion under radiological control or open embolectomy.

The use of vena caval filters in pregnancy has not been properly evaluated. Although there have been reports of the successful use of vena caval filters in pregnancy, many authors feel that their use is not justified because of the high risk of angulation and movement as a result of the pressure of the gravid uterus. However, they could be of use in women in whom anticoagulation is contraindicated or in those with recurrent VTE despite pharmacological treatment.

Thromboprophylaxis in pregnancy

Increasing numbers of women are being given prophylaxis against arterial or venous thrombosis in pregnancy. In the 2018 CEMD, one-third of deaths occurred in the antenatal period; it is therefore recommended that risk assessment for VTE should be undertaken at booking and repeated at any hospital admission, intrapartum or immediately postpartum and before discharge from hospital.

Some women have a hereditary or acquired thrombophilia or a past medical history of thrombosis. In addition, some obstetricians treat women with a history of stillbirth, intrauterine death and miscarriage with prophylactic doses of antithrombotics such as aspirin, heparin or both. Other women, for example those with prosthetic heart valves, require continuation of pre-pregnancy therapeutic doses of antithrombotics. Warfarin is teratogenic when used in the first trimester, and it is now rarely used in pregnancy. Women with metal heart valves are at particular risk of valve thrombosis and are therefore an exception (see Chapter 97, *Valvular heart disease*). Evaluation of women who may require anticoagulation should ideally be done before pregnancy.

Thromboprophylaxis following caesarean section

VTE occurs in around 1% of women following vaginal delivery and 2–3% following caesarean section. A significant proportion of fatal PE occurs 2–6 weeks postpartum. Guidance on the prophylaxis of VTE following caesarean section lists risk factors for which prophylactic low-molecular-weight heparin should be given. Many units prefer to treat all women as high-risk and give prophylaxis routinely unless there is a contraindication, in order to reduce the chance of omitting prophylaxis accidentally.

Increased doses of heparin are required in pregnancy and especially in obesity (Table 104.1). Neither warfarin nor heparin is excreted in breast milk.

Table 104.1 Recommended daily doses of low-molecular-weight heparin for thromboprophylaxis in pregnancy and the puerperium

Weight	Enoxaparin	Dalteparin	Tinzaparin
< 50 kg	20 mg od	2500 units od	3500 units od
50–90 kg [a]	40 mg od	5000 units od	4500 units od
91–130 kg	60 mg od or 30 mg bd	7500 units od	7000 units od or 3500 units bd
131–170 kg	80 mg od or 40 mg bd	10,000 units od	9000 units od or 4500 units bd
> 170 kg	0.6 mg/kg/day	75 units/kg/day	75 units/kg/day

[a] bd if at particularly high risk.

Adapted with permission from Royal College of Obstetricians and Gynaecologists. *Reducing the Risk of Venous Thromboembolism during Pregnancy and the Puerperium*. Green-top Guideline 37a. London: RCOG, 2015. www.rcog.org.uk/en/guidelines-research-services/guidelines/gtg37a.

Key points

- Venous thromboembolism (VTE) carries a high mortality if untreated.
- Low-molecular-weight heparin is the treatment of choice for VTE.
- Prophylaxis against VTE should be considered in all women undergoing caesarean section.

Further reading

Durán-Mendicuti A, Sodickson A. Imaging evaluation of the pregnant patient with suspected pulmonary embolism. *Int J Obstet Anesth* 2011; **20**: 51–9.

Guimicheva B, Czuprynska J, Arya R. The prevention of pregnancy-related venous thromboembolism. *Br J Haematol* 2015; **168**: 163–74.

Knight M, Bunch K, Tuffnell D, *et al.*; MBRRACE-UK. *Saving Lives, Improving Mothers' Care: Lessons learned to inform maternity care from the UK and Ireland Confidential Enquiries into Maternal Deaths and Morbidity 2014–16*. Oxford: National Perinatal Epidemiology Unit, University of Oxford, 2018.

Nelson-Piercy C, on behalf of the MBRRACE-UK thrombosis and thromboembolism chapter writing group. Prevention and treatment of thrombosis and venous thromboembolism. In Knight M, Tuffnell D, Kenyon S, *et al.*; MBRRACE-UK. *Saving Lives, Improving Mothers' Care: Surveillance of maternal deaths in the UK 2011–13 and lessons learned to inform maternity care from the UK and Ireland Confidential Enquiries into Maternal Deaths and Morbidity 2009–13*. Oxford: National Perinatal Epidemiology Unit, University of Oxford, 2015, pp. 42–52.

Royal College of Obstetricians and Gynaecologists. *Reducing the Risk of Venous Thromboembolism during Pregnancy and the Puerperium*. Green-top Guideline 37a. London: RCOG, 2015. www.rcog.org.uk/en/guidelines-research-services/guidelines/gtg37a (accessed December 2018).

Royal College of Obstetricians and Gynaecologists. *Thromboembolic Disease in Pregnancy and the Puerperium: Acute Management*. Green-top Guideline 37b. London: RCOG, 2015. www.rcog.org.uk/en/guidelines-research-services/guidelines/gtg37b (accessed December 2018).

Thrombophilia

Thrombophilia has been defined as a familial or acquired abnormality of haemostasis likely to predispose to thrombosis. Up to 30–50% of patients with a history of venous thromboembolism may have a congenital thrombophilia, and others may have a detectable phospholipid autoantibody. This is a developing area, which may yet demonstrate further congenital or acquired factors explaining a propensity to thrombosis.

Problems and special considerations

Pregnancy is associated with a physiological hypercoagulable state. When a pre-existing thrombophilia is present, thrombosis may occur within the uterus causing failure of implantation; within the placenta causing fetal loss, abruption, pre-eclampsia, fetal growth restriction and fetal distress in labour; or in the systemic circulation. Patients with thrombophilia may thus present with subfertility, with a personal or family history of venous and arterial thromboses, or with thromboses in pregnancy or in the puerperium.

Diagnosis is difficult in pregnancy because of the changes in clotting-factor profile associated with pregnancy.

The usual treatment of thrombophilia complicating pregnancy is prophylactic subcutaneous low-molecular-weight heparin combined with low-dose aspirin. This has implications for the timing of regional analgesia and anaesthesia (see Chapter 106, *Coagulopathy*).

Thrombophilias can be classified into congenital and acquired.

Congenital thrombophilias

These deficiencies are heterogeneous; factors may be reduced quantitatively or qualitatively, underlying the importance of haematological input in their management. Subtle, subclinical deficiencies of these factors are very much more common than the figures quoted below (around 1 in 200):

- **Activated protein C resistance (APCR).** The circulating anticoagulant protein C, when activated by thrombin, inactivates factors V and VIII. APCR occurs normally in pregnancy, associated with an increase in factor VIII. This makes diagnosis in pregnancy difficult. In congenital APCR, factor V is more resistant to cleavage by protein C. Factor V Leiden occurs in about 5–7% of the European population and is associated with a rate of thrombosis in pregnancy of about 1 in 400–500. Factor V Leiden is much more sinister when in the homozygous form or when combined with another thrombophilia. In the absence of other risk factors such patients should not need thromboprophylaxis in pregnancy.

- **Antithrombin III (ATIII) deficiency.** This is a rare defect occurring in 1 in 5000 women, but it may account for up to 12% of thromboembolic events in pregnancy. In untreated affected women, 55–68% of pregnancies are complicated by venous thromboembolism. Anticoagulant prophylaxis may be required throughout pregnancy and for at least 3 months postpartum. Discontinuation of heparin at the time of delivery and administration of ATIII concentrate has been advocated by some authors, but this is controversial.
- **Protein C or protein S deficiency.** This occurs in 1 in 15,000 pregnancies and is associated with a rate of venous thrombosis of up to 25% (protein S is a cofactor for protein C). Treatment with heparin throughout pregnancy and the puerperium is controversial. The risk of thrombosis is greatest postpartum in both protein C and S deficiencies, and several authors suggest thromboprophylaxis for this period only.
- **Other causes.** These include hyperhomocystinaemia and mutations of the prothrombin gene.

Acquired thrombophilia

The antiphospholipid syndrome is the most common cause of acquired thrombophilia. Autoantibodies against cell membrane phospholipids, including lupus anticoagulant and anticardiolipin antibodies, may lead to intravascular thrombosis which may lead to fetal loss. There is some evidence that other as yet unidentified autoantibodies may also cause thrombosis and miscarriage.

The lupus anticoagulant is so called because it causes a prolongation of the activated partial thromboplastin time even when diluted (because the autoantibody binds to phospholipid in the assay). However, it is associated with a thrombotic tendency. It may occur on its own (hence antiphospholipid syndrome) but may also occur as part of various autoimmune diseases such as systemic lupus erythematosus. Anticardiolipin antibodies are detected by using an immunoassay.

Of women with recurrent miscarriage (three or more), 15% have persistently positive results for phospholipid antibodies. If untreated, 90% will have spontaneous abortions or stillbirths in subsequent pregnancies. Lupus anticoagulant is detected in ~30% of cases and anticardiolipin antibodies in ~70%. Clinical features of the antiphospholipid syndrome are recurrent fetal loss, thrombosis (arterial and venous), thrombocytopenia, haemolytic anaemia, hypertension, pulmonary hypertension and livedo reticularis. Antiphospholipid syndrome is associated with a 5% incidence of thromboembolism or cerebrovascular accident in pregnancy. Rarely, a severe generalised thrombotic state may lead to multi-organ failure.

Management options

Women with a strong personal or family history of thrombosis and a poor obstetric history should be screened for known causes of thrombophilia.

Patients are at high risk of obstetric intervention in labour and may benefit from epidural analgesia and regional anaesthesia for delivery and caesarean section. The decision to site an epidural should be based on the dose and interval after heparin administration and the potential benefit to the patient. Ideally, women who are likely to be receiving heparin at the time of delivery should discuss a management plan with an anaesthetist in an assessment clinic. In the majority of cases the benefits of regional analgesia and anaesthesia far outweigh the risk of epidural haematoma.

Key points

- Thrombophilias are a significant cause of fetal loss in pregnancy.
- The adverse effects on maternal and fetal health are treatable.
- The risks and benefits of regional analgesia and anaesthesia should be considered antenatally if possible.

Further reading

Bates SM, Greer IA, Middeldorp S, *et al.* VTE, thrombophilia, antithrombotic therapy, and pregnancy: antithrombotic therapy and prevention of thrombosis, 9th edn: American College of Chest Physicians Evidence-based Clinical Practice Guidelines. *Chest* 2012; **141** (2 Suppl): e691S–736S.

Danza A, Ruiz-Irastorza G, Khamashta M. Antiphospholipid syndrome in obstetrics. *Best Pract Res Clin Obstet Gynaecol* 2012; **26**: 65–76.

Gray G, Nelson-Piercy C. Thromboembolic disorders in obstetrics. *Best Pract Res Clin Obstet Gynaecol* 2012; **26**: 53–64.

Royal College of Obstetricians and Gynaecologists. *Reducing the Risk of Thromboembolism During Pregnancy and the Puerperium.* Green-top Guideline 37a. London: RCOG, 2015. www.rcog.org.uk/en/guidelines-research-services/guidelines/gtg37a (accessed December 2018).

Coagulopathy

Normal coagulation is important to the obstetric anaesthetist for two reasons: firstly because of the potential risk of spinal haematoma following regional analgesia and anaesthesia, and secondly because of the risk of antepartum and postpartum haemorrhage.

Problems and special considerations

In general terms, increased bleeding may arise from defects in the function of:

- **Blood vessels** – e.g. caused by severe infections, metabolic disease (such as hepatic failure, renal failure) or congenital structural abnormalities.
- **Platelets** – caused by reduced numbers (e.g. thrombocytopenia, disseminated intravascular coagulation (DIC)) or impaired function (e.g. antiplatelet drugs).
- **The coagulation system** – caused by congenital disorders (e.g. haemophilia, von Willebrand's disease), acquired coagulation factor dysfunction (e.g. anticoagulant therapy, hepatic failure, vitamin K deficiency, DIC) or increased fibrinolysis.

Management options

Specific disorders should be managed according to the underlying pathology and in conjunction with haematologists. In the absence of a known or potential haemostatic disorder that may be suggested by eliciting a history, coagulation studies are not generally indicated as screening tools in healthy parturients. It has been suggested that regional blockade can be performed as long as the activated partial thromboplastin time ratio (APTTR) or international normalised ratio (INR) is less than 1.5, although this is controversial. Symptoms of excessive bruising or bleeding should be sought, since they may signify increased risk of bleeding in borderline cases.

In recent years, more research has been directed at establishing the usefulness of point-of-care coagulation tests such as thromboelastography/thromboelastometry (TEG/ROTEM) in the assessment of coagulation status in pregnant women. Information provided by these techniques may aid decision making in major obstetric haemorrhage, especially as part of a validated transfusion protocol algorithm. Other tools such as platelet function analysis have been described, but their role in clinical practice is yet to be established.

Increasing numbers of women are presenting in pregnancy taking anticoagulant therapy. Whereas full anticoagulation is a contraindication to regional analgesia and anaesthesia, it should be possible to time regional analgesia and anaesthesia for prophylactic regimens. Low-dose aspirin is generally felt to pose minimal risk, although the numbers of mothers who have been studied (receiving both aspirin and regional blockade) are small considering the rarity of the outcome (spinal haematoma). Other antiplatelet drugs are less commonly used in pregnancy, and experience with them is limited.

Prophylactic heparin (especially low-molecular-weight heparin) has been associated with spinal haematoma in non-pregnant patients who receive regional analgesia and anaesthesia, although many of these cases have been associated with relatively large doses in high-risk patients. The risk of therapeutic levels of heparin activity following a supposedly prophylactic dose in pregnancy is unknown. In addition, heparin pharmacokinetics are altered in pregnancy and larger doses are required than in non-pregnant patients, so data from series in which standard (non-pregnant) doses of heparin were used may be misleading. It must be remembered that the duration of action of these agents may be prolonged in women with renal dysfunction.

Most obstetric anaesthetists would follow the guidelines recommended for non-pregnant patients, as shown in Table 106.1. In particular cases where the risks of general anaesthesia are increased (e.g. obesity, cardiac disease), regional anaesthesia may still represent a safer option than general anaesthesia, even within these time limits.

Key points

- Specific coagulation disorders should be managed with the involvement of haematologists.
- Low-dose aspirin therapy is considered to represent minimal risk.
- The risks and benefits of regional analgesia and anaesthesia should be considered for women who are receiving prophylactic heparin therapy. In general, guidelines prohibiting regional blockade or catheter removal within certain periods of heparin administration should be followed.

Further reading

Association of Anaesthetists of Great Britain and Ireland; Obstetric Anaesthetists' Association; Regional Anaesthesia UK. Regional anaesthesia and patients with abnormalities of coagulation. *Anaesthesia* 2013; **68**: 966–72.

Gonzalez-Fiol A, Eisenberger A. Anesthesia implications of coagulation and anticoagulation during pregnancy. *Semin Perinatol* 2014; **38**: 370–7.

Katz D, Beilin Y. Disorders of coagulation in pregnancy. *Br J Anaesth* 2015; **115**: ii75–88.

Pacheco LD, Costantine MM, Saade GR, *et al.* von Willebrand disease and pregnancy: a practical approach for the diagnosis and treatment. *Am J Obstet Gynecol* 2010; **203**: 194–200.

Table 106.1 Relative risk of neuraxial blockade in obstetric patients with abnormalities of coagulation

Risk factor	Normal risk	Increased risk	High risk	Very high risk
LMWH – prophylactic dose	> 12 h	6–12 h	< 6 h	< 6 h
LMWH – therapeutic dose	> 24 h	12–24 h	6–12 h	
UFH – infusion	Stopped > 4 h and APTTR ≤ 1.4			APTTR above normal range
UFH – prophylactic bolus dose	Last given > 4 h	Last given < 4 h		
NSAID + aspirin	Without LMWH	With LMWH dose 12–24 h	With LMWH dose < 12 h	
Warfarin	INR ≤ 1.4	INR ≤ 1.4–1.7	INR ≤ 1.7–2.0	INR > 2.0

General anaesthesia	Starved, not in labour, antacids given		Full stomach or in labour	
Pre-eclampsia	Platelets > 100 × 10⁹/l Within 6 h of block	Platelets 75–100 × 10⁹/l (stable) and normal coagulation tests	Platelets 75–100 × 10⁹/l (decreasing) and normal coagulation tests	Platelets < 75 × 10⁹/l or abnormal coagulation tests with indices ≥ 1.5 or HELLP syndrome
Idiopathic thrombocytopenia	Platelets > 75 × 10⁹/l within 24 h of block	Platelets 50–75 × 10⁹/l	Platelets 20–50 × 10⁹/l	Platelets < 20 × 10⁹/l
Intrauterine fetal death	FBC and coagulation tests normal within 6 h of block	No clinical problems but no investigation results available		With abruption or overt sepsis
Cholestasis	INR ≤ 1.4 within 24 h	No other clinical problems but no investigation results available		

APTTR, activated partial thromboplastin time ratio; FBC, full blood count; HELLP, haemolysis, elevated liver enzymes and low platelet count; INR, international normalised ratio; LMWH, low-molecular-weight heparin; NSAID, non-steroidal anti-inflammatory drug; UFH, unfractionated heparin.
Reproduced with permission from Association of Anaesthetists of Great Britain and Ireland, Obstetric Anaesthetists' Association and Regional Anaesthesia UK. Regional anaesthesia and patients with abnormalities of coagulation. Anaesthesia 2013; **68**: 966–72.

Von Willebrand's disease and haemophilia

Von Willebrand's disease (vWD) is a heterogeneous group of mainly autosomal dominant disorders in which there is reduced or abnormal circulating von Willebrand factor (vWF); it is the most common inherited bleeding disorder.

Von Willebrand factor has two functions. Firstly, it combines with factor VIII in vivo to produce a procoagulant complex (VIIIc) that protects factor VIII from premature destruction. Hence, factor VIII activity may be reduced in vWD. Secondly, vWF assists platelet adhesion to exposed sub-endothelium of damaged capillaries and is excreted by endothelium and activated platelets. Deficiency of vWF therefore affects platelet adherence and the clotting cascade itself. It ranges from a mild disease of little significance, seen in up to 1% of the population, to a very severe form in which vWF is absent.

Haemophilia A and B (factor VIII and IX deficiency respectively) are X-linked disorders and classically do not affect the female population. As many as a third of female carriers, however, will have sub-threshold factor levels.

Problems and special considerations

Von Willebrand's disease

This is classified into three main variants:

- **Type I** (80–90% of cases). vWF is normal but present in diminished quantities.
  In pregnancy, vWF increases and may even return to normal, although this may not be the case in patients with severe disease. Following delivery, VIIIc levels can fall dramatically (though this change may be delayed until late in the puerperium), and there is an increased incidence of postpartum haemorrhage. Levels of VIIIc can be increased by the administration of desmopressin (DDAVP) intravenously.
- **Type II** (9–15% of cases). There is an abnormal vWF; hence additional release of abnormal vWF following administration of DDAVP does not generally improve the coagulopathy. Clotting does not improve in pregnancy. Several subtypes have been described, including IIA, IIB, IIM, and IIN. In the IIB subtype, abnormal vWF clumps inactivated platelets and causes thrombocytopenia. In this variant, DDAVP exacerbates the coagulopathy because increased amounts of abnormal vWF worsen the thrombocytopenia. In IIN (Normandy), there is an isolated decrease in factor VIII concentration because of decreased affinity of the abnormal vWF for factor VIII, which results in increased factor VIII consumption. Thus it can be confused with haemophilia A.

- **Type III** (autosomal recessive; < 1% of cases). vWF is undetectable and VIIIc concentration is very low. The bleeding abnormality is severe and does not respond to DDAVP.

No consensus exists regarding the safe levels of VIIIc and vWF for using neuraxial techniques, and the literature consists only of case reports and series.

Haemophilia

Levels of factor VIII may normalise by the end of pregnancy; however, factor IX does not increase and will require supplementation. Half of all fetuses will be affected, and therefore fetal blood sampling and forceps or ventouse deliveries should be avoided unless chorionic villous sampling or amniocentesis has shown the fetus to be unaffected. After delivery, factor VIII level can fall abruptly, resulting in secondary haemorrhage.

Management options

Close liaison with haematologists is necessary throughout pregnancy. A management plan, including treatment for significant haemorrhage, is essential. An epidural is rarely contra-indicated in type I vWD, but specialist interpretation of laboratory tests (particularly VIIIc concentration) is required. Because of the sometimes precipitous drop in vWF and VIIIc following delivery, removal of the epidural catheter postpartum may be more of a problem; it is advisable either to remove epidural catheters immediately or to wait until the bleeding diathesis can be assessed.

The usual dose of DDAVP is 20 mg (0.3 mg/kg) in 50 ml of saline given over 30 minutes. DDAVP also stimulates fibrinolysis, so tranexamic acid is often given simultaneously. DDAVP can cause fluid retention and therefore hyponatraemia.

Patients with type I disease may deliver vaginally. Patients with type II or III disease frequently have an elective caesarean section, with correction of their coagulopathy. In this situation, regional anaesthesia has been used if clotting is corrected. Where DDAVP is contraindicated, fresh frozen plasma, cryoprecipitate or infusions of vWF and factor VIII may be given.

In haemophilia, close monitoring of factor VIII or IX levels as appropriate is required. The aim is to bring peripartum factor VIII or IX levels to > 50 IU/dL, which may be achieved by the administration of factor concentrates. DDAVP may be used in some patients with haemophilia A carrier status. Regional analgesia/anaesthesia is generally contraindicated unless haematological advice suggests a fully corrected coagulation profile and the possible risks are outweighed by the benefits particular to the case concerned.

Factor VIII levels rapidly decline in the postpartum period. Supplementation is there-fore required in these women and in those with low vWF or factor IX for 3–5 days after delivery, in order to reduce the risk of secondary postpartum haemorrhage.

Key points

- Von Willebrand's disease is a heterogeneous condition that ranges in severity.
- The commonest form of von Willebrand's disease is usually improved by pregnancy.
- Coagulation may rapidly deteriorate after delivery in both von Willebrand's disease and haemophilia.
- In haemophilia, the fetus should be assumed to be affected.
- Specialist advice is necessary before, during and after delivery.

Further reading

Chi C, Kadir RA. Inherited bleeding disorders in pregnancy. *Best Pract Res Clin Obstet Gynaecol* 2012; **26**: 103–17.

Katz D, Beilin Y. Disorders of coagulation in pregnancy. *Br J Anaesth* 2015; **115**: ii75–88.

Pavord S, Rayment R, Madan B, *et al.*; Royal College of Obstetricians and Gynaecologists. Management of inherited bleeding disorders in pregnancy. Green-top Guideline 71. *BJOG* 2017; **124**: e193–263.

Peyvandi F, Garagiola I, Young G. The past and future of haemophilia: diagnosis, treatments, and its complications. *Lancet* 2016; **388**: 187–97.

Disseminated intravascular coagulation

In disseminated intravascular coagulation (DIC) the coagulation process is activated, causing widespread thrombosis and vascular occlusion, and resulting in consumption of clotting factors and platelets with concomitant activation of the fibrinolytic pathway. Conventional treatment of this consumptive coagulopathy is removal of the underlying trigger and support of the patient with replacement of clotting factors and platelets. In many respects, DIC can be seen as the haematological manifestation of a multi-organ disease such as sepsis or pre-eclampsia.

Problems and special considerations

The common triggers for DIC in the obstetric population are listed in Table 108.1. Many of these conditions have their own particular implications for analgesia and anaesthesia. The coagulopathy usually precludes regional anaesthesia.

Diagnosis of DIC depends on clinical features and laboratory tests. Presentation may be of rapid collapse, with shock, respiratory failure, renal impairment, acidosis, hypoxaemia and bleeding from venepuncture sites and the respiratory, gastrointestinal and urogenital tracts (the last including the uteroplacental bed). Coagulation studies show prolonged coagulation times, decreased fibrinogen concentration and platelet count and raised titres of fibrin degradation products. Some authors favour thromboelastography/thromboelastometry because it demonstrates changes in both coagulation and thrombolysis.

In some cases there may be a more insidious progression; initially, increased circulation of activated clotting factors may even shorten coagulation times. It is important to

Table 108.1 Triggers of disseminated intravascular coagulation (DIC) in obstetrics

Placental abruption

Pre-eclampsia/eclampsia

HELLP (haemolysis, elevated liver enzymes and low platelet count) syndrome

Acute fatty liver of pregnancy

Intrauterine death (DIC may occur after 3–4 weeks)

Amniotic fluid embolism

Massive blood transfusion (produces a dilutional coagulopathy; however, tissue factors released)

Drug reactions

Placenta accreta

remember that, owing to the procoagulant physiological changes of pregnancy, changes in the prothrombin time (PT) and activated partial thromboplastin time (APTT) in DIC may not be immediately apparent, and that mild prolongation of these tests or even prolongation within their normal range should be regarded as significant.

The platelet count may initially be normal or mildly reduced, although a progressive decrease may aid diagnosis.

Fibrin degradation products have an anticoagulant effect by interfering with platelet function and reducing the efficiency of myometrial contraction, exacerbating blood loss. Levels are increased in pregnancy and may confuse the picture; trends are therefore more informative than absolute values.

Management options

Management of DIC requires timely recognition and removal of the precipitating factor. This usually involves delivering the fetus if antepartum.

In fulminant DIC there may be no time to wait for laboratory results in the face of massive blood loss, haemostatic failure and multi-organ failure. Patients often require hysterectomy. The successful management of fulminant DIC requires input from senior obstetricians, obstetric anaesthetists, haematologists, laboratory staff and intensivists (see Chapter 78, *Major obstetric haemorrhage*).

Conventional treatment of DIC is to correct the consumptive coagulopathy by administering exogenous clotting factors: fresh frozen plasma to treat prolongation of the APTT or PT, cryoprecipitate or fibrinogen concentrate to treat a low fibrinogen concentration (< 1.5 g/dl), and platelet concentrates.

Some authors have attempted to break the cycle of thrombosis and fibrinolysis by giving heparin, antithrombin or antifibrinolytic drugs. However, giving such agents to a bleeding patient is fraught with danger.

Transfer to an intensive care unit may be necessary to treat the multisystem dysfunction.

Key points

- Coagulopathy may coexist with other organ failures.
- Treatment includes removing the cause of the coagulopathy.
- Aggressive treatment is required to treat fulminating disseminated intravascular coagulation.
- Management of massive obstetric haemorrhage requires coordinated care with haematologists, obstetricians, obstetric anaesthetists and intensivists.

Further reading

Erez O. Disseminated intravascular coagulation in pregnancy: clinical phenotypes and diagnostic scores. *Thromb Res* 2017; **151**: S56–60.

Erez O, Mastrolia SA, Thachil J. Disseminated intravascular coagulation in pregnancy: insights in pathophysiology, diagnosis and management. *Am J Obstet Gynecol* 2015; **213**: 452–63.

Martí-Carvajal AJ, Comunián-Carrasco G, Peña-Martí GE. Haematological interventions for treating disseminated intravascular coagulation during pregnancy and postpartum. *Cochrane Database Syst Rev* 2011; (3): CD008577.

Squizzato A, Hunt BJ, Kinasewitz GT, *et al.* Supportive management strategies for disseminated intravascular coagulation: an international consensus. *Thromb Haemost* 2016; **215**: 896–904.

Chapter 109

Thrombocytopenia

A low platelet count ($< 150 \times 10^9$/l) is seen in around 7–10% of pregnant women and may occur for a variety of reasons, ranging from the relatively benign (gestational thrombocytopenia) to the frankly sinister (HELLP syndrome).

Problems and special considerations

Conditions involving reduced platelet numbers or function include:

- **Gestational thrombocytopenia (GT).** This is the most common cause of low platelet count in pregnancy, accounting for 70% of all cases. It is seen in around 6% of parturients and manifests in late pregnancy. The reduction in platelet count is likely to be secondary to haemodilution and accelerated platelet destruction, and the level rarely drops below $70–75 \times 10^9$/l. In 75% of cases the condition is clinically unimportant, and in its mild form it may not need investigation. It does not appear to increase the risk of maternal or fetal haemorrhage and is usually not regarded as a contraindication to regional analgesia. Spontaneous resolution occurs within 6–8 weeks post-delivery, and the condition may recur in future pregnancies.

- **Immune thrombocytopenia (ITP).** This represents around 5% of the cases of thrombocytopenia in pregnancy and is seen in around 0.01–0.5% of pregnancies. It is characterised by the production of platelet autoantibodies that may cross the placenta, putting the fetus at risk of intracranial haemorrhage during delivery. The development of thrombocytopenia in early pregnancy or the existence of a pre-pregnancy low platelet count may favour the diagnosis of ITP over GT. Although the platelet count is often below 100×10^9/l, coagulation is rarely affected because the young platelets, which make up a higher than usual proportion of the platelet mass, are more aggressively haemostatic. Treatment is by corticosteroid therapy, administration of immunoglobulin (IgG), or a combination of both in severe cases, and this should be considered when the platelet count is below $20–30 \times 10^9$/l, in the presence of bleeding manifestations, or to achieve a platelet count of at least 50×10^9/l before delivery or obstetric interventions. Platelet transfusion may stimulate autoantibody production and is generally ineffective, but may be considered in combination with IgG in the presence of bleeding in severely thrombocytopenic parturients. Splenectomy may be considered in refractory cases. A number of drugs may induce thrombocytopenia (Table 109.1).

- **Thrombotic thrombocytopenic purpura (TTP) and haemolytic uraemic syndrome.** Thrombotic thrombocytopenic purpura is a rare condition that, if untreated, may be associated with a maternal mortality rate of 90%. TTP manifests with haemolytic anaemia, thrombocytopenia and widespread vascular occlusion, often resulting in

Table 109.1 Drugs that may impair platelet function or cause thrombocytopenia

Impaired platelet function	Thrombocytopenia
Aspirin	Heparin
Non-steroidal anti-inflammatory drugs	Thiazide diuretics
Colloid plasma substitutes	Hydralazine
H_2 blockers	
Digoxin	
Cocaine	

neurological disturbance and renal failure. A deficiency in von Willebrand factor cleaving protease has been identified as a causative factor. Unlike HELLP syndrome (haemolysis, elevated liver enzymes and low platelet count; see below), TTP usually presents in the second trimester. The high morbidity and mortality associated with this condition warrants aggressive intervention, and exchange transfusions and plasmapheresis may be employed. Haemolytic uraemic syndrome presents clinically in a similar way to TTP but the renal problems tend to be more severe.

- **Pre-eclampsia.** This is accompanied by a low platelet count in about 20% of cases. Around 10% of women with severe pre-eclampsia will progress to develop its most malignant version, HELLP syndrome. Mothers with evidence of pre-eclampsia must have their platelet count monitored frequently, and a fall should be regarded as evidence that the condition is worsening. The thrombocytopenia of pre-eclampsia is often accompanied by clotting defects; therefore, regular coagulation tests should also be done. Management should be targeted at treatment of the underlying condition, ultimately by delivery, but specific therapy may be needed, including platelet transfusion and fresh frozen plasma in severe cases.

- **Others.** Reduced platelet concentration may also result from other causes of impaired production, such as bone marrow depression, viral infections, vitamin B_{12}/folate deficiency, hereditary defects, paroxysmal nocturnal haemoglobinuria or alcohol toxicity; or from causes of shortened survival of platelets, such as malignancy, drugs (including heparin and methyldopa) or disseminated intravascular coagulation.

Management options

The obstetric anaesthetist is often called upon to make a decision regarding the advisability of regional analgesia and anaesthesia in these cases. In general, patients with a platelet count above 75×10^9/l in the absence of pre-eclampsia are unlikely to have significantly altered platelet function. Some authorities have even suggested that there is a very low risk of adverse outcomes following a neuraxial technique in women with platelet counts as low as 50×10^9/l. Current guidance suggests a stable platelet count of 75×10^9/l or higher as an acceptable cut-off point for the performance of regional anaesthesia in women with no risk factors or abnormal coagulation. The mother with a rapidly falling count should, however, be regarded with more suspicion than the one with a low, but stable, platelet level. In a patient with a platelet count below $75–80 \times 10^9$/l, the decision to perform a neuraxial technique should be taken by a senior anaesthetist and should be individualised, taking into account the underlying pathology, the general state of the patient (including any new bruising), and the underlying trend and rate of decline of the platelet count, with the risk of the procedure (epidural/spinal haematoma) balanced against the benefits (pain relief, better blood pressure control, avoidance of general anaesthesia).

Tests of platelet function, such as bleeding time, are very operator-dependent and therefore of limited predictive value. Commonly seen phenomena in pregnancy such as clumping of platelets or variability in platelet size, seen in GT and ITP, may cause under-reading of the true count by automated devices. Genuine thrombocytopenia may be verified by examination of a peripheral blood smear, or by analysis of blood samples collected in tubes containing citrate anticoagulant rather than ethylene diamine tetra-acetic acid (EDTA). Routine coagulation studies are usually indicated in thrombocytopenia, in case any other defect should be present. The mother should always be questioned about excessive bruising or bleeding, since the presence of these may signify impaired platelet function in borderline cases.

Key points

- All patients with thrombocytopenia must be fully investigated.
- Trends in platelet count are more important than absolute values.
- There is no fixed cut-off point for the platelet count when regional analgesia is being considered.
- Patients should be asked about excessive bruising or bleeding.

Further reading

American College of Obstetricians and Gynecologists. Practice Bulletin No. 166: Thrombocytopenia in pregnancy. *Obstet Gynecol* 2016; **128**: e43–53.

Association of Anaesthetists of Great Britain and Ireland; Obstetric Anaesthetists' Association; Regional Anaesthesia UK. Regional anaesthesia and patients with abnormalities of coagulation. *Anaesthesia* 2013; **68**: 966–72.

Cines DB, Levine LD. Thrombocytopenia in pregnancy. *Blood* 2017; **130**: 2271–7.

Myers B. Diagnosis and management of maternal thrombocytopenia in pregnancy. *Br J Haematol* 2012; **158**: 3–15.

Lymphoma and leukaemia

Haematological malignancies in pregnant women are rare, with an incidence of 2 in 10,000 pregnancies. Nonetheless, lymphomas are now the fourth most common malignancy in pregnancy. In the UK, this increase in prevalence is associated with increased maternal age, whereas in the developing world it is associated with AIDS-related non-Hodgkin's lymphoma. Successful pregnancy has been described with chemotherapy for both acute and chronic leukaemia and lymphoma.

Increasing numbers of patients are surviving childhood or adult treatment of haematological malignancies. However, such treatment can leave both physical and psychological problems associated with chemotherapeutic treatment.

Problems and special considerations

Treatment of haematological malignancies often involves intense periods of chemotherapy or radiotherapy followed by maintenance doses. The most aggressive forms of therapy result in permanent ablation of bone marrow. Bone marrow rescue is achieved by transplantation of stored autologous bone marrow or donated allogeneic bone marrow. Patients may require repeated lumbar punctures to test for disease and to administer chemotherapeutic agents (e.g. methotrexate).

The limiting factor in administration of most chemotherapeutic agents is short- and long-term toxicity. Short-term problems include malaise, nausea and vomiting, anorexia and acute organ impairment, especially of the liver and kidneys. Toxicity may also arise from antimicrobial therapy (e.g. gentamicin and vancomycin). Bone marrow depression may result in anaemia, neutropenia with increased risk of infection and coagulopathy. Long-term toxicity may include neurotoxicity, neuropathies (e.g. vincristine) and arachnoiditis (e.g. methotrexate). Cardiomyopathy may occur as a dose-dependent result of anthracycline antibiotics such as daunorubicin. Pulmonary toxicity and fibrosis may follow busulfan and bleomycin administration. Although sterility often occurs following high-dose chemotherapy, many survivors do conceive spontaneously or following infertility treatments. Central and peripheral venous access may be a persisting problem.

The long-term effects of chemotherapy on children exposed in utero is unknown. Although there are concerns regarding neurodevelopment, childhood malignancy and fertility, the current data suggest that chemotherapy exposure in utero does not have significant impact.

The psychological effects of a cancer diagnosis in a young person followed by prolonged periods of therapy and isolation may include flashbacks, phobias or features of a post-traumatic stress syndrome. Frequently, these psychological aspects influence management far more than physical aspects.

Patients with Hodgkin's lymphoma or who have had a stem cell transplant require irradiated blood, so additional time is required to ensure its availability.

Management options

All patients who have or have had haematological malignancies require a detailed assessment by a multidisciplinary antenatal team. Wherever possible, the treatment records should be obtained, preferably with a haematological summary. The patient may find it distressing to recall details of her treatment or of unpleasant experiences such as general anaesthesia or lumbar puncture, and this may induce unexpected irrational behaviour. A careful sensitive approach is required.

Commonly performed laboratory investigations include renal and liver function tests and a full blood count. Assessment of cardiorespiratory status may require studies such as chest radiography, echocardiography or pulmonary function tests.

The spectrum of such patients varies from some that can be treated as normal to those with significant hepatic, renal and cardiopulmonary disease. In the last group, regional analgesia and anaesthesia are usually recommended, depending on the pattern of disease. Concerns over the introduction of circulating blast cells into the cerebrospinal fluid by a traumatic dural puncture (either intentional or accidental) and subsequent central nervous system involvement may contraindicate the use of regional anaesthesia in some patients. Consultation with the haematologist and oncologist is advised if a regional technique is being considered.

Key points

- Organ impairment may arise from the haematological malignancy itself or from its treatment.
- Regional anaesthesia may not be recommended in some patients.
- Survivors of leukaemia and lymphoma need support and sensitive, carefully planned care.

Further reading

Amit O, Barzilai M, Avivi I. Management of hematologic malignancies: special considerations in pregnant women. *Drugs* 2015; **75**: 1725–38.
Elterman KG, Meserve JR, Wadleigh M, Farber MK, Tsen LC. Management of labor analgesia in a patient with acute myeloid leukemia. *A A Case Rep* 2014; **3**: 104–6.
Lishner M, Avivi I, Apperley JF, *et al.* Hematologic malignancies in pregnancy: management guidelines from an international consensus meeting. *J Clin Oncol* 2016; **34**: 501–8.
Owsiak JN, Bullough AS. Chronic myeloid leukemia in pregnancy: an absolute contraindication to neuraxial anesthesia? *Int J Obstet Anesth* 2016; **25**: 85–8.

Haemoglobinopathies

Haemoglobin abnormalities result from either synthesis of abnormal haemoglobin (e.g. sickle cell anaemia) or reduced rate of synthesis of normal haemoglobin chains (the thalassaemias).

Problems and special considerations

Sickle cell disease

Patients with sickle cell disease are homozygotes for an abnormal haemoglobin (haemoglobin S). Heterozygotes have a significantly attenuated form (sickle cell trait), which is not normally of clinical significance except when combined with another abnormal haemoglobin (e.g. haemoglobin C). Haemoglobin S is poorly soluble in its deoxygenated form and therefore crystallises at a variable oxygen concentration dependent on relative concentrations of normal and abnormal haemoglobin within the red cell.

Haemoglobin S in heterozygotes appears to have some protective action against malaria and is therefore more common in Africa, Asia, Arabia and southern Europe, particularly coastal Greece and Turkey. The disease is characterised by haemolysis, reticulocytosis, anaemia, recurrent sepsis, vaso-occlusive and sequestration crises and hypersplenism followed by splenic infarction. Diagnosis is based on demonstration of sickling (Sickledex test) followed by haemoglobin electrophoresis.

Sickle cell disease (homozygous SS) is a particularly aggressive disease. Affected patients may not survive into their third decade. Maternal and perinatal mortality rates are variable and in some countries may reach 11% and 20%, respectively. Careful management can, however, significantly reduce the morbidity and mortality associated with the disease.

Problems in pregnancy include vaso-occlusive and thromboembolic phenomena, infection and an increased risk of obstetric complications such as preterm labour, pre-eclampsia, placental infarction and fetal loss. Cardiorespiratory morbidity includes systemic and pulmonary hypertension, and cardiomyopathy. Despite earlier evidence to the contrary, recent work has demonstrated that sickle cell trait is not associated with a higher incidence of pre-eclampsia, although these women may be at an increased risk of venous thromboembolism.

Thalassaemias

This disease is classified according to the haemoglobin chain affected (α or β). It is common in Mediterranean countries and also occurs in a narrow band of distribution crossing Africa, the Middle East, India, Myanmar and Southeast Asia. Its distribution therefore closely follows that of sickle cell disease, and both diseases are said to give some protection against *falciparum* malaria.

α-Thalassaemia

The α-haemoglobin gene is encoded twice on each chromosome 16, giving a total of four genes controlling its production. When all four genes are deleted, α-chain synthesis is completely suppressed and death occurs in utero (hydrops fetalis). Three α-gene deletions lead to a moderately severe microcytic, hypochromic anaemia with splenomegaly (HbH disease). Precipitation of relatively insoluble HbH within cells induces mild haemolysis. Crises of haemolysis associated with infection may occur. Patients with two (thalassaemia trait) and one (silent carriers) α-chain deletions are asymptomatic.

Pregnancies complicated by hydrops fetalis (Bart's hydrops) are associated with pre-eclampsia, retained placenta and ante- and postpartum haemorrhage.

β-Thalassaemia

In contrast to α-thalassaemia, the β-haemoglobin gene is coded by a single gene; thus patients can be homozygous or heterozygous for the faulty gene. However, about 125 individual mutations of the β-gene have been described, which can markedly affect the clinical picture. Hence the terms thalassaemia major, intermedia and minor have been used to describe clinical pictures of varying severity. Furthermore, the geographical distribution of thalassaemia and sickle cell trait means that it is possible to have a mixed sickle cell–thalassaemia genotype.

In thalassaemia major either no β-haemoglobin chains are produced or small amounts are produced (5–30%). Anaemia results from ineffective erythropoiesis and haemolysis and inadequate supplies of haemoglobin for formed red cells. Features include skeletal abnormalities because of bone marrow hyperactivity and chronic multi-organ failure including the pancreas, liver and heart. Patients may be thrombocytopenic because of hypersplenism or thrombocythaemic following splenectomy. Thrombocythaemic patients require thromboembolic prophylaxis and may also develop arterial thrombosis including cerebral thrombosis. Frequent cannulation may make venous access difficult (many patients have permanent indwelling intravenous catheters). There is a high incidence of blood transfusion reactions and a small incidence of transfusion-related HIV and hepatitis C. Splenectomised patients are at risk of infection.

Treatment of β-thalassaemia includes frequent transfusion, with iron chelation therapy to reduce iron overload. Modern haematological management means that more women with thalassaemia major are becoming pregnant. There is an increased incidence of fetal growth restriction, fetal loss and obstetric intervention because of cephalopelvic disproportion resulting from skeletal abnormalities.

In thalassaemia intermedia there are usually few symptoms. Women may have chronic anaemia and require folate therapy in pregnancy. In severe cases, however, they may develop iron overload, with a clinical syndrome that lags behind the progression seen in thalassaemia major.

Women with thalassaemia minor have few symptoms but may have a higher incidence of fetal growth restriction.

Management options

In sickle cell disease, the haemoglobin concentration is usually maintained above 80 g/l (optimum haematocrit 0.26) with blood transfusion. Exchange transfusion may decrease the rate of maternal complications in pregnancy but does not change fetal or obstetric outcome. A detailed plan made in collaboration with a haematologist is essential for delivery. In general, patients should be warm, well hydrated, not acidotic or hypercarbic, and venous stasis should be avoided. Around a third of parturients with a history of multiple transfusions will have atypical red cell antibodies; cross-matched blood must therefore be made available for delivery. It must be noted that the use of cell salvage is not advised in women with homozygous sickle cell disease because of the potential for reinfusing sickle cells and the precipitation of sickle cell crisis. Its use in women with sickle cell trait remains controversial.

Management of a sickling crisis is by correction of the precipitating factors, organ support, analgesia and blood transfusion if required. The clinical picture of acute chest syndrome may overlap with that of pneumonia or pulmonary embolism, and therefore a high index of suspicion must be maintained.

Parenteral opioids may be used for labour analgesia but pethidine is not recommended due to its epileptogenic potential. An epidural provides analgesia without respiratory depression, although mobility is beneficial. Regional anaesthesia is preferable for operative delivery. Oxygen administration is essential postoperatively, especially after general anaesthesia. The safety of blood patch in sickle cell disease has not been assessed, but colloid patches have been used successfully.

α-Thalassaemia rarely results in maternal disease sufficient to cause significant problems with anaesthesia. Related problems such as haemorrhage and pre-eclampsia are covered elsewhere. In β-thalassaemia, haemoglobin should be kept above 100 g/l with transfusion. Complications such as thrombocytopenia, diabetes, hypothyroidism, cardiomyopathy and facial and vertebral abnormalities require the choice of anaesthesia and analgesia to be assessed on an individual basis.

Key points

- Patients with sickle cell disease should be kept warm, well hydrated, mobile and well oxygenated.
- Haemoglobin should be kept above 80–90 g/l in sickle cell disease.
- Exchange transfusion reduces maternal and fetal complications of sickle cell disease.
- Thalassaemia major causes significant multisystem compromise including cardiac, endocrine and skeletal abnormalities; it may cause intrauterine death and concomitant maternal disease.
- Non-fatal α-thalassaemias are of variable significance.

Further reading

Boga C, Ozdogu H. Pregnancy and sickle cell disease: a review of the current literature. *Crit Rev Oncol Hematol* 2016; **98**: 364–74.

Royal College of Obstetricians and Gynaecologists. *Management of Sickle Cell Disease in Pregnancy.* Green-top Guideline 61. London: RCOG, 2011. www.rcog.org.uk/en/guidelines-research-services/guidelines/gtg61 (accessed December 2018).

Royal College of Obstetricians and Gynaecologists. *Management of Beta Thalassaemia in Pregnancy.* Green-top Guideline 66. London: RCOG, 2014. www.rcog.org.uk/en/guidelines-research-services/guidelines/gtg66 (accessed December 2018).

Connective tissue disorders

The connective tissue disorders are a diffuse group of diseases that include the rheumatoid diseases (rheumatoid arthritis, ankylosing spondylitis), the collagen vascular diseases (systemic lupus erythematosus (SLE), scleroderma, the vasculitides), granulomatous diseases and inherited connective tissue disease (e.g. Ehlers–Danlos syndrome).

The factors of importance to the anaesthetist are firstly, the widespread systemic nature of the diseases, and secondly, the drug treatment that is used.

Problems and special considerations

With the exception of the rheumatoid diseases, connective tissue disorders are rare in the antenatal population. Although many are autoimmune disorders, which tend to have an increased incidence in females, the onset of significantly symptomatic disease is frequently towards the end of reproductive life. Both spontaneous abortion and late pregnancy loss are increased in women who do become pregnant. Preterm delivery is also increased.

Drug treatment

Drug treatment frequently includes long-term oral corticosteroids, which may be associated with gestational diabetes and fetal adrenal suppression, and may also include immunosuppressive agents such as azathioprine, chlorambucil, cyclophosphamide or methotrexate. Low-dose aspirin and subcutaneous heparin are often used in SLE. In arthritic conditions, non-steroidal anti-inflammatory drugs (NSAIDs) are invariably used. Monoclonal antibody therapy is used in severe forms of rheumatoid arthritis.

Cardiopulmonary involvement

Pericardial effusions are common, especially in rheumatoid and collagen disorders. A restrictive pericarditis may ensue. Valvular dysfunction can occur. Any unexplained dyspnoea or tachycardia should therefore prompt further investigation. A miscellany of electrocardiographic changes may be seen, and echocardiography is useful in assessing both valvular and ventricular function. Connective tissue disorders may also be associated with hypertension, and seem to be associated with an increased incidence of pre-eclampsia.

Pleural effusions and impaired pulmonary function of both restrictive and obstructive patterns may occur, and pulmonary vasculitis may be a feature of both collagen and vasculitic disorders, rarely leading to spontaneous pulmonary haemorrhage. Pulmonary hypertension may also be present.

Women with scleroderma may be at increased risk of chronic aspiration because of impaired gastrointestinal motility. These women may also have significant airway problems.

Haematological involvement

Thrombocytopenia and anaemia may be present or occur anew, and may be difficult to differentiate from the typical gestational picture or conditions such as HELLP syndrome.

Multiple antibody formation

This is a significant problem in women with SLE, although it may also occur in other autoimmune connective tissue disorders. Maternal antibodies cause difficulty and delay in obtaining adequately cross-matched blood for transfusion. In severe cases, there may be maternal coagulation disorders that may be thrombotic or may increase risk of bleeding.

Anticardiolipin antibodies are associated with increased pregnancy loss and increased maternal morbidity. Treatment with aspirin combined with heparin has been associated with a decrease in miscarriage rate. Anti-Ro antibodies may cross the placenta and cause fetal cardiac conduction defects, rendering the fetus bradycardic and unable to mount a tachycardic response to stress; this may occur in 2% of neonates whose mothers have anti-Ro antibodies. If present, Doppler echocardiography is recommended every 1–2 weeks between 16 and 28 weeks, as this is considered the vulnerable stage for the fetus. Expedited delivery and neonatal pacing may be required.

Musculoskeletal problems

Musculoskeletal involvement is a feature of several connective tissue disorders. Women with scleroderma classically have very tight perioral skin and may also have involvement of the temporomandibular joints; both may limit mouth opening.

Cervical arthritis and consequent reduction of neck mobility is a feature of several connective tissue disorders. Kyphoscoliosis may also be seen, which may complicate neuraxial analgesia/anaesthesia.

Tissue fragility and skin involvement

Several conditions (e.g. certain forms of Ehlers–Danlos syndrome) may be associated with increased fragility of tissues including blood vessels, leading to an increased susceptibility to trauma and bleeding; even frequent non-invasive blood pressure reading may cause bruising. Uterine rupture and delayed wound healing have both been reported.

Bullous diseases such as pemphigus and epidermolysis bullosa are characterised by formation of large bullae on the skin and mucous membranes in response to minor trauma. Although extremely rare, cases have been reported in pregnancy, and there are significant implications for the anaesthetist. Any airway instrumentation (including pressure from a facemask) can provoke bullous formation, and bullae may also form in the trachea. Regional anaesthesia is recommended in these cases.

Management options

Early antenatal assessment is vital, and pre-conception counselling is ideal. If pregnancy has occurred unexpectedly, expert advice should be sought about the relative risks of teratogenicity of immunosuppressive drugs, and the patient counselled appropriately.

Many women with connective tissue disorders have multisystem involvement, and disease activity may change during pregnancy. Detailed history and examination is necessary, with particular reference to drug treatment and symptoms or signs suggestive of cardiac or pulmonary disease. The possibility of difficulty with airway management and cardiopulmonary involvement should be remembered if anaesthesia is required for termination of pregnancy. Maternal mobility may be limited by the underlying disease. The skin should be examined for fragility and ease of intravenous access, which may be facilitated by the use of ultrasound guidance. Investigations should include electro- and echocardiography, pulmonary function tests, chest radiography and full biochemical and haematological investigation.

Women who continue with pregnancy should be regarded as high-risk and receive consultant obstetric care. Serial monitoring of the mother should include assessment of cardiac, pulmonary and renal reserve. Mothers needing maintenance NSAIDs throughout pregnancy will require fetal cardiac monitoring during the third trimester, because of the risk of premature closure of the ductus arteriosus and potential fetal renal compromise.

An individualised, multidisciplinary plan is required, depending on the particular disorder involved. There should be provision for high-dependency level of care during and after delivery. In the absence of coagulation disorder, regional analgesia is not contraindicated; however, recent coagulation studies and a platelet count must be reviewed. Regional anaesthesia is considered unwise by some authorities because of the risk of major haemorrhage during surgery, but a risk–benefit analysis must be made for each patient. Both increased and decreased efficacy of local anaesthetic techniques have been reported in patients with connective tissue disorders, possibly due to altered uptake of local anaesthetic; a history of previous problems should be discussed. If difficulty with the airway is considered to be a major potential risk, relative contraindications to regional anaesthesia are usually outweighed by the benefits. There are no absolute contraindications to regional anaesthesia in these circumstances. A plan for a difficult airway should be made and equipment available; awake fibreoptic intubation may be necessary. Published case reports indicate successful management of individual cases using both general and regional techniques.

Key points

- Connective tissue disorders encompass a wide variety of clinical conditions. Each woman must be assessed on an individual basis.
- Many connective tissue disorders are associated with cardiac, pulmonary and renal dysfunction.
- Drug treatment frequently includes corticosteroids.
- Early and detailed antenatal assessment with serial monitoring during pregnancy are essential.
- Regional analgesia and anaesthesia are not contraindicated, but careful assessment of the balance of risks and benefits is necessary.

Further reading

Clowse ME, Jamison M, Myers E, James AH. A national study of the complications of lupus in pregnancy. *Am J Obstet Gynecol* 2008; **199**: 127:e1–6.

Marder W, Littlejohn EA, Somers EC. Pregnancy and autoimmune connective tissue diseases. *Best Pract Res Clin Rheumatol* 2016; **30**: 63–80.

Märker-Hermann E, Fischer-Betz R. Rheumatic diseases and pregnancy. *Curr Opin Obstet Gynecol* 2010; **22**: 458–65.

Saar P, Hermann W, Muller-Ladner U. Connective tissue diseases and pregnancy. *Rheumatology* 2006; **45**: 30–2.

Rheumatoid arthritis

Rheumatoid arthritis (RA) is three times more common in women than in men, and although the peak time of onset is not until the mid-thirties, it is reported to complicate approximately 1 in 1000 pregnancies. It is a non-specific autoimmune disease. A proportion of patients are seropositive for rheumatoid factor, an anti-IgG antibody.

RA tends to run a course of remissions and relapses. Pregnancy usually has a beneficial effect on disease progress, though relapses during the puerperium are common (but may be delayed by lactation). New-onset rheumatoid arthritis is also more common in the post-partum period.

Problems and special considerations

The pregnant woman with RA poses several concerns for the anaesthetist.

Effects of the disease on the joints

RA tends to affect primarily the small joints of the hands and wrists, and although this can be disabling for the patient, it is not usually a problem for the anaesthetist. In more severe cases there may be involvement of the hips, knees and lumbar spine, which may make positioning for regional analgesia or anaesthesia difficult. In very severe cases there may be kyphosis of the thoracic spine and fixed deformity of the ribs, causing restrictive lung disease.

RA affects the cervical spine in up to 45% of cases, and it is important to remember that the cervical spine may be unstable and prone to subluxation. The temporomandibular joint (TMJ) may also be affected, and tracheal intubation may be difficult or impossible. Cricoarytenoid arthritis may be present, causing glottic constriction.

Systemic effects of the disease

These are widespread. Both pericardial and pleural effusions may occur (often asymptoma-tically). Systemic granulomas can form in the lungs, myocardium, heart valves, aortic root and coronary arteries. Deposits in the cardiac conducting system may occur. A vasculitic process may rarely cause coronary or pulmonary arteritis.

Syndromes associated with RA include Felty's and Sjögren's, in both of which peripheral neuropathies may occur.

Long-term medication

The general principle of drug management during pregnancy is to reduce medication to a minimum and to restrict it to those drugs with the best safety record.

Women with symptomatic RA are usually maintained on high-dose aspirin, nonsteroidal anti-inflammatory drugs and corticosteroids. Although these are all relatively contraindicated during pregnancy, it may be impossible to stop them. Serial ultrasound examination of the fetal heart helps to give early warning of closure of the fetal ductus arteriosus or of developing fetal pulmonary hypertension.

Gold, penicillamine and most immunosuppressive drugs are avoided during pregnancy where possible. The degree of risk from the newer immunomodulatory preparations (e.g. tumour necrosis factor inhibitors/antibodies) is unclear.

Management options

The mother with RA may have several anaesthetic risk factors and should be identified as early as possible during pregnancy and referred for anaesthetic assessment. History taking should include a drug history, and questioning about any previous anaesthetics, especially if these involved tracheal intubation. A history of hoarseness or stridor may suggest cricoarytenoid arthritis; nasendoscopy can be performed if further investigation is necessary. A full airway assessment is mandatory, including jaw protrusion (TMJ involvement) and neck movement (cervical spine involvement). Where appropriate, cervical spine x-rays should be taken in extension and flexion – for example, if neck symptoms are present, or the disease has been present for a long duration. A detailed cardiorespiratory history is essential. Pulmonary function tests may be considered, and electrocardiography should be performed to exclude conduction defects. If there is suspicion of a rheumatoid cardiomyopathy, echocardiography should be requested. The extent of any peripheral neuropathy must be documented.

The mother should be advised to accept early epidural analgesia. If this is precluded by coagulopathy or absolute maternal refusal, patient-controlled opioid analgesia may be offered. If caesarean section is necessary, a graduated epidural top-up or combined spinal–epidural is often recommended in preference to single-shot spinal anaesthesia, in order to reduce the risk of an unexpectedly high motor or sensory block compromising the airway, and to provide greater haemodynamic stability in the event of undiagnosed cardiac problems. There is some anecdotal evidence to suggest that neuraxial anaesthesia may result in a more extensive spread of block than expected in patients with RA.

If there are known cervical spine problems and general anaesthesia is essential, the anaesthetist must have access to fibreoptic equipment and awake intubation. Indirect video laryngoscopy may be useful to avoid excessive cervical spine movement, even if the airway is not predicted to be difficult. Even if there is severe fetal distress, general anaesthesia should not be induced without additional aids for difficult intubation (and the presence of an anaesthetist who is familiar with their use). Careful attention is required to positioning throughout labour and delivery, particularly in the presence of regional analgesia/anaesthesia or during general anaesthesia, to avoid forcing joints beyond their normal range.

Key points

- Rheumatoid arthritis is a multisystem autoimmune disease.
- Pregnancy tends to be associated with remission of the disease.
- The anaesthetist should expect difficulty with tracheal intubation.
- Cardiac and respiratory manifestations of the disease may be present.

- Peripheral neuropathy may infrequently occur.
- The mainstay of drug treatment is non-steroidal anti-inflammatory drugs, which the mother may need to continue throughout pregnancy.

Further reading

Elliott AB, Chakravarty EF. Management of rheumatic diseases during pregnancy. *Postgrad Med* 2010; **122**: 213–21.

Märker-Hermann E, Fischer-Betz R. Rheumatic diseases and pregnancy. *Curr Opin Obstet Gynecol* 2010; **22**: 458–65.

Samanta R, Shoukrey K, Griffiths R. Rheumatoid arthritis and anaesthesia. *Anaesthesia* 2011; **66**: 1146–59.

Smolen JS, Aletaha D, McInnes IB. Rheumatoid arthritis. *Lancet* 2016; **388**: 2023–38.

Chapter 114

Cervical spine disorders

Women may have limited cervical spine movement because of rheumatoid arthritis, ankylosing spondylitis, cervical disc disease, trauma, accessory cervical ribs or cervical spondylosis, although the last is extremely uncommon in women of childbearing age.

A rare but important cause of cervical scoliosis is Klippel–Feil syndrome, in which there is fusion of two or more cervical vertebrae. In extreme cases, the patient may present with severe webbing of the neck, marked scoliosis and virtually no neck movement, but milder cases may pass unnoticed until the woman presents to the anaesthetist in the obstetric theatre.

Problems and special considerations

The major concern of the obstetric anaesthetist is reduced flexibility of the neck and the likelihood of difficulty with tracheal intubation. In addition, there may be other features of the underlying cause of the neck problems (e.g. rheumatoid arthritis). Obstetric management is further complicated by the uncertain mode, timing and urgency of delivery; antenatal review and planning for all possibilities are prudent.

Management options

Whenever possible, women should be identified and assessed antenatally. The woman with limited cervical spine movement should be advised of the potential hazards associated with general anaesthesia and advised to accept epidural analgesia for labour and regional anaesthesia for any proposed operative procedure.

Obstetric and midwifery staff must be aware that patients with potentially difficult airways represent increased anaesthetic risk, and that the anaesthetist should be involved early in any decision that might lead to operative delivery.

If general anaesthesia is essential, the anaesthetist must fully assess the patient preoperatively (including women presenting for emergency surgery). Basic assessment must include neck movement and mouth opening. If difficulty with intubation is anticipated, senior assistance must be sought before proceeding with induction of general anaesthesia. Local protocols should be followed in the event of unexpected failed intubation (see Chapter 38, *Failed and difficult intubation*).

All obstetric theatres should have a difficult intubation trolley readily available, with a variety of laryngoscopes, including McCoy and polio blades, and a video laryngoscope. Awake fibreoptic intubation is now thought by many to be the management of choice when general anaesthesia is required in a woman who is known to have significant cervical spine abnormality, although elective preoperative tracheostomy has also been suggested.

Key points

- The main problem posed by cervical spine disorders is potentially difficult tracheal intubation.
- Regional techniques are usually considered best.

Kyphoscoliosis

Kyphoscoliosis may be congenital, associated with neuromuscular disorders (e.g. muscular dystrophies, neurofibromatosis, poliomyelitis or cerebral palsy) or idiopathic. Idiopathic kyphoscoliosis is much more common in females than males (ratio of 4:1) and accounts for 80% of all cases of kyphoscoliosis.

Progressive kyphoscoliosis is almost invariably accompanied by progressive symptoms and signs of restrictive pulmonary disease, and ultimately, if left uncorrected, it leads to pulmonary hypertension and death.

Severe uncorrected kyphoscoliosis is extremely uncommon in the UK, and most women presenting to the antenatal clinic will either have mild deformity or will have had corrective orthopaedic surgery.

Problems and special considerations

Although kyphoscoliosis in pregnant women is likely to be idiopathic, alternative causes are important to eliminate. Neurofibromatosis is associated with other serious complications (intracranial tumours, congenital heart disease), and familial dysautonomia, characterised by massive swings in blood pressure and generalised autonomic dysfunction, is associated with kyphoscoliosis in 90% of cases. If kyphoscoliosis is associated with neuromuscular disease, respiratory function may be compromised by the underlying disorder in addition to the structural abnormality.

The bony pelvis is normal in women with idiopathic scoliosis, and there is no increase in the incidence of malpresentation or prolonged labour; caesarean delivery should be reserved for obstetric indications. However, if spinal instrumentation extends near the lumbosacral junction, this may impair sacral movement and interfere with descent of the fetus within the pelvis.

Women who have had corrective surgery have two major sources of potential morbidity: firstly residual cardiorespiratory disease, and secondly limited access to the thoracolumbar spine.

Management options

Antenatal assessment is important, and access to previous medical records, x-ray films and magnetic resonance imaging scans, where available, should be sought as early as possible in the pregnancy. Respiratory function tests can readily be performed on an outpatient basis and may be repeated later in the pregnancy to assess any deterioration. It has been suggested that correction of scoliosis improves respiratory function, whereas in women with uncorrected scoliosis, cardiorespiratory function is likely to deteriorate further as a result of pregnancy. Increased cardiorespiratory demand, coupled with reduced functional residual capacity and the inability to increase minute ventilation because of restrictive lung disease, may lead to respiratory compromise.

In women with corrected scoliosis, the major problem for the anaesthetist is provision of regional analgesia and anaesthesia. The most common means of correction of kyphoscoliosis is with Harrington rods or with the newer adaptations, Luque and Cotrel–Dubousset instrumentation. Each technique involves metal instrumentation and bone grafting. Thoracoplasty is sometimes also offered as an additional surgical procedure in order to reduce the rib 'hump' that affects some patients. This is also used to obtain bone grafts from the ribs instead of the pelvis. Although preservation of the L5/S1 interspace is a cardinal orthopaedic rule, instrumentation and grafting may extend down to L4/5 in up to 20% of cases. The level of skin scar is a poor guide to the level of fixation, and therefore operation notes and/or imaging results are extremely helpful during antenatal assessment. If there is no pre-pregnancy imaging available, and there is doubt about the extent of instrumentation of the lumbar spine, relevant radiography may be performed during the third trimester of pregnancy. Assessment and written documentation of any existing neurological deficit and any pre-existing back pain is important.

Successful insertion of both epidural and spinal needles is well described in women with Harrington rod fixation, but women should be warned that the procedure may be technically difficult. Neuraxial techniques are unlikely to be successful at the site of fixation owing to the presence of metalwork, bone graft material and scar tissue; insertion above or below is recommended. False loss of resistance has been described, and the risk of accidental dural puncture is increased. There is an increased risk of patchy analgesia or anaesthesia with epidural techniques, thought to be caused by epidural adhesions and scarring following disruption of the ligamentum flavum.

Because of the potential problems of epidural analgesia and anaesthesia, spinal techniques may offer significant advantages. Spinal needle insertion at the L5/S1 interspace is more likely to be successful, even in very low fusions. There is a definite endpoint, which overcomes the problem of false loss of resistance, and deliberate dural puncture with an appropriate needle avoids the risks of accidental dural puncture with an epidural needle. Spread of local anaesthetic within the cerebrospinal fluid is unlikely to be affected by previous surgery, and therefore anaesthesia for operative delivery is more reliable with spinal than with epidural techniques. There are theoretical reasons to recommend continuous spinal catheter analgesia for labour as an alternative to epidural analgesia, depending on local expertise and familiarity with the technique.

In cases of uncorrected scoliosis, technical difficulty and an increased incidence of complications should be anticipated for neuraxial techniques; however, a review of patients with scoliosis having neuraxial anaesthesia found that patients with uncorrected scoliosis were more likely to have a successful block than those who had had corrective surgery (79% versus 69%). The anaesthetist should consider that vertebral rotation is likely to be present, making identification of anatomical landmarks and location of the epidural/subarachnoid space more challenging. A paramedian approach may be more successful. Those experienced in the use of ultrasound for neuraxial techniques may find it to be a useful adjunct. Once the correct space is reached, scoliosis may cause pooling and affect spread of local anaesthetic.

It is important to discuss in advance alternative methods of analgesia such as Entonox and patient-controlled intravenous opioids, and the potential need for general anaesthesia in case regional techniques fail. If general anaesthesia is required, the airway may be more difficult due to fixed deformity or reduced mobility of the spine, and care should be given to positioning and padding of pressure points. Combined spinal–epidural techniques are advisable in women with an anticipated difficult airway in whom a regional technique is undertaken.

Key points

- Although at least 80% of kyphoscoliosis is idiopathic, association with other diseases such as neurofibromatosis and familial dysautonomia should not be forgotten.
- Uncorrected progressive kyphoscoliosis leads to severe restrictive pulmonary disease and pulmonary hypertension.
- The major anaesthetic problem in pregnant women with corrected kyphoscoliosis is provision of regional anaesthesia and analgesia. Spinal techniques offer several advantages over epidural.
- Lumbar fusions are unlikely to involve the L5/S1 interspace.
- Radiography of the lumbar spine may be performed during the third trimester to aid management of regional analgesia.

Further reading

Ko JY, Leffert L. Clinical implications of neuraxial anesthesia in the parturient with scoliosis. *Anesth Analg* 2009; **109**: 1930–4.

Smith PS, Wilson RC, Robinson AP, Lyons GR. Regional blockade for delivery in women with scoliosis or previous spinal surgery. *Int J Obstet Anesth* 2003; **12**: 17–22.

Low back pain in pregnancy

Low back pain, sacroiliac pain and sciatic pain are common during pregnancy, affecting between 50% and 90% of women. Symptoms vary from mild 'normal' backache to severe pain that may render the woman bed-bound and necessitate early delivery.

The prevalence of low back pain during pregnancy increases with increasing maternal age. Numerous other risk factors have been investigated, but reports are contradictory about the relevance of maternal weight, socioeconomic class, number of pregnancies and previous history of back pain, although it is thought that women with a previous history of spinal surgery are not necessarily at increased risk of back pain during pregnancy.

Retrospective studies significantly under-report low back pain, usually quoting an incidence of 20–25%. This accounts for the conflicting data concerning any putative relationship between epidural analgesia and backache, which is now considered not to be causal (see Chapter 50, *Backache*).

Problems and special considerations

Non-specific back pain

The majority of back pain in pregnancy is directly attributable to the physiological changes that occur. The influence of relaxin, which is produced by the corpus luteum, leads to generalised ligamentous laxity. Serum levels of relaxin are highest during the first trimester of pregnancy. The pelvis widens, which may lead to sacroiliac joint instability. This may in turn allow anterior displacement of the sacrum, causing stretching of the lumbosacral plexus and subsequent pain. The expanding uterus alters the woman's centre of gravity and causes an increased lumbar lordosis and pelvic tilt, and this, combined with the additional weight carried as pregnancy progresses, contributes to development of back pain. Some women complain of night-time back pain, for which a vascular mechanism has been proposed. It is suggested that inferior vena caval compression and increased intravascular volume occurring during recumbency may lead to distension in the vertebral venous plexus and subsequent stagnant hypoxia in the nerve roots and vertebral bodies, producing radicular and low back pain.

Pelvic girdle pain

Some women have symptoms relating specifically to the sacroiliac joints or the symphysis pubis. These women complain of pain localised to the pelvis and pubic symphysis, with radiation to the buttocks and thighs but not to the calf or foot, and commonly complain of pain when turning over in bed at night. In extreme cases there may be separation of the pubic symphysis, in which case the woman may become unable to walk or weight bear at all.

Abduction of the legs and external rotation of the hips may be difficult, and women may have anxieties about their ability to cope with labour and vaginal delivery. Pelvic girdle pain may persist for up to 2 years after delivery and has an increased incidence in future pregnancies.

Acute disc prolapse

Central disc herniation occurs in about 1 in 10,000 pregnancies and may require surgical decompression. Large central disc herniations can occur during pregnancy and at the time of delivery, and if there is an associated significant neurological deficit, surgical decompression is indicated. If magnetic resonance imaging (MRI) is used, disc bulges and herniations can be demonstrated in approximately half of all pregnant women, which is the same incidence as in asymptomatic non-pregnant women. Low back pain with sciatic radiation is common in pregnancy, and careful history taking and examination are needed to ensure that the availability of MRI does not lead to unnecessary surgical intervention.

Other causes

Less common causes of back pain should not be overlooked. Spinal cord tumours are extremely rare, and most of those reported during pregnancy are angiomas, presumed to be present before pregnancy. The increased vascularity of pregnancy is assumed to cause the tumours to become symptomatic. Secondary metastasis to the spine of primary malignancies such as breast can occur during pregnancy.

Management options

General management

Back care advice early in pregnancy has been reported to reduce the incidence and severity of low back pain during pregnancy. This may be particularly important for women with a history of pre-pregnancy back pain, who may be at increased risk of worsening pain during pregnancy. Simple physiotherapy, exercise programmes and the use of lumbosacral corsets have all been reported to provide symptomatic pain relief during pregnancy, although evidence for treatment of pelvic pain is less clear.

Simple analgesics such as paracetamol and codeine-based preparations are acceptable during pregnancy, but non-steroidal anti-inflammatory drugs should be avoided whenever possible. If their use is considered essential, treatment should be agreed with the obstetrician, and fetal cardiac ultrasound monitoring arranged because of the risk of premature closure of the ductus arteriosus. Amitriptyline may be prescribed as a co-analgesic, especially if pain is disrupting normal sleep patterns. In cases of severe back pain, strong opioid analgesia may be required.

Transcutaneous electrical nerve stimulation for back pain during the second half of pregnancy is not recommended by the manufacturers of the machines but is used in clinical practice, frequently with good effect. Injection of local anaesthetic and steroid into the epidural space, the sacroiliac joints or the symphysis pubis may be considered necessary if symptomatic control of pain cannot be achieved by other methods. The safety of such procedures during pregnancy is unknown, and a risk–benefit analysis must be undertaken for each woman.

Delivery before term may be considered when pain control is difficult to achieve.

Anaesthetic management

Women with pre-existing musculoskeletal pathology should be fully assessed during the antenatal period. Previous spinal surgery is not a contraindication to regional analgesia and anaesthesia, although women may have been told by their midwife, general practitioner or orthopaedic surgeon that they will be unable to have epidural analgesia (see Chapter 115, *Kyphoscoliosis*). There may be respiratory impairment following significant corrective surgery, and some postoperative neurological deficit, and if so these must be documented antenatally. Women should be told that epidural analgesia for labour does not increase the likelihood of experiencing postnatal backache. If neuraxial analgesia/anaesthesia is administered, both the obstetric team and patient must be careful not to over-extend relaxed joints or adopt positions that would not have been accepted before analgesia/anaesthesia.

Regional anaesthesia and analgesia in women who have had discectomy or laminectomy is not usually technically difficult, but there may be a slightly increased risk of accidental dural puncture or poor spread of local anaesthetic, and patients should be warned about this. There is some evidence to suggest that women with severe chronic back pain with associated neurology may have a delayed onset of epidural analgesia. This may be due to increased time for diffusion of local anaesthetic to the affected nerve root because of scarring that develops secondary to disc injury, or mechanical obstruction by disc prolapse.

There is no contraindication to vaginal delivery, nor to the use of regional analgesia in women with pregnancy-related back pain, although many women request (and some obstetricians suggest) delivery by elective caesarean section to avoid any risk of exacerbating existing back symptoms.

The management of women who have had surgery is considered in Chapter 115, *Kyphoscoliosis*.

Key points

- Low back pain is common in pregnancy; it is usually mechanical and should be treated symptomatically.
- Although rare, acute disc prolapse with neurological deficit may occur and require surgical treatment.
- There is no contraindication to epidural or spinal analgesia or anaesthesia in women with low back pain.
- Serious spinal and neurological pathology may, rarely, present during pregnancy, and should always be considered in the differential diagnosis of new-onset back pain.

Further reading

Liddle SD, Pennick V. Interventions for preventing and treating low-back and pelvic pain during pregnancy. *Cochrane Database Syst Rev* 2015; (9): CD001139

Orlikowski CE, Dickinson JE, Paech MJ, McDonald SJ, Nathan E. Intrapartum analgesia and its association with post-partum back pain and headache in nulliparous women. *Aust N Z J Obstet Gynaecol* 2006; **46**: 395–401.

Vermani E, Mittal R, Weeks A. Pelvic girdle pain and low back pain in pregnancy: a review. *Pain Pract* 2010; **10**: 60–71.

The parturient with chronic pain

Chronic pain, which may be defined as pain that persists or recurs for longer than 3 months, is not uncommon in the obstetric population. The physiological stresses of pregnancy, such as musculoskeletal or pelvic girdle strain, may trigger a chronic pain disorder or exacerbate a pre-existing one. Chronic pain in the parturient poses particular challenges to the maternity team and has significant implications for both maternal and fetal wellbeing.

Problems and special considerations

Management of women with chronic pain may be hindered by a lack of awareness among maternity staff of the medical and pharmacological issues involved, such that patients may be denied effective analgesia or placed at risk if monitoring is inadequate. If there is a background of drug misuse, this situation may be compounded by any underlying psychological issues on the part of the mother, and/or by any judgemental attitudes on the part of the staff.

Women with chronic pain syndromes may be on long-term opioids and/or adjuvant medication. Long-standing opioid therapy may cause tolerance and/or hyperalgesia, and hence these women may experience difficulty with the control of postpartum pain and are likely to require higher doses of postoperative analgesia – which may be up to five times higher than in their opioid-naive counterparts. Despite exhibiting tolerance to some opioid-related side effects, these patients remain at risk of respiratory depression, particularly with escalating opioid requirements in the peripartum period.

Chronic opioid use is associated with adverse obstetric and neonatal outcomes including miscarriage, fetal growth restriction and placental abruption. Sudden interruption of opioid intake may lead to the development of acute withdrawal syndrome in the mother, which manifests as agitation, haemodynamic changes and uterine contractions. Infants who have been chronically exposed to opioids in utero may suffer with neonatal abstinence syndrome after birth.

Some women with neuropathic pain disorders that are refractory to conventional pharmacological or surgical treatment may require the placement of a spinal cord stimulator (SCS) or an intrathecal drug delivery device. The former consists of a pulse generator and electrode leads that are placed in the epidural space and acts by delivering electrical stimulation to the dorsal column, thus reducing the perception of pain, while the latter consists of an indwelling intrathecal catheter and an external or implantable pump that enables the delivery of a fixed or variable dose of drug. The presence of these devices has implications for regional anaesthesia as there is a risk of damage to the leads or catheter by the regional block needle or epidural catheter, or introduction of infection. In addition, previous instrumentation of the epidural space for device placement may result in scarring, with subsequent failed or patchy epidural analgesia.

Management

The successful peripartum management of women with chronic pain disorders should be a multidisciplinary effort and must include input from a specialist pain team and neonatologist. Antenatally, a plan should be made and referral routes established in case acute intervention is required at any time during pregnancy or postpartum.

As a rule, baseline opioid maintenance therapy should continue throughout labour and delivery. Antenatal involvement of an acute pain specialist can help to form a strategy. Multimodal analgesia should be utilised, and adjuvant drugs such as ketamine may be useful to supplement opioid therapy in the postoperative period. Abdominal field blocks such as a transversus abdominis plane (TAP) block may be used to supplement parenteral analgesia after caesarean section, although their reported efficacy in opioid-dependent parturients is variable. These patients should be closely monitored for respiratory depression, and some may best be observed in a high-dependency setting in the postnatal period.

In parturients with an implanted pain management device, the location of the leads or catheter must first be verified before attempting regional anaesthesia, in order to minimise the risk of damage to the device's components. Post-implantation images should be obtained, and antenatal consultation with the chronic pain or neurosurgery team is required. Where previous images of the spine cannot be acquired, ultrasound guidance may be used to confirm the position of the leads and guide insertion. Strict procedural asepsis is particularly important, and must be observed and clearly documented. An SCS is sensitive to the electromagnetic interference that may be generated by the use of diathermy, so appropriate precautions, similar to those taken with cardiac implantable electronic devices, must be observed to reduce this (see Chapter 92, *Arrhythmias*).

It is recommended that the baseline infusion rate of an intrathecal pump remains active during labour and delivery alongside regional analgesia. Utilisation of the access port to administer spinal anaesthesia is generally not advised; if it were to be used, then initial aspiration of the intrathecal catheter must be performed, to dispose of the drug in situ. If epidural placement is attempted, the point of entry should avoid the site of the dural puncture.

Key points

- Pregnant women on treatment for chronic pain syndromes are at risk of adverse maternal and fetal outcomes.
- Opioid maintenance therapy should be continued throughout the peripartum period.
- Chronic opioid therapy is unlikely to provide useful analgesia, and should be considered a patient's baseline; multimodal analgesic regimens with significant additional opioid administration are likely to be required.
- High-dependency monitoring may be necessary.
- The presence of an implanted pain management device requires special precautions with the performance of neuraxial blocks and the use of diathermy.
- Multidisciplinary input is required at intervals throughout pregnancy and postpartum.

Further reading

Sommerfield D, Hu P, O'Keeffe D, McKeating K. Caesarean section in a parturient with a spinal cord stimulator. *Int J Obstet Anesth* 2010; **19**: 114–17.

Souzdalnitski D, Snegovskikh D. Analgesia for the parturient with chronic nonmalignant pain. *Tech Reg Anesth Pain Manag* 2014; **18**: 166–71.

Young AC, Lubenow TR, Buvanendran A. The parturient with implanted spinal cord stimulator: management and review of the literature. *Reg Anesth Pain Med* 2015; **40**: 276–83.

Young JL, Lockhart EM, Baysinger CL. Anesthetic and obstetric management of the opioid-dependent parturient. *Int Anesthesiol Clin* 2014: **52**: 67–85.

Chapter 118

Neurological disease

The pregnant woman may have suffered (and/or recovered) from a neurological condition before she became pregnant, or she may develop neurological disease while pregnant (Table 118.1).

Problems and special considerations

Traditionally, regional analgesia and anaesthesia have been avoided in most chronic neurological diseases because of the fear of making the woman's condition worse or being blamed should a worsening occur. Since randomised controlled trials are lacking for most of these conditions, traditional prejudices persist, although such evidence that there is supports regional techniques in many cases.

Table 118.1 Neurological conditions that may be seen in pregnancy

Pre-existing		
Previous history	Trauma	Head injury
		Spinal cord injury
	Infection	Meningitis
		Acute post-infective neuropathy
	Tumour	
Established neurological disease	Cerebrovascular disease	
	Migraine	
	Myasthenia gravis	
	Spina bifida	
	Epilepsy	
	Multiple sclerosis	
	Idiopathic intracranial hypertension	
Arising during pregnancy		
	Trauma	Acute head injury
		Acute spinal cord injury
	Infection	Meningitis
		Acute post-infective neuropathy
	Tumour	

Acute neurological conditions may put both the mother and the fetus at risk. Anaesthetic input may be required for peripartum analgesia or anaesthesia, acute medical management of critically ill patients, or surgery indicated by the neurological condition.

Management options

The management of both groups of women depends on the nature of the disease, its effects on pregnancy and delivery and the implications of the physiological changes of pregnancy.

Ideally, women who have a diagnosed neurological disease should be counselled before conception, so that they are aware of the possible problems that may be associated with their disease during pregnancy and delivery. In practice, the majority of women are seen after conception, and the aim should be early antenatal assessment. The effect of maintenance therapy and the necessity to change treatment to avoid teratogenic effects must also be considered. Good communication between the clinicians involved is essential in the management of these women. Clear guidelines for care should be written in the medical record and should be revised and updated as necessary.

Neuroimaging may occasionally be required during pregnancy. Magnetic resonance imaging is generally perceived to be a safe modality in pregnant women; the risks of harm to the fetus secondary to tissue heating or exposure to high levels of noise are considered largely theoretical. Some authors, however, advise caution with its use in the first trimester. Ionising radiation is associated with the potential risks of pregnancy loss, fetal malformations or an increased incidence of childhood malignancy, and the risk is related to the stage of gestation and the total dose of radiation delivered. If computerised tomography is deemed essential in pregnancy, measures to minimise fetal radiation exposure should be taken. Gadolinium or iodinated contrast media may be associated with adverse fetal effects and should be reserved for situations where there is a strong clinical indication for their use.

Key points

- Neurological conditions may already be present before pregnancy or may arise acutely during pregnancy.
- Management depends on the condition, the effects on pregnancy and the effects of pregnancy on the condition.
- Early assessment and drawing up of management plans should take place whenever possible.

Further reading

American College of Obstetricians and Gynecologists' Committee on Obstetric Practice. Opinion no. 656. Guidelines for diagnostic imaging during pregnancy and lactation. *Obstet Gynecol* 2016; **127**: e75–80.

Hopkins AN, Alshaeri T, Akst SA, Berger JS. Neurologic disease with pregnancy and considerations for the obstetric anesthesiologist. *Semin Perinatol* 2014: **38**: 359–69.

Ng J, Kitchen N. Neurosurgery and pregnancy. *J Neurol Neurosurg Psychiatry* 2008; **79**: 745–52.

Meningitis

Acute infections of the nervous system may occur at any time during pregnancy or the peripartum period. The most important infection for the anaesthetist to consider is meningitis, as this can (rarely) occur as a sequel to spinal anaesthesia and confuse the differential diagnosis of a postdural puncture headache.

Women may also present having previously had meningitis.

Problems and special considerations

Meningitis may be:

- **Infective,** caused by bacteria, viruses and, rarely, as a complication of other diseases such as tuberculosis or fungal infections
- **Aseptic,** caused by topical chemical agents (e.g. disinfectants) and, rarely, systemic drugs, e.g. H_2-blockers, non-steroidal anti-inflammatory drugs and antibiotics

Meningitis that occurs as a complication of regional anaesthesia may be either of the above, and in each case prevention is better than cure. Meticulous attention to aseptic technique is an essential part of minimising the risk of infection or chemical contamination at the time of performing the regional block.

The classic signs of meningitis are headache, neck stiffness, photophobia, vomiting, fever and raised white cell count. Many of these symptoms are also produced by an accidental dural puncture, and so the exclusion of meningitis is essential in the differential diagnosis of any headache that develops after a regional anaesthetic.

Almost all women with a history of previous meningitis have had a diagnostic lumbar puncture, which may have been a frightening experience, leading to apprehension of any further similar procedures. Some may have residual neurological impairment, although this is uncommon with modern management.

Management options

Preventive measures include full aseptic precautions (including the use of a facemask to prevent droplet spread) during the performance of neuraxial techniques, and bacterial filters must be used with epidural catheters. Disconnected epidural systems may carry an increased risk of contamination, and obstetric units should have local guidance on their management. If within 15–30 minutes of witnessed disconnection, this may include wiping the epidural catheter with alcohol, letting it dry and cutting the catheter with a sterile blade, 5–10 cm proximal to the fluid meniscus, before reconnecting. Some may advocate re-siting of the catheter; however, the risk of repeated instrumentation of the epidural space,

Table 119.1 Typical cerebrospinal fluid (CSF) findings in postdural puncture headache and meningitis

	Postdural puncture headache	Viral meningitis	Bacterial meningitis	Aseptic meningitis
CSF	Clear, normal	Clear, normal	May be cloudy	May be cloudy
CSF protein	–	↑	↑	↑
WBC in CSF	–	↑ Lymphocytes	↑	↑ [a]
Glucose	Normal	↓	↓	Normal
Culture	Negative	Negative	May be positive	Negative

WBC, white blood cells.
[a] Variable, usually leucocytes.

particularly in obese women or those in whom the initial placement was technically difficult, must be weighed against that of introducing infection into the neuraxis.

The performance of regional anaesthesia in women in labour with features of bacteraemia is controversial, and the decision should be based on an individual risk–benefit assessment (see Chapter 144, *Pyrexia during labour*).

Meningitis should be considered as a possible diagnosis in any patient who has a raised temperature or white cell count associated with a headache. Differentiation between meningitis and accidental dural puncture as the cause of the headache may be difficult. When there is any doubt, a neurological consultation is essential, and where appropriate a diagnostic lumbar puncture should be performed (Table 119.1). Antibiotics are usually prescribed empirically while awaiting the results of microbiological investigation.

Ideally, women with a previous history of meningitis should be seen antenatally by the obstetric anaesthetist for assessment and reassurance. In general, most women can be reassured that they are not at extra risk from regional analgesia and anaesthesia.

Key points

- Meningitis is the most important acute neurological infection in obstetrics.
- Meningitis should always be considered in a woman with severe postpartum headache.
- Adherence to aseptic technique during the performance of regional anaesthesia is essential, to minimise the risk of introducing contaminants into the neuraxial space.

Further reading

American Society of Anesthesiologists, American Society of Regional Anaesthesia and Pain Medicine. Practice advisory for the prevention, diagnosis, and management of infection complications associated with neuraxial techniques: an updated report by the American Society of Anesthesiologists Task Force on infectious complications associated with neuraxial techniques and the American Society of Regional Anaesthesia and Pain Medicine. *Anesthesiology* 2017; **126**: 585–601.

Association of Anaesthetists of Great Britain and Ireland, Obstetric Anaesthetists' Association, Regional Anaesthesia UK, Association of Paediatric Anaesthetists of Great Britain and Ireland. Safety guideline: skin antisepsis for central neuraxial blockade. *Anaesthesia* 2014; **69**: 1279–86.

Horlocker TT, Wedel DJ. Infectious complications of regional anesthesia. *Best Pract Res Clin Anaesthesiol* 2008; **22**: 451–75.

McGill F, Heyderman RS, Michael BD, *et al.* The UK joint specialist societies guideline on the diagnosis and management of acute meningitis and meningococcal sepsis in immunocompetent adults. *J Infect* 2016; **72**: 405–38.

Chapter 120

Acute post-infective peripheral neuropathy (Guillain–Barré syndrome)

Acute post-infective peripheral neuropathy (Guillain–Barré syndrome; Landry's paralysis) is a rare condition that usually follows an acute respiratory infection, although it may follow clostridial diarrhoea or surgery, and more recently has been linked to infection with the Zika virus. In pregnant women, the disease may have a rapid course and an increased risk of maternal mortality. There may be a slight increase in incidence in the early postpartum period. The symptoms usually commence some days after the infection, which triggers an autoimmune acute demyelinating neuropathy. The first symptoms are peripheral sensory paraesthesiae followed by a loss of motor power. The neuropathy ascends and may affect respiratory muscles. Generally, the disease is short-lived, and full recovery is usual over a period of weeks or months.

Problems and special considerations

Respiratory reserve in pregnant women is reduced, making these patients especially prone to respiratory impairment.

Autonomic dysfunction may be present and may cause significant haemodynamic fluctuations in response to regional anaesthesia, blood loss or tracheal intubation.

Women with a past history of Guillain–Barré syndrome who present for obstetric analgesia and anaesthesia may have concerns about whether regional techniques will cause a recurrence of the disease. Some may be anxious about having a needle in their back if they have had a bad experience with a lumbar puncture during investigation of the acute episode, or they may be worried about a significant motor block (e.g. when a caesarean section is performed).

Residual neurological impairment is rare after an acute episode.

Management options

Management of the acute illness should take into account the physiological changes of pregnancy and the wellbeing of the growing fetus. Careful monitoring of respiratory function is required, with ventilatory support when necessary. Particular attention must be paid to the avoidance of aortocaval compression and thromboprophylaxis in the immobilised parturient.

General and regional anaesthetic techniques have both been employed for the delivery of women with Guillain–Barré syndrome. If general anaesthesia is required, suxamethonium should be avoided because of the risk of hyperkalaemia, and neuromuscular function should be monitored. The mother should be closely observed for features of respiratory compromise in the immediate postpartum period.

There is no contraindication to regional analgesia or anaesthesia, when there is a past history of Guillain–Barré syndrome, and the woman can be reassured that it will not cause a recurrence of the acute episode. The risks and benefits of regional blocks should be discussed before the woman is in pain, preferably at an antenatal consultation. The woman's fears of a motor block need to be considered by the anaesthetist, particularly if she has required ventilation for her acute illness. If there is any neurological deficit, this should be assessed and documented before a regional block is performed.

Key points

- Acute Guillain–Barré syndrome is rare in pregnancy but carries an increased risk of maternal morbidity and mortality.
- Antenatal assessment of women with a previous history of Guillain–Barré syndrome is advisable, since they may be very worried about regional analgesia and anaesthesia.
- Regional analgesia and anaesthesia are not contraindicated.

Further reading

Pacheco LD, Saad AF, Hankins GDV, Chiosi G, Saade G. Guillain–Barré syndrome in pregnancy. *Obstet Gynecol* 2016; **128**: 1105–10.
Willison HJ, Jacobs BC, van Doom PA. Guillain–Barré syndrome. *Lancet* 2016; **388**: 717–27.

Past history of neurological trauma

It is not uncommon for patients with previous head or spinal cord injury to become pregnant. Many of these women will seek pre-conception advice, but others will present in the antenatal period.

Problems and special considerations

The extent of the problems depends on the neurological deficit. For head-injured patients, the main concerns are related to:

- **The presence of upper motor neurone lesions** (causing difficulties with positioning and mobility; possible hyperkalaemic response to suxamethonium)
- **Immobility** (increasing the risk of thromboembolism, pressure sores and atelectasis following general anaesthesia)
- **Any associated injuries**, especially neck (affecting the airway) and pelvis or vertebral column (affecting mode of delivery and regional analgesia/anaesthesia)
- **Difficulties in communication**

For spinal-cord-injured patients, the above concerns may also exist. The level of the neurological deficit is the most important issue; the major considerations are:

- **Pulmonary function and the effect of pregnancy and delivery.** If the level is above T4, there is likely to be some reduction in respiratory reserve. The phrenic nerve supply to the diaphragm arises from cervical roots 3–5, so this muscle is usually spared in paraplegics. However, the intercostal nerves, which contribute to ventilation and which may be particularly important in pregnancy, will be affected.
- **Risk of autonomic hyperreflexia.** This is usually associated with injuries above T4–6 and results in increased sensitivity of sympathetic reflexes in response to cutaneous or visceral stimulation below the level of the lesion, leading to exaggerated sympathetic nervous activity and release of catecholamines. There is resultant labile blood pressure, typically causing massive vasoconstriction and hypertension that may be severe enough to cause seizures or stroke. Arrhythmias may occur, and there may be a compensatory bradycardia. Susceptibility usually develops within a few weeks of injury.
- **Mode of delivery.** A sensory level above T10 is usually associated with a painless labour, and these women are also more likely to deliver prematurely. This may result in a painless precipitous delivery. Some of these women will suffer from muscle spasms, and many will need an assisted delivery.

Management options

These women should be seen antenatally, and any neurological deficit should be carefully assessed. A thorough history should seek to elicit symptoms and triggers of autonomic hyperreflexia, and details of previous spinal surgery should be obtained. The delivery plan should take the above points into consideration, with epidural analgesia part of the management in most cases.

Epidural analgesia has been shown to be effective in prophylaxis and treatment of autonomic hyperreflexia. The epidural should be carefully managed to minimise any cardiovascular changes, and a low concentration of local anaesthetic combined with an opioid is usually considered the method of choice, although the need for more concentrated local anaesthetic has been suggested in order to block the powerful afferent triggers of autonomic hyperreflexia. Autonomic hyperreflexia is difficult to treat pharmacologically, and α- and β-blocking drugs and nifedipine are of limited value. The use of magnesium sulfate has been described, although experience is limited.

Regional anaesthesia is the anaesthetic of choice for operative delivery in most cases. If general anaesthesia is used, alternatives to suxamethonium should be considered if within the period of risk of hyperkalaemia (10 days to 6–7 months after injury). Care must be taken to avoid autonomic hyperreflexia, and deep anaesthesia is needed.

Key points

- Any patient who has had a past neurological trauma requires individual assessment of her neurological deficit and associated injuries in order to estimate her risk factors.
- Regional analgesia and anaesthesia are indicated in most cases.
- Autonomic hyperreflexia is best prevented or controlled by epidural block.

Further reading

Vercauteren M, Waets P, Pitkänen M. Neuraxial techniques in patients with pre-existing back impairment or prior spine interventions: a topical review with special reference to obstetrics. *Acta Anaesthesiol Scand* 2011; **55**: 910–17.

Idiopathic intracranial hypertension

Idiopathic intracranial hypertension (previously termed benign intracranial hypertension or pseudotumour cerebri) is defined as raised intracranial pressure (> 20 mmHg) that is not associated with intracranial pathology. It is a rare but well-recognised syndrome that typically affects young to middle-aged overweight females, causing headache and visual disturbances. The aetiology is unclear and there are no focal neurological signs. In pregnancy, it is more common in the first two trimesters.

Problems and special considerations

General treatment is weight control and diuretics if necessary. In more severe cases, lumbar puncture and cerebrospinal fluid (CSF) removal may be recommended. Insertion of lumbo-peritoneal shunts and optic nerve sheath decompression have been performed in very severe cases.

Headache and visual disturbances may also occur in pre-eclampsia and postdural puncture headache, possibly posing a diagnostic challenge.

Although CSF pressure is increased, dural puncture (deliberate or accidental) will not lead to coning in this group of patients, and it may even be temporarily beneficial in relieving CSF pressure.

Management options

Epidural and spinal analgesia/anaesthesia (single-shot or via an intrathecal catheter) have been successfully used for labour and caesarean section in this patient group. Concerns have been raised over the possibility of excessive increases in intracranial pressure with bolus injection of epidural solutions; slow administration or the use of infusions has been suggested. Spinal anaesthesia may be potentially difficult, as the CSF is under pressure, and some CSF may need to be withdrawn before injection of the local anaesthetic. Recent CSF drainage may precipitate a block level that is higher than expected.

Regional anaesthesia in women with lumboperitoneal shunts carries a potential risk of damage to the shunt catheter or dissipation of the injectate into the peritoneal cavity. Radiographic imaging may demonstrate the exact location of the shunt; if this is unavailable, epidural catheter insertion should be performed using a midline approach in the intervertebral space above or below the skin scar.

General anaesthesia is not contraindicated, but the technique must be modified to ensure the maintenance of adequate cerebral perfusion and the avoidance of factors that may cause a rise in intracranial pressure.

Key points

- Idiopathic intracranial hypertension may present with severe headache and visual disturbances.
- Regional analgesia and anaesthesia (including spinal block) are not contraindicated.

Further reading

Anson JA, Vaida S, Giampetro DM, McQuillan PM. Anesthetic management of labor and delivery in patients with elevated intracranial pressure. *Int J Obstet Anesth* 2015; **24**: 147–60.

Hopkins AN, Alshaeri T, Akst SA, Berger JS. Neurologic disease with pregnancy and considerations for the obstetric anesthesiologist. *Semin Perinatol* 2014; **38**: 359–69.

Chapter 123

Intracranial tumour

Obstetric anaesthetists may be involved in the care of women who present with a previous history of intracranial tumour, or in whom a brain tumour is diagnosed for the first time during pregnancy, labour and delivery, or in the postpartum period.

Problems and special considerations

Previous history of tumour

Women with a past history of a brain tumour may have residual neurological impairment, as for a past history of neurological trauma. A small number of women have residual tumour left, and this may be affected by the pregnancy. There may be a shunt to maintain normal cerebrospinal fluid (CSF) pressures. Generally, these shunts drain from the brain into the peritoneal cavity; however, some drain CSF around the spinal cord into the peritoneum. The latter may be placed in the lumbar region and thus cause a problem if regional block is to be considered (see Chapter 122, *Idiopathic intracranial hypertension*). The risk of introducing infection at the time of a regional block is very small but may be a deterrent to regional block in these women. Most patients will be particularly anxious about the effects of both regional and general anaesthesia on their neurological function.

Tumour diagnosed during pregnancy

Particular problems may be related to:

- The nature of the tumour
- The treatment the patient is receiving, e.g. steroids or anticonvulsants
- The presence of raised intracranial pressure (ICP), its severity and the associated risk of coning
- The effect of pushing in the second stage of labour on ICP and the tumour
- The presence of any other medical problems
- The risks of regional analgesia or anaesthesia and general anaesthesia

Tumour manifesting itself in the peripartum period

The woman may present with neurological signs or symptoms that may be related to the position of the tumour or to the development of raised ICP. The obstetric anaesthetist may be asked to see the woman, particularly if she has had a regional anaesthetic.

Presentation may be with altered consciousness, focal signs, a convulsion or a headache. The differential diagnosis includes eclampsia, epilepsy, meningitis, posterior reversible encephalopathy syndrome, cerebral venous thrombosis and postdural puncture headache. The headache associated with raised ICP is usually present when the patient is supine and, unlike postdural puncture headache, does not worsen on standing; typically it is made worse by stooping, coughing and straining. The associated symptoms and signs of photophobia, vomiting and neck stiffness may be present both in raised ICP and following dural puncture.

Management options

If a tumour has been diagnosed during pregnancy, the obstetric anaesthetist should be consulted about the management of the labour and the provision of regional analgesia/ anaesthesia to help minimise the stress of labour and delivery. The benefits of regional techniques in these patients must be balanced against the risk of dural puncture and of coning. Decision making should take into account the size and location of the tumour, the presence of mass effect, any clinical or radiological evidence of raised ICP and the potential risks of general anaesthesia. The advice of a neurologist or neurosurgeon should also be sought. If epidural analgesia is indicated, a senior anaesthetist should be involved.

Slow, titrated boluses or a continuous infusion of epidural solution is advisable to reduce the sharp rise in ICP that may result from compression of the dural sac with injection. Pushing in the second stage should be minimised, to reduce the possibility of bleeding into the tumour or acute increases in ICP. If the patient is suffering from a significant increase in ICP and the obstetrician advises urgent delivery, caesarean section under general anaesthesia may be the technique of choice. General anaesthesia may need to be modified to give a 'neuro' anaesthetic that would minimise raised ICP at the time of induction of and emergence from anaesthesia. Nausea and vomiting should be well controlled. It is important to remember that decreased arterial partial pressure of carbon dioxide from the normal value in pregnancy (approximately 4 kPa) in the mother will reduce placental perfusion and this may compromise the fetus.

When new headaches, convulsions or other neurological symptoms and signs present in the peripartum period, it is easy to assume more common conditions such as postdural puncture headache and eclampsia, rather than think of intracranial tumour. A careful history and examination (where appropriate by a neurologist) is important in reaching the correct diagnosis, with cranial imaging as appropriate. Once diagnosed, treatment is as for any non-pregnant patient.

The majority of women who have had previous intracranial tumours are entirely normal and have no residual problems. Neurological/neurosurgical advice will be necessary to establish whether the pregnancy will affect any residual tumour.

Key points

- In women who have or have had an intracranial tumour, regional analgesia is usually indicated during labour, but an accidental dural puncture may be catastrophic; thus the decision should depend on the individual features of each case.
- Underlying intracerebral pathology should always be considered when new symptoms or signs present postpartum.
- A neurologist should be consulted if in doubt.

Further reading

Anson JA, Vaida S, Giampetro DM, McQuillan PM. Anesthetic management of labor and delivery in patients with elevated intracranial pressure. *Int J Obstet Anesth* 2015; **24**: 147–60.

Leffert LR, Schwamm LH. Neuraxial anesthesia in parturients with intracranial pathology: a comprehensive review and reassessment of risk. *Anesthesiology* 2013; **119**: 703–18.

Verheecke M, Halasaka MJ, Lok CA, *et al.* Primary brain tumours, meningiomas and brain metastases in pregnancy: report on 27 cases and review of literature. *Eur J Cancer* 2014; **50**: 1462–71.

Wang LP, Paech MJ. Neuroanesthesia for the pregnant woman. *Anesth Analg* 2008; **107**: 193–200.

Chapter 124

Neurofibromatosis

Neurofibromatosis (NF) is an inherited systemic disease with an autosomal dominant pattern of transmission. It is caused by mutation of the genes that encode for the secretion of proteins that inhibit abnormal cell growth. The multisystem nature of the disease has several implications for peripartum anaesthetic and obstetric management.

The disorder is commonly classified into NF-1 or NF-2, but other forms/subtypes have been described. NF-1 is the most prevalent type and typically presents with widespread pigmented skin lesions, nerve sheath tumours (neurofibromas) in variable locations including the airway and mediastinum, and ocular manifestations. Patients may have associated cardiovascular dysfunction such as hypertension, cardiomyopathy, structural heart disease or vasculopathy. Other features may include scoliosis or kyphoscoliosis, learning difficulties, epilepsy and an association with phaeochromocytoma. NF-2 is a much less common form that predominantly affects the central nervous system and is characterised by the development of bilateral acoustic neuromas and cranial, meningeal or spinal tumours.

Problems and special considerations

Neurofibromas may show a hormone-mediated proliferation and/or an increase in number during pregnancy. Intracranial lesions may be associated with raised intracranial pressure (ICP) and an increased risk of brain herniation with dural puncture. Unintentional instrumentation of a spinal tumour during regional anaesthesia may result in dissemination of tumour cells or bleeding into the neuraxis. Regional anaesthesia may be difficult to perform in the presence of scoliosis or with extensive lesions on the lumbar spine.

Previously, it was thought that patients with NF-1 were sensitive to neuromuscular blocking drugs, but this is no longer thought to be the case. Nonetheless, caution is required because of the associated renal complications that may occur with the disease.

Tumours infrequently develop in the oral cavity, tongue, larynx or lower airways, and may complicate airway management.

Previous studies have reported an increased incidence of obstetric complications in women with NF-1, including pre-eclampsia, fetal growth restriction and preterm labour.

Management options

Pregnant women with neurofibromatosis require advance planning of their mode of delivery and anaesthetic management. The decision to administer regional anaesthesia in these patients should be guided by the severity of the disease, the distribution of the fibromas and the presence of cranial/neuraxial or airway tumours. A thorough history and clinical examination is essential, but it is important to remember that the absence of symptoms does not exclude the presence of spinal neuromas. Appropriate imaging of the spine and cranium, as guided by radiologist advice, enables the detection of tumours and is recommended before proceeding with central neuraxial blocks. Patients with raised ICP should be managed in the appropriate way (see Chapter 122, *Idiopathic intracranial hypertension*). Advanced airway management techniques may be required in the presence of a potential difficult airway (see Chapter 38, *Failed and difficult intubation*).

Key points

- Neurofibromatosis is a multisystem disease with a variable clinical presentation.
- Regional anaesthesia may have deleterious effects in these women, and antenatal neuroimaging is recommended.
- A thorough airway assessment is required.

Further reading

Fox CJ, Tomajian S, Kaye AJ, *et al.* Perioperative management of neurofibromatosis type 1. *Ochsner J* 2012; **12**: 111–21.

Hirbe AC, Gutmann DH. Neurofibromatosis type 1: a multidisciplinary approach to care. *Lancet Neurol* 2014; **13**: 834–43.

Sakai T, Vallejo MC, Shannon KT. A parturient with neurofibromatosis type 2: anesthetic and obstetric considerations for delivery. *Int J Obstet Anesth* 2005; **14**: 332–5.

Stroke

Stroke may occur during pregnancy and delivery and may be caused by intracranial haemorrhage or thrombosis. The incidence varies but is thought to be between 11 and 26 per 100,000 deliveries.

Problems and special considerations

Stroke presenting during pregnancy or peripartum

Pregnancy and labour increase the risk of stroke. This risk will be further increased if there is associated obesity, smoking or hypertensive disease of pregnancy.

Intracerebral haemorrhage may occur at any stage during the pregnancy; the risk is increased in the third trimester and is highest during the intra- and postpartum periods. The most common problem is subarachnoid haemorrhage (SAH), which presents as an acute onset of severe headache, often with associated neck stiffness, photophobia and vomiting. There may be neurological deficits or loss of consciousness. SAH is often associated with an underlying berry aneurysm or arteriovenous malformation, and is also a cause of death associated with pre-eclampsia. Haemorrhagic stroke was identified as one of the most common causes of death in women with hypertensive disease of pregnancy. Intracranial haemorrhage may also be a consequence of reversible cerebral vasoconstriction syndrome or may be caused by venous bleeding associated with cerebral venous thrombosis.

Ischaemic stroke usually occurs in the territory of the middle cerebral arteries and can be associated with an underlying structural cardiac or vascular cause. Pregnancy predisposes to cerebral thrombosis, including cortical vein thrombosis. More than three-quarters of all pregnancy-associated cases of cerebral venous thrombosis occur postpartum. Other predisposing factors include dehydration and other hypercoagulable states (e.g. thrombophilias). Although cortical vein thrombosis is rare, it is important to the obstetric anaesthetist in the differential diagnosis of postdural puncture headache. The patient may present with focal neurological signs, seizures or other signs of raised intracranial pressure.

Sudden collapse carries the risk of airway obstruction and hypoxaemia, aspiration of gastric contents, aortocaval compression and fetal compromise. As for many acute medical emergencies in the maternity suite, staff may be unfamiliar with basic resuscitative measures unless these are regularly practised.

Previous history of stroke

The most common presentation in the childbearing age group is a previous history of SAH. Some of these women will have made a complete recovery and others will have a neurological deficit of which the anaesthetist should be aware. They may be frightened by the thought of a needle in their back after a bad experience with lumbar puncture. There may be an exaggerated hyperkalaemic response to suxamethonium 10 days to 6–7 months after stroke. Women with a previous cerebral thrombosis may be taking heparin or aspirin.

Management options

Prevention

The risk of SAH is one reason for ensuring adequate blood pressure control in pre-eclampsia, particularly in the peripartum period and in parturients who receive general anaesthesia. The intense sympathetic stimulation associated with tracheal intubation may precipitate a sharp rise in systemic blood pressure and intracranial pressure, and appropriate modification of the anaesthetic technique is required to attenuate this pressor response.

Simple preventive measures for intracranial venous thrombosis include avoidance of dehydration and prompt treatment of infection, especially in women with a recognised risk factor such as thrombophilia.

Diagnosis

Diagnosis of stroke is by computerised tomography or magnetic resonance imaging of the brain; if the diagnosis is suspected, it is wise to involve the neurologists early. The use of lumbar puncture has largely been superseded by imaging techniques for the diagnosis of SAH, partly because of the risk of coning.

Therapy

In pregnant women who suffer a stroke with loss of consciousness, basic resuscitation must be performed, with particular attention to uterine displacement and avoidance of aspiration. There is a significant risk of rebleeding following SAH, so assessment by neurosurgeons with a view to surgical treatment is essential. The indication for surgical intervention should not be altered by the fact that the woman is pregnant, and the procedure should generally be managed as for non-pregnant patients.

In addition to supportive treatment, thrombolysis should be considered in women with acute ischaemic strokes. Cerebral venous thrombosis in pregnancy requires systemic anti-coagulation for the remainder of the gestation and for the initial postpartum period.

Management of delivery depends on the clinical condition of the patient, who may still have a significant neurological deficit. If the patient is well recovered, a stress-free vaginal delivery with epidural analgesia is the management of choice, taking care to avoid significant fluctuations in blood pressure and exercising caution in the presence of anticoagulation. The indications for caesarean section should only be obstetric. However, if the patient is confused or has a problem with cognitive function, the wisest course of action may be delivery by caesarean section under general anaesthesia, which should be carefully managed to minimise the hypertensive response to tracheal intubation. Each patient will need to be considered individually in consultation with the obstetrician and neurosurgeons, and other disciplines where appropriate. Combined caesarean section and neurosurgery has been performed.

The management of women with previous SAH depends on whether the underlying pathology has been surgically treated. If so, the woman can be regarded as relatively normal. The risk of a further bleed is increased if there is hypertension, and in particular if there are sudden surges in blood pressure. The control of blood pressure and the avoidance of stress during labour or delivery are therefore important. Generally, regional analgesia should be recommended for labour. If a caesarean section is required, regional anaesthesia is appropriate. This should, however, be preceded by a detailed discussion with the woman, ideally in the antenatal period, when a clearly documented plan for the management of analgesia and anaesthesia should be made. If general anaesthesia is necessary, strict pharmacological control of blood pressure is required, and alternatives to suxamethonium should be used if within the period of risk.

Rarely, stroke (usually subdural or subarachnoid haemorrhage) has followed spinal anaesthesia or accidental dural puncture.

Key points

- Control of blood pressure in hypertension is important in pregnancy, whether or not it is pregnancy-related.
- Headaches are not always caused by dural puncture.
- Pregnancy is not a contraindication to neurosurgery.
- Regional analgesia or anaesthesia is usually indicated unless there is significant neurological impairment.

Further reading

Edlow JA, Caplan LR, O'Brien K, Tibbles CD. Diagnosis of acute neurological emergencies in pregnant and post-partum women. *Lancet Neurol* 2013; **12**: 175–85.

Frontera JA, Ahmed W. Neurocritical care complications of pregnancy and puerperum. *J Crit Care* 2014; **29**: 1069–81.

Scott CA, Bewley S, Rudd A, *et al.* Incidence, risk factors, management, and outcomes of stroke in pregnancy. *Obstet Gynecol* 2012; **120**: 318–24.

Shainker SA, Edlow JA, O'Brien K. Cerebrovascular emergencies in pregnancy. *Best Pract Res Clin Obstet Gynaecol* 2015; **29**: 721–31.

Chapter 126

Epilepsy

Epilepsy is the most common neurological disease in pregnant women and a risk factor for increased maternal mortality. The condition may be idiopathic or secondary to intracranial insult, such as previous surgery or tumour. Convulsions may develop for the first time in pregnancy and cause a problem in differential diagnosis.

Problems and special considerations

It is generally thought that pre-existing epilepsy is affected by the hormonal changes of pregnancy, and that the frequency of seizures may increase in 14–32% of women during pregnancy. However, in an equal proportion of women, the symptoms improve. Lack of pre-pregnancy advice and the woman's anxiety over the teratogenic effects of antiepileptics may lead to poor compliance with medication. In addition, the pharmacodynamics and pharmacokinetics of antiepileptic drugs may be affected by the physiological changes of pregnancy. Hyperventilation, dehydration and the pain and stress of labour may lower the threshold for convulsions.

In recent reports of the Confidential Enquiries into Maternal Deaths, epilepsy (especially poorly controlled) has been a major factor in deaths from neurological disease. The majority of the reported deaths were classed as sudden unexpected death in epilepsy (SUDEP) or were associated with drowning.

Convulsions occurring during labour, delivery, and the early postpartum period may be particularly hazardous to maternal and fetal health. Immediate problems include aortocaval compression, hypoxaemia, stroke, aspiration of gastric contents and trauma. In addition, the differential diagnosis may include a number of conditions both related and unrelated to pregnancy (see Chapter 127, *Convulsions*).

Management options

Ideally, the woman with diagnosed epilepsy should have had pre-conception counselling to discuss the management of her epilepsy during pregnancy, with the aim of simplifying the drug regimen. Medication may be stopped in a woman who has been convulsion-free for a long time. Assessing the risks and benefits of changing the treatment requires specialist advice for each individual.

During pregnancy, normal medication should be maintained. This may necessitate alternative routes of administration when gastric absorption is affected. Regular monitoring of drug levels during pregnancy is not routinely recommended but may be warranted in some cases. Antiepileptic medication should be continued through labour and delivery, and women at high risk of developing peripartum seizures may require additional anticonvulsants during this period.

When carefully managed, women with epilepsy do not usually experience problems during pregnancy, and most can be offered any form of pain relief that they wish. Pethidine is not recommended, as its active metabolite norpethidine has epileptogenic potential; diamorphine may be a more suitable alternative. A woman with poorly controlled epilepsy will benefit from epidural analgesia to reduce the stress of labour and hyperventilation. General anaesthesia is not associated with increased risk in women with epilepsy in comparison with pregnant women without epilepsy, and thiopental remains a good anticonvulsant. Alfentanil has greater proconvulsant properties than other opioids, and avoidance in these patients has been suggested.

Convulsions are managed in the standard way, taking into account the risk of aortocaval compression and aspiration of gastric contents (see Chapter 127, *Convulsions*).

Key points

- Epilepsy is the commonest neurological disease in pregnancy and a risk factor for poor maternal outcomes.
- Eclampsia is not the only cause of convulsions in pregnancy.
- Epilepsy may become poorly controlled in pregnancy.
- Management of women whose epilepsy is well controlled is as for normal women.

Further reading

Hart LA, Sibai BM. Seizures in pregnancy: epilepsy, eclampsia and stroke. *Semin Perinatol* 2013; 37: 207–24.

Kelso A, Wills A, on behalf of the MBRRACE-UK neurology chapter writing group. Learning from neurological complications. In Knight M, Kenyon S, Brocklehurst P, *et al.*; MBRRACE-UK. *Saving Lives, Improving Mothers' Care: Lessons learned to inform future maternity care from the UK and Ireland Confidential Enquiries into Maternal Deaths and Morbidity 2009–12*. Oxford: National Perinatal Epidemiology Unit, University of Oxford, 2014, pp. 73–9.

Royal College of Obstetricians and Gynaecologists. *Epilepsy in Pregnancy*. Green-top Guideline 68. London: RCOG, 2016. www.rcog.org.uk/en/guidelines-research-services/guidelines/gtg68 (accessed December 2018).

Convulsions

Convulsions occurring ante-, peri- or postpartum are uncommon but important causes of collapse on the labour ward; they may herald significant maternal disease or reflect a transient disturbance, but in either case management must be prompt and appropriate. Although petit mal (absence seizures) and focal seizures may occur, they are less common in the maternity suite than grand mal (tonic–clonic seizures).

Problems and special considerations

The diagnosis may be uncertain if the event is not witnessed by an experienced observer – for example, a simple faint may be labelled as a 'fit'. A history of a tonic–clonic seizure may not always be obtained. Furthermore, collapse from non-neurological causes may itself lead to convulsions if severe hypotension or hypoxaemia occurs.

Physiological effects include increased cerebral and whole-body oxygen requirements, with increased carbon dioxide production. Together with hypoventilation arising from airway obstruction and chest wall rigidity, this may result in hypoxaemia, acidosis, hypercapnia and increased sympathetic activity. These effects may be exacerbated by the increased cardiac output and metabolic requirements of the pregnant woman compared with the non-pregnant one.

Convulsions in pregnancy may be more likely to lead to stroke than in the non-pregnant state. Aortocaval compression further exacerbates the situation before delivery. If inadequately treated, convulsions may merge into each other without breaks in between (status epilepticus).

As for collapse generally, the labour ward staff may be less familiar with emergency equipment and drugs than staff elsewhere. Although most of the possible causes of convulsions are the same as outside of the maternity suite (Table 127.1), the emphasis is different in this setting.

Management options

Initial management includes avoidance of aortocaval compression, protection of the airway (remembering the risk of aspiration) and support of ventilation and circulation.

The differential diagnosis (Table 127.1) is usually one of exclusion; the initial task is to distinguish between a primary convulsion and one resulting from hypoxaemia and/or cardiovascular collapse, hence the importance of a careful history from the patient and observer(s). Since eclampsia is such an important and relatively common cause in the peripartum period, it should be assumed until proven otherwise. Although 'pre-eclampsia screening' investigations are commonly performed, eclampsia may precede other evidence

Table 127.1 Causes of convulsions on the labour ward

Neurological disease	Pre-existing epilepsy
	Stroke
	Cerebral venous thrombosis
	Infection
	Migraine
	Posterior reversible encephalopathy syndrome
	Reversible cerebral vasoconstriction syndrome
	Incidental disease, e.g. tumours
Hypoxaemia	Cardiovascular collapse, e.g. haemorrhage
	Pulmonary embolus
Obstetric	Eclampsia
	Amniotic fluid embolism
Metabolic	Hypoglycaemia
	Hypocalcaemia
	Hyponatraemia [a]
	Uraemia
Autoimmune	Thrombotic thrombocytopenia purpura
Drugs	Anaesthetic, e.g. local anaesthetics
	Others, e.g. intoxication, overdoses, acute withdrawal (including alcohol)
Other	Psychogenic non-epileptic seizures

[a] Hyponatraemia is especially important in the delivery suite, where it may follow prolonged infusion of oxytocin diluted in dextrose solutions.

of pre-eclampsia. A thorough neurological examination should be performed and baseline laboratory investigations and a toxicology screen should be done. A computerised tomography (CT) or magnetic resonance imaging (MRI) scan of the head is generally advised unless a clear history of epilepsy is obtained or the picture is consistent with eclampsia in pregnancy. Blood gas analysis may be useful in guiding management but not in the differential diagnosis; it may reveal marked metabolic and respiratory acidosis resulting from the seizure itself, although this may also represent cardiorespiratory collapse preceding the convulsion. Hypoxaemia may be apparent if aspiration has occurred. Further investigations are guided by the results of preliminary testing and the clinical course.

Drug treatment is with standard anticonvulsant drugs (e.g. diazepam 5–10 mg boluses intravenously; phenytoin 10–15 mg/kg slowly intravenously, preferably with electrocardiographic monitoring), although magnesium sulfate has been shown to be more effective in preventing recurrent eclamptic seizures and should be the first choice unless eclampsia can be excluded. Thiopental, tracheal intubation and controlled ventilation may be required if convulsions are severe and continuous; however, this does prevent further neurological assessment.

Prolonged seizures may cause fetal hypoxia, and fetal monitoring should not be forgotten. Once control of the convulsion has been achieved and the mother is stabilised, delivery should be considered, depending on the aetiology of the convulsions, the gestation and the state of the mother and fetus. In eclampsia, delivery is usually expedited as soon as the stability of the mother allows.

Key points

- Convulsions on the labour ward should be considered as eclampsia until proven otherwise, although other causes should not be overlooked.
- Immediate management is with support of the airway, breathing and circulation, and avoidance of aortocaval compression; magnesium sulfate is the treatment of choice in eclampsia to prevent further convulsions.
- Continuous fetal monitoring is essential.

Further reading

Hart LA, Sibai BM. Seizures in pregnancy: epilepsy, eclampsia and stroke. *Semin Perinatol* 2013; 37: 207–24.

Migraine

The classic presentation of migraine is with a paroxysmal unilateral headache preceded by visual and sensory phenomena, accompanied or followed by nausea and vomiting. Migraine may present for the first time during or shortly after pregnancy.

Problems and special considerations

Migraine often improves in pregnancy but recurs in more than 50% of women postpartum. Many women are anxious about how labour and the pain-relieving drugs given in labour will affect them, and may seek advice as to whether regional analgesia is a problem.

Many drugs used for migraine cross the placenta, and drug therapy may need altering during pregnancy.

Stress, including pain and starvation, can precipitate an attack of migraine.

An acute migraine attack presenting with severe headache and visual disturbances may be confused with pre-eclampsia. Rarely, migraine may be associated with other neurological symptoms.

In the postpartum period, migraine may be confused with postdural puncture headache (PDPH); indeed, the cerebral vasodilatation that is thought to cause the headache of migraine may in part be responsible for the headache that follows dural puncture.

Management options

There is no contraindication to epidural or spinal analgesia or anaesthesia.

Migraine can usually be easily distinguished from PDPH. In migraine, the headache is usually unilateral and frontal, whereas in PDPH the headache is usually bilateral, occipital and frontal. The dramatic improvement in PDPH on lying down is not present with migraine. New-onset severe headache should always alert medical staff to the possibility of other underlying conditions (see Chapter 45, *Postdural puncture headache*).

Key points

- Migraine is common but often improves during pregnancy.
- Migraine may resemble pre-eclampsia and postdural puncture headache.
- Anaesthetic management is routine.

Further reading

Contag SA, Bushnell C. Contemporary management of migrainous disorders in pregnancy. *Curr Opin Obstet Gynecol* 2010; **22**: 437–45.

Goadsby PJ, Goldberg J, Silberstein SD. Migraine in pregnancy. *BMJ* 2008; **336**: 1502–4.

Klein AM, Loder E. Postpartum headache. *Int J Obstet Anesth* 2010; **19**: 422–30.

Pearce CF, Hansen WF. Headache and neurological disease in pregnancy. *Clin Obstet Gynecol* 2012; **55**: 810–28.

Multiple sclerosis

Multiple sclerosis is a disease of unknown aetiology in which the clinical symptoms are caused by patches of damage to the myelin sheath of the central, but not peripheral, neurones. The onset of the disease is generally between the ages of 20 and 40 years and it is usually a disease of relapse and remission. The prevalence of the disease is around 110 per 100,000 in the UK, and it is more common in females (two out of three patients will be female). Therefore, it is not uncommon in women who present for obstetric care.

The condition may manifest with varying degrees of sensory abnormalities, visual disturbance, motor weakness, cranial nerve or bladder and/or bowel dysfunction. Cognitive impairment or epilepsy may be present in some patients. The rate of relapse may decrease during pregnancy, especially in the third trimester, and pregnancy is usually well tolerated, although the rate of relapse may increase in the first three months post-partum before returning to the basal rate

Problems and special considerations

Anaesthetists might feel reluctant to perform regional analgesia in these women, since a relapse may occur after a stressful event such as delivery of a baby. The regional anaesthetic may then erroneously be blamed. Previous studies have suggested an increased incidence of relapse if higher concentrations of bupivacaine are used, although subsequent evidence has not confirmed this.

Women who are very disabled may have impairment of laryngeal reflexes and ventilation. Those with kyphosis, scoliosis or muscle spasticity may be unable to position themselves for regional blockade, and some may be physically unable to achieve a vaginal delivery without assistance.

Women will be concerned about any possible effect of regional analgesia and anaesthesia on their disease.

Management options

Antenatal counselling is advised if possible, to enable a plan for analgesia and anaesthesia to be drawn up and documented in the mother's notes. Time should be taken to discuss the risks and benefits of regional techniques so that the woman may give informed consent where appropriate. It is good practice to assess and document any pre-existing neurological deficit before performing a regional block.

There is no logical reason why these women should not have regional analgesia, and there may be benefits in reducing the stress of labour caused by pain while maintaining as much motor power as possible. Similarly, both spinal and epidural anaesthesia are suitable if operative delivery is necessary. If general anaesthesia is required, standard techniques are used. Suxamethonium may cause exaggerated hyperkalaemia in patients with severe progressive debilitating disease and should be avoided. Measures to minimise the risk of infection must be observed and maternal temperature must be monitored, as a small rise may exacerbate existing symptoms or trigger a relapse.

Key points

- Epidural analgesia should not be denied to women with multiple sclerosis.
- Relapse is not more common with regional anaesthesia than without.
- Routine techniques are used, taking into account any pre-existing neurological deficit.

Further reading

Hopkins AN, Alshaeri T, Akst SA, Berger JS. Neurologic disease with pregnancy and considerations for the obstetric anesthesiologist. *Semin Perinatol* 2014; **38**: 359–69.
Tsui A, Lee MA. Multiple sclerosis and pregnancy. *Curr Opin Obstet Gynecol* 2011; **23**: 435–9.

Myasthenia gravis

Myasthenia gravis is an autoimmune disease affecting the neuromuscular junction, at which circulating antibodies compete with acetylcholine, interfering with neuromuscular transmission and causing skeletal muscle weakness. It has an incidence of around 1 per 100,000 and is more common in females, with an onset at any age. The muscles that are most commonly involved are the oculomotor, facial, pharyngeal and respiratory. The weakness is generally made worse by stress, physical exertion, minor infections and fatigue and is improved by rest.

The disease is treated with acetylcholinesterase inhibitor therapy. The treatment of choice is pyridostigmine in a dose range of 30–90 mg orally given at regular intervals through the day. The side effects of treatment may include bradycardia, sweating and increased salivary secretion.

Problems and special considerations

Pregnancy has a variable effect on the disease, with roughly similar proportions of women showing improvement, deterioration or no change in clinical condition. The increased volume of distribution in pregnant women and altered renal clearance of drugs may cause aggravation of symptoms in some women, and dose modification may be required.

As with many neurological diseases, women with myasthenia gravis may be very worried about regional analgesia and anaesthesia and any adverse effect on their disease.

During labour, an increase in weakness can be expected, which may cause a marked reduction in maternal expulsive efforts in advanced labour and an increased need for instrumental delivery. Parturients with severe disease are also at risk of respiratory insufficiency and aspiration of gastric contents, which may increase as labour progresses.

Requirements for acetylcholinesterase inhibitors may be difficult to estimate during labour because of worsening weakness and possibly reduced gastric absorption of oral pyridostigmine (especially if opioids have been administered). Inadequate dosage may lead to severe weakness (myasthenic crisis), whereas overdosage with acetylcholinesterase inhibitors may lead to a cholinergic crisis (muscle weakness and fasciculation, sweating, miosis, lacrimation, abdominal colic, etc.).

There is increased sensitivity to non-depolarising neuromuscular blocking drugs, with the risk of prolonged neuromuscular blockade during and after general anaesthesia. Resistance to suxamethonium has been reported, although most authorities recommend a normal dose. Magnesium sulfate worsens muscle weakness and is not recommended for the prophylaxis of eclampsia in these patients. It may be used for the treatment of an eclamptic seizure, although caution must be exercised and the need for respiratory support must be anticipated.

Table 130.1 Oral and parenteral anticholinesterase inhibitors (*all the following dosages are equivalent in clinical effect*)

Neostigmine	15 mg oral
	0.7–1.0 mg intramuscular
	0.5 mg intravenous
Pyridostigmine	60 mg oral
	3–4 mg intramuscular
	2 mg intravenous

Some women will be taking long-term steroid therapy and will require supplementation in labour.

Placental transfer of maternal antibodies may cause neonatal myasthenia.

Management options

There should be a team approach to the management of a woman with myasthenia gravis during the antenatal period. The extent of her muscle weakness, and whether this affects the bulbar and respiratory muscles, should be carefully assessed, and the disease should be regularly monitored during the pregnancy.

Treatment will need to be adjusted to maintain muscle strength, and pulmonary function tests may be useful in assessing the strength of the respiratory muscles. Although vaginal delivery is preferred in this patient group, the mode of delivery should be decided on obstetric grounds, taking into account the severity of the illness and the ability of the woman to tolerate the work of labour.

Regional analgesia is advisable, to minimise the stress of labour and to avoid the sedative effects of pethidine or Entonox. If opioids have not been given, gastric function can be considered to be near-normal and oral medication continued. If in doubt in severe cases, equivalent doses of parenteral acetylcholinesterase inhibitors can be given (Table 130.1). Atropine should also be given to reduce unwanted cholinergic effects. If in doubt over whether worsening weakness represents a myasthenic or cholinergic crisis, edrophonium 2 mg intravenously will improve the former but worsen or have no effect on the latter.

In well-controlled myasthenia gravis, caesarean section may be performed under regional anaesthesia. If the disease is not well controlled, the risk of aspiration and respiratory impairment with a high regional block must be weighed against the risks of respiratory impairment following general anaesthesia. Non-depolarising neuromuscular blocking drugs are usually not necessary, but if one is required the dose should be significantly reduced and neuromuscular monitoring should be used to confirm adequate recovery before extubation. Following general anaesthesia, some mothers may require postoperative ventilation while their medication is reintroduced and their muscle power returns to normal.

Key points

- Team management and advance planning are essential for the pregnant woman with myasthenia gravis.
- Regular monitoring of muscle strength throughout pregnancy is essential.

- Oral medication can be continued throughout labour unless the disease is very severe and gastric function is in doubt, when parenteral medication may be substituted.
- Both myasthenic and cholinergic crises may occur.
- Regional analgesia and anaesthesia are indicated in most cases.

Further reading

Gilhus NE. Myasthenia gravis. *N Engl J Med* 2016; **375**: 2570–81.

Norwood F, Dhanjal M, Hill M, *et al.* Myasthenia in pregnancy: best practice guidelines from a U.K. multispecialty working group. *J Neurol Neurosurg Psychiatry* 2014; **85**: 538–43.

Sussman J, Farrugia ME, Maddison P, *et al.* Myasthenia gravis: Association of British Neurologists' management guidelines. *Pract Neurol* 2015; **15**: 199–206.

Chapter 131

Spina bifida

Spina bifida is a congenital neural tube defect with a spectrum of severity. Neural tube defects in survivable form are estimated to occur in 1–3 in 1000 live births; with modern management 25-year survival is over 80%. Many of these survivors will have a significant neurological deficit, in spite of which they will strive to achieve as normal a lifestyle as possible; for women this includes pregnancy and childbirth. Traditionally, spina bifida is categorised as occulta and cystica:

- **Spina bifida occulta.** Its reported prevalence is between 5% and 36% of the population and it is not usually associated with a neurological deficit. It may only be discovered incidentally on radiography or when a woman presents for regional analgesia. It is a vertebral defect and occurs when the two halves of the vertebral arch fail to fuse.
- **Spina bifida cystica.** This is a collective term for the more severe forms of spina bifida, which include spina bifida with meningocoele, myelomeningocoele or myeloschisis. Common to all these malformations is a sac-like protrusion through the defect in the vertebral arch. The neurological deficit depends on the severity and level of the defect and, to an extent, on the effect of subsequent surgery. Some women may have associated cardiac, musculoskeletal or genitourinary anomalies.

Problems and special considerations

Pregnancy in women with spina bifida can prove to be a serious challenge to both obstetric and anaesthetic staff, depending on both the severity of the neurological deficit and any associated skeletal abnormality. Kyphoscoliosis and distortion of the pelvis may make vaginal delivery or positioning for regional anaesthesia difficult. There may be an intraventricular shunt to maintain normal cerebrospinal fluid pressure.

There is an increased risk of accidental dural puncture, particularly when the needle is inserted at the level of the defect. The spinal cord may be tethered and may terminate at an abnormally low level. There is a risk of abnormal spread of local anaesthetic, resulting in either excessive cranial spread or inadequate sacral spread. This may be exacerbated if the woman has had previous corrective surgery. There is also often anxiety regarding the conduct of regional anaesthesia, particularly in patients with an established neural deficit.

Caesarean section, if required, may be difficult because of previous urological surgery, such as ileal conduit.

Latex allergy is more common in patients with spina bifida cystica.

Management options

Ideally, women should be seen by the anaesthetist in the antenatal period, when the nature and level of the lesion and any neurological deficit can be identified and the risks of regional anaesthesia can be assessed and explained. Women who have spina bifida occulta usually have lesions in the low lumbar or sacral areas, with minimal impact on regional techniques, and may be offered regional analgesia or anaesthesia when appropriate. The patient should be warned that there may be an increased risk of an inadequate or failed block, and also of dural puncture as the supporting ligaments (interspinous and ligamentum flavum) may be abnormal at the level of the lesion. It should be remembered that spinal cord tethering may be present in these patients, especially if they give a history of neurological abnormalities and cutaneous manifestations. Occasionally, spina bifida occulta may only be discovered incidentally during siting the epidural or spinal, but this is not a reason to deny appropriate analgesia or anaesthesia.

In spina bifida cystica, there may be significant neurological deficit including skeletal abnormalities and impairment of bladder and bowel function. Some women may be wheel-chair-bound. The aim is to achieve as normal a pregnancy and labour as possible for the individual; for this, effective antenatal consultation and team planning are essential in order that all the options for delivery are discussed and documented. Before regional analgesia is contemplated, baseline clinical findings should be documented in the records, including neurological assessment and, where possible, pre-existing spinal and pelvic x-ray films (pelvic radiography in pregnancy may not be advisable). Magnetic resonance imaging enables the identification of the underlying anatomic abnormality and is recommended in the presence of neurological symptoms that may suggest tethering of the spinal cord, or in women with a history of previous back surgery. Its benefit in asymptomatic patients is controversial, and not all authorities would insist on scanning. The neurological examination is helpful in assessing whether the pain pathways of labour are intact and how regional analgesia can be used to help in labour and delivery. Women may have been told that they will not feel the pain of labour because of their pre-existing sensory deficit. However, this ignores the fact that most are neurologically intact above the lower lumbar segments and therefore will experience the normal pain of the first stage of labour, although it is true that the pain of the second stage may be modified. The increased risk of failed regional analgesia/anaesthesia and dural tap must be explained.

For analgesia in labour, epidural analgesia is generally not contraindicated. However, siting the epidural may be difficult and it is advisable to insert it above the defect and/or the scar from previous surgery. For caesarean section, regional anaesthesia is acceptable. Spinal anaesthesia may be more predictable than epidural anaesthesia, particularly for spread of the block to the sacral roots. Normal volumes of subarachnoid injectate may be used. However, depending on the complexity of the previous surgery and the wishes of the woman, some may opt for general anaesthesia. This usually poses no particular problems, although tracheal intubation and mechanical ventilation may be difficult in some patients with kyphoscoliosis. These patients have a normal response to suxamethonium.

Key points

- Antenatal assessment of women with spina bifida is important.
- Magnetic resonance imaging should be considered in the presence of neurological features or history of previous back surgery.

- Regional analgesia or anaesthesia may be difficult but should not be denied, and women should be warned of the risks of accidental dural tap and inadequate block.
- Spinal anaesthesia may be preferable to epidural anaesthesia for caesarean section.

Further reading

Griffiths S, Durbridge J. Anaesthetic implications of neurological disease in pregnancy. *Contin Educ Anaesth Crit Care Pain* 2011; **11**: 157–61.

May AE, Fombon FN, Francis S. UK registry of high-risk obstetric anaesthesia: report on neurological disease. *Int J Obstet Anesth* 2008; **17**: 31–6.

Murphy CJ, Stanley E, Kavanagh E, Lenane PE, McCaul CL. Spinal dysraphisms in the parturient: implications for perioperative anaesthetic care and labour analgesia. *Int J Obstet Anesth* 2015; **24**: 252–63.

Respiratory disease

The prevalence of respiratory disease in pregnancy is increasing: the incidence of asthma generally is rising, and more women with chronic conditions such as cystic fibrosis are surviving into reproductive life.

Problems and special considerations

Both primarily obstructive and primarily restrictive disease may be exacerbated by the increased respiratory demands of pregnancy (although asthma often improves in pregnancy), with further worsening in labour. In addition, the physiological changes of pregnancy may further hinder respiratory function, in particular airway oedema, upward displacement of the diaphragm and reduced functional residual capacity. It is also important to remember the increased risk factors associated with obesity, smoking and kyphoscoliosis, any of which may complicate the underlying respiratory condition.

Management options

Morbidity and mortality related to respiratory disease were examined in the 2014 and 2017 Confidential Enquiries into Maternal Deaths. Issues highlighted include:

- The importance of pre-pregnancy counselling to prevent maternal cessation of medical therapy due to concerns of adverse fetal effects
- The need to screen for pulmonary hypertension in those with severe respiratory disease prior to pregnancy
- The under-appreciation by healthcare professionals of the severity of the disorder

Clinicians must be familiar with the physiological changes of pregnancy affecting the respiratory system in order to understand the relevant pathophysiology (see Chapter 11, *Physiology of pregnancy*). Early antenatal assessment of the woman, including pulmonary function tests when appropriate, is essential. Ideally, this should be in the first trimester. If the condition is severe, pre-conception counselling may be advisable. The effect of the pregnancy and delivery may then be assessed in light of the physiological changes of pregnancy and the respiratory stresses of delivery. Specifically, pulmonary function tests will give an idea of how the mother might cope with labour.

Women with mild disease can be treated as normal. In more severe disease, regional analgesia and anaesthesia are usually indicated to reduce the stress and demands of labour. Continuous pulse oximetry is advisable throughout labour in severe disease. If operative delivery is required, regional techniques avoid the depressant effects of general anaesthetic drugs, but care must be taken in case of high regional blocks.

Key points

- Respiratory disease may be exacerbated by the physiological changes of pregnancy and the increased demands of the fetus.
- Careful antenatal assessment is important.
- Regional analgesia and anaesthesia are usually indicated.

Further reading

Bonham CA, Patterson KC, Strek ME. Asthma: outcomes and management during pregnancy. *Chest* 2018; **153**: 515–27.

Knight M, Kenyon S, Brocklehurst P, *et al.*; MBRRACE-UK. *Saving Lives, Improving Mothers' Care: Lessons learned to inform future maternity care from the UK and Ireland Confidential Enquiries into Maternal Deaths and Morbidity 2009–12.* Oxford: National Perinatal Epidemiology Unit, University of Oxford, 2014.

Knight M, Nair M, Tuffnell D, *et al.*; MBRRACE-UK. *Saving Lives, Improving Mothers' Care: Lessons learned to inform maternity care from the UK and Ireland Confidential Enquiries into Maternal Deaths and Morbidity 2013–15.* Oxford: National Perinatal Epidemiology Unit, University of Oxford, 2017.

Chapter 133

Asthma

Asthma is one of the most common diseases in the UK, with a prevalence of 15% in children and 10% in adults. Its incidence is increasing. Asthma is both the most common respiratory condition and one of the most common medical conditions seen in pregnancy, occurring in approximately 10% of pregnant women. Of these, around 10% will need hospital admission for an acute exacerbation.

Anaesthetists may be involved in looking after women who have an exacerbation of their asthma during pregnancy or when on the delivery suite.

Problems and special considerations

In pregnancy, asthma remains stable in approximately one-third of patients, worsens in one-third, and improves in another third of patients, an effect thought to be caused by progesterone and cortisol. If symptoms do deteriorate, this is related to both the altered respiratory physiology of pregnancy and increased prostaglandin (PG) $F_{2\alpha}$ secretion, which has bronchoconstrictor effects; this tends to occur in the second and third trimester, with peak deterioration occurring in the sixth month.

In severe cases, patients may be taking a number of bronchodilator and anti-inflammatory drugs, including steroids. If high-dose steroids are being taken (> 7.5 mg prednisolone), steroid replacement should be considered during labour and delivery.

Stress, especially pain and anxiety, may precipitate an acute exacerbation, although viral infections are thought to be the most common cause of an acute exacerbation.

The increased demands of pregnancy make mothers more vulnerable to acute exacerbations of asthma. During an acute attack, physicians not accustomed to the assessment of pregnant patients may misinterpret blood gas results, for example by not appreciating that an arterial partial pressure of carbon dioxide of 5.5–6.0 kPa is grossly abnormal.

Both maternal (hypertensive disorders, haemorrhage and complicated labour) and neonatal (low birth weight, fetal growth restriction, preterm labour) complications are more common in mothers with asthma, especially if poorly controlled.

Pethidine has been implicated in worsening asthma because of its histamine-releasing action, though it is thought to be better than other opioids as it has a smooth muscle relaxant effect.

General anaesthesia in an asthmatic pregnant patient may provoke severe bronchospasm, especially when the airway is instrumented. Thiopental has been implicated in causing bronchospasm, although this is disputed; propofol or ketamine may be considered for induction of anaesthesia. Non-steroidal anti-inflammatory drugs are well known to induce bronchospasm in susceptible patients.

Carboprost (Hemabate) is a $PGF_{2\alpha}$ analogue and should be used with extreme caution in women with asthma. Beta-agonists are usually best avoided when managing hypertensive disorders of pregnancy.

Management options

Ideally, women with moderate or severe asthma should be counselled in the antenatal period and a plan set out for their management in labour. The primary aim of treatment is the maintenance of oxygenation. As asthma sufferers often play down their symptoms, direct questioning about their exercise tolerance and their current treatment, including steroids, is required for the antenatal record. Acute exacerbations should be treated aggressively. Current advice is that influenza vaccinations should not be given until after 12 weeks' gestation.

Caesarean delivery is reserved for obstetric reasons. Induction of labour using prostaglandins is usually avoided. Basic techniques for analgesia and anaesthesia are as for non-asthmatic mothers, bearing the above points in mind. Acute asthma attacks are rare in labour. However, bronchospasm in labour may interfere with effective self-administration of Entonox. The woman should be fully alert and in control during her labour as much as possible, and therefore able to manage her asthma treatment with her inhalers. Epidural analgesia should be recommended generally.

Regional anaesthesia is indicated for operative deliveries, although a high block may reduce the ability to cough. In a woman with unstable asthma, neuraxial techniques may impede use of accessory muscles of respiration, and extreme care is required.

There is no contraindication to the standard treatments for an asthmatic attack in pregnancy or labour, including the use of inhaled or systemic steroids, intravenous theophyllines and magnesium. It is important to remember that peak flow measurements are useful for monitoring the condition, and that respiratory reserve is less during pregnancy, particularly if the mother's attack is precipitated by a respiratory tract infection. Chest radiography and arterial blood sampling may both be needed in the investigation of an acute asthma attack.

Key points

- Both maternal and neonatal complications are more common in mothers with asthma, especially if poorly controlled.
- Epidural analgesia should be encouraged in labour.
- Regional anaesthesia is indicated for operative delivery.
- Acute exacerbations should be treated as for non-pregnant patients.

Further reading

Bonham CA, Patterson KC, Strek ME. Asthma outcomes and management during pregnancy. *Chest* 2018; **153**: 515–27.

British Thoracic Society, Scottish Intercollegiate Guidelines Network. *British Guideline on the Management of Asthma: a National Clinical Guideline.* London: BTS; Edinburgh: SIGN, 2016. www.sign.ac.uk/assets/sign153.pdf (accessed December 2018).

Cystic fibrosis

Cystic fibrosis (CF) is an autosomal recessive genetic disorder with a frequency of approximately 1 in 2000 births. It is primarily a disease of exocrine gland function. As a result of improved medical care, women with CF are increasingly reaching childbearing age and presenting in pregnancy. Pregnancy itself is not thought to increase mortality in women unless pre-pregnancy forced expiratory volume in 1 second (FEV_1) is less than 50–60% of predicted, there is respiratory colonisation with *Burkholderia cepacia*, or she has pancreatic insufficiency. Women with CF will often need an increased level of medical care during and after pregnancy to maintain their clinical status. However, studies have shown that women with CF who become pregnant have a higher 10-year survival rate than those who do not, probably reflecting milder disease severity. Overall mortality has been reported as 5% within 2 years of pregnancy and 10–20% within 5–10 years.

Problems and special considerations

Depending on their pre-pregnant state, women with CF may tolerate the physiological changes of pregnancy poorly.

The main anaesthetic consideration is limited pulmonary reserve. These patients have tenacious secretions that can lead to hypoxaemia secondary to ventilation–perfusion mismatch, and they suffer multiple respiratory infections necessitating intravenous antibiotics. They often have hyperreactive airways, and there is an increased incidence of spontaneous pneumothorax. They may also develop bronchiectasis, for which regular postural drainage is required. Regional blockade may further impair respiratory function, especially if extensive.

Pulmonary hypertension with right heart failure may also occur; it carries with it a poor outcome for both mother and baby.

Diabetes, renal impairment and obstructive jaundice may occur.

Common gastrointestinal symptoms of pregnancy, such as reflux and vomiting, may be particularly prevalent.

Management options

The outcome of the pregnancy will depend on the woman's nutritional status and the degree of pulmonary insufficiency, with more severe disease associated with an increased incidence of respiratory deterioration, preterm delivery and neonatal complications such as low birth weight and perinatal death. Respiratory function is best assessed by performing pulmonary function tests in the first and third trimesters. Careful cardiac assessment is also required to exclude the coexistence of right heart failure.

Vaginal delivery

Oxygenation should be optimal at all times, and continuous oxygen saturation monitoring with supplemental oxygen may be required. Stress and pain during labour will increase the respiratory demands, and it is thus important to reduce these. The respiratory depressant effect of drugs, and in particular opioids, should be considered. Mobility is important to facilitate postural drainage. Low-dose epidural analgesia is the management of choice in most cases in order to satisfy these conditions; the height of block should be monitored closely to reduce the risk of a block height above the T10 dermatome. Physiotherapy may be required after delivery to prevent chest infections, and an increased level of midwifery help with the new baby may be necessary.

Caesarean section

In addition to obstetric indications, caesarean section may also be required for worsening maternal respiratory function. Regional anaesthesia is recommended, although it may be difficult for women with severe respiratory impairment to lie flat. Care should be taken to avoid a high block, and an incremental technique (e.g. using combined spinal–epidural anaesthesia) may be best if impairment is already severe. If general anaesthesia is undertaken, bronchial secretions will need regular suction, particularly before extubation. Techniques to avoid bronchospasm (see Chapter 133, *Asthma*) and ventilatory strategies to avoid development of a pneumothorax should be employed. Postoperative analgesia is particularly important and is best provided by neuraxial opioids. During the recovery period, high-dependency care is essential and should include regular physiotherapy.

Key points

- Antenatal planning, with close liaison with the mother's cystic fibrosis team, is essential.
- Maintenance of oxygenation should be given high priority at all times.
- Regional analgesia and anaesthesia are usually indicated, but care should be taken to avoid high blocks.

Further reading

Edenborough FP, Borgo G, Knoop C, *et al.*; European Cystic Fibrosis Society. Guidelines for the management of pregnancy in women with cystic fibrosis. *J Cyst Fibros* 2008; **7** (Suppl 1): S2–32.

Huffmyer JL, Littlewood KE, Nemergut EC. Perioperative management of the adult with cystic fibrosis. *Anesth Analg* 2009; **109**: 1949–61.

McArdle J. Pregnancy in cystic fibrosis. *Clin Chest Med* 2011; **32**: 111–20.

Pulmonary fibrosis

The most common fibrotic pulmonary lesion in young women is pulmonary fibrosis secondary to radiotherapy. Other causes include idiopathic pulmonary fibrosis, hypersensitivity pneumonitis (formerly known as extrinsic allergic alveolitis), autoimmune/connective tissue disease-related fibrosis, occupational lung disease and drug-induced fibrosis. The progressive alveolar and pulmonary fibrotic conditions tend to occur in later life; the general principles are the same, although these conditions are potentially life-threatening. There are few case reports of pregnancy in women with idiopathic pulmonary fibrosis, as two-thirds of presentations are diagnosed after the age of 60, with a median survival from diagnosis of 3 years; however, successful vaginal and caesarean deliveries have been described.

Problems and special considerations

Many women who have had a successfully treated malignancy expect to have children. Many of them are unaware that their pulmonary function is not normal, as they have no symptoms during ordinary activities, and they may not have been told that there has been any pulmonary damage as a result of treatment of their malignancy. Pulmonary function tests show a reduction in the vital capacity and forced expiratory volume, with no evidence of restrictive lung disease unless there is other pathology. Most of these women tolerate their pregnancy with little or no problem, although they need a plan for their delivery.

Patients who have had a treated malignancy have usually had chemotherapy and may have had drugs that cause myocardial damage, such as bleomycin. It is therefore important that these women have echocardiography to assess their cardiac function.

Women who are symptomatic before pregnancy may find the additional physiological challenges of pregnancy difficult; restrictive lung disease does not allow for the usual increases in minute volume seen in pregnancy.

Management options

It is important to assess these women antenatally so that they may understand their restrictions and how these might affect the management of labour and delivery. The delivery plan will depend on the degree of pulmonary damage. Some women may be treated as entirely normal, whereas others require a clear plan comprising avoidance of general anaesthesia and sedative drugs, epidural analgesia during labour to avoid further increases in minute ventilation and oxygen consumption, and regional anaesthesia for operative delivery.

Key points

- Antenatal assessment of the woman with pulmonary fibrosis is essential, including pulmonary function tests and echocardiography when appropriate.
- Intrapartum management is as for respiratory disease in general.

Further reading

Budev MM, Arroliga AC, Emery S. Exacerbation of underlying pulmonary disease in pregnancy. *Crit Care Med* 2005; **33** (10 Suppl): S313–18.

Wexler ID, Johannesson M, Edenborough FP, Sufian BS, Kerem E. Pregnancy and chronic progressive pulmonary disease. *Am J Respir Crit Care Med* 2007; **175**: 300–5.

Chapter 136

Sarcoidosis

Sarcoidosis is a systemic granulomatous reaction affecting many organs. The main effects of the disease are seen in the peripheral and central nervous systems and in the pulmonary and cardiac systems. An important aspect of the disease for the anaesthetist is pulmonary infiltration, which occurs in up to 80% of cases and produces a restrictive type of lung disease; therefore it is considered with the respiratory diseases.

The disease is treated with high doses of steroids and is not made worse by pregnancy.

Problems and special considerations

Sarcoidosis produces a restriction of the lungs, causing a reduction in the vital capacity and functional residual capacity. These changes, compounded by the physiological changes of pregnancy, mean that these patients may have little or no significant pulmonary reserve and may tolerate pregnancy (and especially labour) poorly. There is also an increased incidence of bronchospasm and airway hyperreactivity.

Cardiac impairment may be related to the primary disease (e.g. causing heart block or heart failure) or secondary to pulmonary involvement (causing pulmonary hypertension and right-sided failure). Patients with cardiac sarcoid may be sensitive to the negatively inotropic effects of anaesthetic agents.

There may also be renal impairment, central nervous system involvement, including isolated cranial nerve lesions, and haematological involvement. Anaemia affects 40% of cases, but thrombocytopenia is rare.

Mucosal infiltration of the upper airways occurs in about 5% of cases, and women may describe hoarseness, stridor, dysphagia or symptoms of obstructive sleep apnoea.

Sarcoidosis has been linked to adverse maternal and neonatal outcomes, including hypertensive disorders of pregnancy, thromboembolic disease, premature and caesarean delivery, and postpartum haemorrhage.

Management options

The main consideration is to assess the pulmonary and cardiac functions of the woman, and the effect of pregnancy and delivery on function. All these women should have pulmonary function tests performed in the first and third trimesters of their pregnancy unless mildly affected, and the management of the labour should be guided by the results. Electrocardiography should also be performed, with echocardiography if pulmonary hypertension or cardiomyopathy is suspected. Antenatal blood tests should include renal function and calcium levels.

In labour, the respiratory challenge of the work of labour and the ventilatory response to pain may be poorly tolerated; therefore epidural analgesia is recommended.

For caesarean section, general anaesthesia is best avoided, regional anaesthesia being the technique of choice. If general anaesthesia is necessary, the airway may be more challenging if there is laryngeal involvement; a smaller-diameter tracheal tube or microlaryngoscopy tube may be necessary. Steroid replacement may need to be considered.

Respiratory, cardiac and renal deterioration may occur in the postpartum period, and a period of close monitoring is advisable.

Key points

- It is important to be aware of the generalised nature of sarcoidosis.
- Pulmonary involvement occurs in up to 80% of cases.
- Pulmonary and cardiac function should be assessed carefully in the antenatal period.
- Regional analgesia and anaesthesia are usually indicated in severe cases.

Further reading

Freymond N, Cottin V, Cordier JF. Infiltrative lung diseases in pregnancy. *Clin Chest Med* 2011; **32**: 133–46.

Sanders D, Rowland R, Howell T. Sarcoidosis and anaesthesia. *BJA Educ* 2016; **16**: 173–7.

Chapter 137

Acute lung injury and acute respiratory distress syndrome

Acute lung injury (ALI) is a syndrome of lung inflammation and increased permeability that is not explained by left atrial or pulmonary capillary hypertension (although they may coexist). The previous term, adult (now acute) respiratory distress syndrome (ARDS), is now reserved for the most severe form of ALI.

Both conditions are characterised by their acute onset, bilateral diffuse infiltrates on chest radiography not explained by cardiac failure or volume overload, pulmonary artery wedge pressure < 18 mmHg or absence of clinical evidence of left atrial hypertension, and arterial hypoxaemia resistant to oxygen therapy alone (ratio of arterial partial pressure/inspired fractional concentration of oxygen < 39.9 kPa [300 mmHg] for ALI, < 26.6 kPa [200 mmHg] for ARDS). Other features include reduced respiratory compliance and lung volumes, increased work of breathing, ventilation–perfusion mismatch and increased shunt.

ALI or ARDS associated with pulmonary oedema is a common feature of deaths associated with pregnancy, and has received special attention in past reports of the Confidential Enquiries into Maternal Deaths; mortality associated with ARDS is elevated in the pregnant population and has been reported as being between 10% and 40%. It has been suggested that ALI may be more likely in the pregnant state, possibly as result of the physiological changes of pregnancy, especially the increased cardiac output, lower colloid osmotic pressure and leaky capillaries. It is also suspected that aggressive fluid therapy, especially in obstetric haemorrhage and pre-eclampsia, has led to many cases of ALI. In the case of haemorrhage, this may be related to rapid transfusion in the presence of high circulating levels of catecholamines and a relatively constricted pulmonary circulation; in pre-eclampsia, over-emphasis on treating oliguria by 'pushing fluids' may lead to pulmonary oedema and ALI.

Problems and special considerations

The causes of ALI in pregnancy are generally the same as those in the non-pregnant state, with sepsis the most common cause, although pre-eclampsia, haemorrhage, aspiration of gastric contents, presence of a dead fetus or retained products of conception and amniotic fluid embolism are also important. Use of β_2-agonists in premature labour may also contribute by causing pulmonary oedema (although whether this in itself leads to ALI and ARDS is uncertain). It is important to consider other causes of respiratory failure, especially peripartum cardiomyopathy, as this is more common than ARDS.

The increased demands on the maternal cardiovascular and respiratory systems make the obstetric patient with ALI less able to cope with hypoxaemia, especially in the third trimester. The decreased functional residual capacity increases the likelihood of airway closure and ventilation–perfusion mismatch. However, established ALI has a similar mortality in both pregnant and non-pregnant women.

The fetus is particularly at risk from hypoxaemia, and this is compounded by any associated cardiovascular instability and the risk of aortocaval compression.

Management options

Management requires early referral to the intensive care unit and involves increasing levels of respiratory support as ALI increases in severity; non-invasive ventilatory support may be considered in pregnancy, but if there is no clinical improvement, invasive ventilation using lung protective strategies may be necessary. Extracorporeal membrane oxygenation (ECMO) has been used successfully in pregnant patients with ARDS and refractory hypoxaemia. Management of the predisposing condition should continue as for any acutely ill patient, and a conservative fluid strategy is usually recommended. The fetus should be monitored for signs of distress that might prompt delivery. The physiological changes of pregnancy pose particular problems for the critically ill obstetric patient (see Chapter 155, *Critical care in pregnancy*).

Key points

- Obstetric patients may be especially prone to acute lung injury.
- Acute lung injury is a common feature in deaths caused by pre-eclampsia, sepsis and massive obstetric haemorrhage.
- The increased physiological demands of pregnancy make obstetric patients especially susceptible to hypoxaemia.

Further reading

Duarte AG. ARDS in pregnancy. *Clin Obst Gynecol* 2014; **57**: 862–70.
Schwaiberger D, Marcz M, Menk M *et al.* Respiratory failure and mechanical ventilation in the pregnant patient. *Crit Care Clin* 2016; **32**: 85–95.

Pneumonia

The incidence of pneumonia in pregnant women overall is thought to be similar to that in the non-obstetric population, although it is more common in women with underlying respiratory disease, anaemia or immunosuppression (e.g. HIV infection, corticosteroids), and in advanced pregnancy. Pneumonia is the commonest cause of sepsis necessitating critical care admission in the obstetric population in the UK, but it is a relatively uncommon cause of death in the Confidential Enquiries into Maternal Deaths reports. However, during the H1N1 influenza ('swine flu') pandemic of 2009–10, the deaths of 32 pregnant women were attributed to H1N1.

The increased mortality from certain pneumonias in pregnancy, compared with non-pregnant women, is thought to arise from the altered immune responses, combined with the decreased functional residual capacity, decreased residual volume and increased oxygen consumption, that are part of the normal physiological changes of pregnancy. Anaesthetists are likely to be involved in the care of women with chest infection through the need for analgesia/anaesthesia around delivery, or for supportive/intensive care should a parturient become critically ill.

Problems and special considerations

Signs and symptoms may be similar to the changes of respiratory physiology in pregnancy and may be non-specific, e.g. fever, rigors, nausea/vomiting, chest discomfort/pain and shortness of breath. Thus, diagnosis may be delayed.

Medical staff are often reluctant to perform a chest x-ray to confirm a diagnosis in a pregnant woman, because of anxiety over fetal exposure to radiation. However, the risks from a single x-ray are small and usually considered to be outweighed by the advantages if pneumonia is suspected.

Sputum and blood cultures should be taken, although their usefulness has been debated, and in a significant proportion of patients the aetiological agent may not be identified.

Pneumonia in the mother is associated with significant fetal morbidity, for example premature labour, fetal growth restriction and premature birth.

Viral pneumonia may be associated with a high risk of infecting staff, increasing spread and hampering the ability of healthcare services to cope in an epidemic or pandemic. The severe acute respiratory syndrome (SARS) epidemic of 2002–03 and the H1N1 pandemic of 2009–10, in particular, carried significant risk to staff.

Bacterial pneumonia

This is usually community-acquired. Common bacterial agents include *Streptococcus pneumoniae* and *Haemophilus influenzae*, but others such as *Mycoplasma*, *Staphylococcus*,

Legionella, *Klebsiella* and *Pseudomonas* may also be responsible. Management involves supportive therapy with the appropriate antibiotics. Guidelines from the American Thoracic Society suggest administering a macrolide antibiotic for mild disease and adding a β-lactam if the pneumonia is more severe. These antibiotics are safe for use in pregnancy and have coverage for most of the microorganisms associated with bacterial pneumonia in pregnancy.

Viral pneumonia

The most common causative agents in pregnancy are the influenza A (the strain most commonly affecting humans) and varicella (chickenpox) viruses. Viral pneumonia may lead to severe acute respiratory failure, secondary bacterial infection and acute lung injury.

Influenza

Seasonal flu is more likely to cause severe illness in pregnant women than in non-pregnant women, and annual vaccination is recommended unless there are contraindications. Recently, a number of newer influenza viral strains have been identified, all of which have been associated with significant maternal and perinatal morbidity. In 2009, the World Health Organization declared a pandemic when H1N1 caused over 18,000 deaths world-wide (over 450 in the UK). Severe disease was notably more common in young people, unlike seasonal influenza, with other risk factors being diabetes, obesity, immunosuppression and particularly pregnancy, with an estimated increased mortality risk of 4–6 times that in the non-pregnant population.

Signs and symptoms are similar to those in non-obstetric women and range from mild illness, typically with high fever, to severe and progressive hypoxaemia. Diagnosis is by nasal/pharyngeal swabs. The mortality rate for those admitted to the intensive care unit is approximately 20–25%, and is thought to be greater in those not receiving antiviral therapy within 2 days of the onset of symptoms. There is an increased risk of premature delivery (times three) and stillbirth/early neonatal death (times five) in pregnant women admitted to hospital.

Varicella

Chickenpox is an illness usually seen in childhood, but primary varicella may also occur in adults, 16% of whom develop complications – one of which is varicella pneumonia. The diagnosis is usually clinical, based on the history, rash and/or previous contact, but may be helped by the presence of granular infiltrates seen on chest x-ray combined with the presence of serum antibodies, although these may not be seen for 2 weeks. Pneumonia occurs in up to 10% of pregnant women with chickenpox; risk factors include smoking, pre-existing lung disease, immunosuppression (e.g. with steroid therapy) and late pregnancy. With appropriate modern therapy (antiviral drugs and intensive care), mortality is thought to be under 1% (approximately five times the rate in non-pregnant adults), though historical rates of up to 45% have been reported.

Fungal pneumonia

This is not commonly seen in pregnancy, but if it is, it may be associated with immunosuppression. Signs and symptoms are as in the non-obstetric population, but, as for viral infection, severe respiratory disease may ensue. The diagnosis may be made with sputum culture or serum antigens and chest x-ray changes (usually a nodular pattern is seen on the x-ray). Treatment is with intravenous amphotericin in the peripartum period and flucanozole in the postpartum period, as there has been an association with flucanozole and fetal malformations.

Management options

Several strategies exist to prevent pneumonia in this high-risk population. Risk factors should be identified and modified where possible; if the mother has a coexisting respiratory disease, this should be optimised. Vaccinations are available for influenza, varicella and pneumococcus and are associated with fewer complications, including pneumonia and mortality. The influenza vaccination in pregnancy has been shown to reduce maternal morbidity and mortality, and improve fetal outcomes including risk of perinatal death, prematurity and low birth weight.

Management of pneumonia in pregnancy includes admission, appropriate investigation (including white blood cell count, C-reactive protein, arterial blood gas analysis and chest x-ray), initiation of antimicrobial/antiviral/antifungal therapy, fetal evaluation and respiratory support when required. Supplemental oxygen is usually required, to improve both maternal and fetal oxygenation.

In swine flu, antivirals such as oseltamivir and zanamivir have been used in pregnancy with success, particularly when administered within the first 48 hours of symptoms; treatment should be administered on clinical grounds rather than on diagnostic testing, owing to the latter's low sensitivity. In chickenpox, aciclovir is usually the treatment of choice. Delivery during varicella viraemia may be associated with maternal coagulopathy and hepatitis and severe neonatal infection, and should be delayed if possible. Respiratory failure may require tracheal intubation and ventilation, although non-invasive methods (e.g. mask-delivered continuous positive airway pressure) may be effective, at least in the short term. Respiratory failure is a result of intrapulmonary shunting rather than hypoventilation, and so ventilation with positive end-expiratory pressure (PEEP) may be beneficial. Hypoxia may not be responsive to therapies such as PEEP, nitric oxide or use of the prone position. High-frequency ventilation/oscillation, extracorporeal membrane oxygenation (ECMO) and intravenacaval membrane oxygenation have been described for refractory cases, and experience in pregnancy is increasing. Early referral to a specialist centre capable of ECMO has been shown to be of benefit to survival in non-obstetric patients with severe respiratory failure. However, consideration must be given to whether obstetric services are available on site.

Delivery of the fetus may be necessary to improve the functional status of the mother, but whether improvement in clinical status really results is debatable; some advocate that delivery should be only for obstetric reasons. If caesarean section is required, the choice of regional or general anaesthesia requires careful consideration of the relative risks and benefits, including the likelihood that the mother's condition may worsen after delivery.

Units should have a clear policy on caring for women with potentially contagious respiratory infections, including the provision of protective masks and training in their use.

Key points

- The effects of pneumonia may be exacerbated by the physiological changes of pregnancy and the increased demands of the fetus.
- Careful antenatal assessment is important.
- Regional analgesia and anaesthesia are usually indicated.

Further reading

Brito V, Niederman MS. Pneumonia complicating pregnancy. *Clin Chest Med* 2011; **32**: 121–32.

Knight M, Kenyon S, Brocklehurst P, *et al.*; MBRRACE-UK. *Saving Lives, Improving Mothers' Care: Lessons learned to inform future maternity care from the UK and Ireland Confidential Enquiries into Maternal Deaths and Morbidity 2009–12*. Oxford: National Perinatal Epidemiology Unit, University of Oxford, 2014.

Lamont RF, Sobel JD, Carrington D, *et al.* Varicella-zoster virus (chickenpox) infection in pregnancy. *BJOG* 2011; **118**: 1155–62.

Rasmussen S, Jamieson D. 2009 H1N1 influenza and pregnancy: 5 years later. *N Engl J Med* 2014; **371**: 1373–5.

Sepsis

Chapter **139**

Sepsis is the sixth leading cause of death in the 2018 Confidential Enquiries into Maternal Death (CEMD) report. While deaths from indirect causes of sepsis such as influenza and pneumonia seem to be decreasing, the incidence of deaths from pregnancy-related sepsis appears fairly constant.

In recent years there has been a drive for increased awareness of sepsis, and in conjunction with the National Institute for Health and Care Excellence (NICE), the UK Sepsis Trust has released clinical toolkits to aid early recognition and management of sepsis in pregnant women, both in the community and in hospital.

Sepsis in the pregnant population may occur at any time; it may arise from a number of sources and not just the genital tract, and it may range from mild sepsis to severe systemic infection leading to multi-organ failure and maternal or fetal demise. In non-pregnant patients, sepsis is a clinical syndrome manifested by infection and a systemic inflammatory response (which is identified by deviations from normal temperature, heart rate, respiration rate and white blood cell count). Current diagnosis of sepsis is based on the sepsis-related organ failure assessment (SOFA) score, which includes respiratory function, coagulation, liver function, blood pressure, conscious level and renal function. Applying such diagnostic criteria to pregnant patients is difficult, as many of these parameters change in pregnancy; the UK Sepsis Trust has defined sepsis 'red flags' to be used in the maternal population (Table 139.1).

Pregnancy is associated with certain risk factors for sepsis, which can be divided into:

- **Patient factors**, e.g. diabetes, obesity, history of streptococcal B infection or of pelvic infection
- **Obstetric factors**, e.g. prolonged rupture of membranes, caesarean section, retained products

The most common organisms associated with bacteraemia or sepsis in pregnancy include *Escherichia coli*, enterococci, *Klebsiella*, *Staphylococcus aureus*, *Streptococcus pneumoniae*, H1N1 and β-haemolytic streptococci. The recognition and aggressive management of developing sepsis, involving a multidisciplinary approach, is thought to be key in preventing morbidity and mortality from a potentially very rapidly evolving condition.

Problems and special considerations

Severe sepsis in obstetrics is usually associated with bacterial infection. Rather than the traditional view that pregnant women are more predisposed to infection owing to a general reduction in immunity during pregnancy, it is now thought that pregnancy may exhibit

Table 139.1 Maternal sepsis 'red flags' (UK Sepsis Trust, 2016)

Responds only to voice or pain/unresponsive
Systolic BP ≤ 90 mmHg (or drop > 40 mmHg from normal)
Heart rate > 130/minute
Respiratory rate ≥ 25/minute
Needs oxygen to keep SpO$_2$ ≥ 92%
Non-blanching rash, mottled/ashen/cyanotic
Not passed urine in last 18 h or urine output < 0.5 ml/kg/h
Lactate ≥ 2 mmol/l

Adapted with permission from UK Sepsis Trust, Inpatient maternal sepsis tool: https://sepsistrust.org/wp-content/uploads/2018/06/Inpatient-maternal-NICE-Final-1107-2.pdf.

a modified response to infection owing to an altered reactivity of the immune system that serves to protect both mother and baby.

The physiological changes that occur in pregnancy, such as vasodilatation and increased blood volume and heart rate, mean that the signs and symptoms of sepsis are often masked; thus, diagnosis and management may be delayed. Severe sepsis associated with bacteraemia may present with non-specific signs such as abdominal pain and diarrhoea, with or without pyrexia. Typically it is rapidly progressive, and when death occurs it may do so within hours of presentation.

A raised white blood cell count, which might support a diagnosis of infection in the non-pregnant population, is less useful in the obstetric setting, since the white cell count is commonly increased by labour and by steroids given to aid fetal lung maturation in prematurity. Thus counts of up to 30×10^9/l are not uncommon in the absence of infection.

Institution of an epidural or spinal block in the presence of systemic infection is potentially very hazardous since cardiovascular compensation, which may be just adequate to maintain blood pressure within normal limits, may be abolished, with catastrophic results as sympathetic blockade develops. In addition, there is a risk of epidural or meningeal infection arising from blood-borne organisms. A more common occurrence is a request for regional analgesia in an otherwise asymptomatic woman with pyrexia (see Chapter 144, *Pyrexia during labour*).

The fetus is at increased risk from many infections during pregnancy, whether manifested by increased incidence of congenital malformations, premature delivery, the consequences of general maternal illness or neonatal infection. Chorioamnionitis itself has been implicated in causing premature labour; thus prophylactic antibiotics have been studied as a means of delaying onset of labour in premature rupture of membranes.

Management options

Prophylactic intraoperative antibiotic therapy has been shown to reduce the incidence of sepsis following caesarean section and should be routine. Usually this is given by the anaesthetist. Administration has traditionally been delayed until after delivery to avoid passage of drugs to the fetus, and because, should an allergic reaction occur, the baby will already have been delivered. However, recent guidance from NICE recommends administration before skin incision, on the basis of greater efficacy. Great care must be taken when following this advice, since thiopental/antibiotic syringe-swap drug errors are easily made, especially in emergencies.

Developing sepsis is easily missed, even by experienced medical staff. A high index of suspicion is therefore important. Use of a modified early obstetric warning score chart can help identify the deteriorating parturient (see Chapter 156).

It is recommended that the management of septic obstetric patients follows the guidelines of the Surviving Sepsis Campaign, a collaboration between the European Society of Intensive Care Medicine, the Society of Critical Care Medicine and the International Sepsis Forum. These aim to standardise care and improve the outcome in sepsis generally; the main points of care are aggressive resuscitation, adequate oxygenation and appropriate and prompt antibiotic treatment.

Resuscitation with fluids and vasopressors is necessary to ensure oxygenation and prevent tissue hypoxia; noradrenaline is usually the first vasopressor of choice. Appropriate resuscitation before organ failure occurs is thought to improve survival by approximately 20%. Fluid overload is always a concern in obstetric patients because of the haemodynamic changes of pregnancy, especially those that occur in the peripartum period, and because of the use of uterotonic drugs (e.g. oxytocin), which are associated with fluid retention. Thus, some clinicians advocate invasive monitoring with central venous lines, but these are not without hazard (see Chapter 157, *Invasive monitoring*). Successive CEMD reports have stressed the importance of involving intensivists early in the care of critically ill women, and that 'intensive care' can be provided outside the intensive care unit.

Blood culture samples should be taken and intravenous antibiotics administered within the first hour of diagnosis, which is considered the 'golden hour'. This is thought to be key to improving maternal and fetal outcome; from the recognition of sepsis, each hour's delay in antibiotic treatment has been associated with an increase in mortality of 8%. It is good practice to seek advice from the microbiology department regarding the most appropriate choice of antibiotics. If there is a focus of infection that can be removed surgically, then this should be done.

When and how to deliver the baby is an obstetric decision, but the discussion should involve the anaesthetist with regard to timing and whether the mother's clinical condition has been or can be stabilised. The choice of anaesthetic is dependent on each individual case; the presence of systemic infection and a developing coagulopathy secondary to sepsis may preclude the use of a neuraxial technique. Moreover, the risk of cardiovascular block secondary to sympathetic blockade caused by a regional technique should also be considered. General anaesthesia may be the preferred choice of anaesthesia for delivery; however, it must be remembered that general anaesthesia may also result in cardiovascular instability. Invasive blood pressure monitoring and central venous access are useful, regardless of the mode of anaesthesia.

Transfer of the patient to a more appropriate environment, such as the high-dependency or intensive care unit, should be discussed between the obstetrician, anaesthetist and intensivist. Decision to extubate will be influenced by the patient's condition.

Key points

- Sepsis is the one of the leading causes of death in pregnancy.
- Diagnosis is not always immediate because of the physiological changes in pregnancy, and clinical deterioration may therefore not be recognised until too late.

- Management involves aggressive treatment with fluid resuscitation and cardiovascular support, appropriate antibiotic treatment and adequate oxygenation.
- Early transfer to high-dependency or intensive care facilities may be advisable.

Further reading

Galvagno SM, Camann W. Sepsis and acute renal failure in pregnancy. *Anesth Analg* 2009; **108**: 572–5.

Knight M, Bunch K, Tuffnell D, *et al.*; MBRRACE-UK. *Saving Lives, Improving Mothers' Care: Lessons learned to inform maternity care from the UK and Ireland Confidential Enquiries into Maternal Deaths and Morbidity 2014–16.* Oxford: National Perinatal Epidemiology Unit, University of Oxford, 2018.

Levy MM, Dellinger RP, Townsend SR, *et al.*; Surviving Sepsis Campaign. The Surviving Sepsis Campaign: results of an international guideline-based performance improvement program targeting severe sepsis. *Crit Care Med* 2010; **38**: 367–74.

Lucas DN, Robinson N, Nel MR. Sepsis in obstetrics and the role of the anaesthetist. *Int J Obstet Anesth* 2012; **21**: 56–67.

Paruk F. Infection in obstetric critical care. *Best Pract Res Clin Obstet Gynaecol* 2008; **22**: 865–83.

Chapter

140

Hepatitis

Hepatitis may predate pregnancy or may occur coincidentally during or after pregnancy. The diagnosis of acute viral hepatitis is made from the history and from blood tests of liver function (increased conjugated bilirubin, markedly increased transaminases, and slightly increased alkaline phosphatase). Chronic hepatitis (active, persistent, drug- or alcohol-induced) also causes abnormality of liver function tests, but definitive diagnosis is made by liver biopsy.

Problems and special considerations

Viral hepatitis

Viral hepatitis accounts for 40% of all liver disease associated with pregnancy, and in its acute form is the most common cause of jaundice in pregnant women. The disease may be caused by the hepatitis viruses, cytomegalovirus, Epstein–Barr virus or herpes simplex virus. It is thought that pregnant women might be more susceptible to viral hepatitis because of their relatively immunosuppressed state.

Hepatitis A is highly contagious and spread by the faecal–oral route. The incidence in pregnancy is unknown, since many infections are mild, but is thought to be low in the UK. The disease course is similar to that in non-pregnant patients, although infection may carry an increased risk of fetal morbidity and preterm labour.

Hepatitis B is thought to infect up to 1 in 50 pregnant women in UK inner cities, in which there is a large immigrant population. It is readily spread by contact with blood and body fluids. Women who are intravenous drug users and those who have had multiple sexual partners or are sex workers should be assumed to be at high risk of having hepatitis B, and appropriate precautions should be taken. There is a ~10% risk of developing chronic liver disease; this may be increased by co-infection with hepatitis D. The risk of transmission to the fetus is 10–20% if the mother is positive for the hepatitis B surface antigen (HbsAg) and around 90% if she is positive for the hepatitis B envelope antigen (HBeAg), and so pregnant women have been screened for hepatitis B in the UK since 2000. Measures to reduce maternofetal transmission of infection include administration of hepatitis B immunoglobulin to the mother during pregnancy and to the baby at birth, and vaccination of the baby at birth, 1 month, 2 months and 12 months of age. Some women with high viral loads may require additional treatment with antivirals in late pregnancy.

Hepatitis C is unusual in pregnancy in the UK; its prevalence in inner-city parturients is thought to be 0.5–1%. It is spread mainly by contact with blood, although sexual transmission may also occur. There is a 50–80% risk of developing chronic liver disease, and a ~5%

risk of transmission to the baby during pregnancy and delivery. There is currently no preventive treatment to decrease the risk of transmission to the fetus.

Hepatitis E is similar to hepatitis A, but is unusual in the UK. Infections occurring during the last trimester may have a fulminant course with a maternal mortality up to 50%.

Symptoms of viral hepatitis are non-specific, and include fatigue, general malaise, loss of appetite, nausea, vomiting, headache and pyrexia. There may be some abdominal discomfort. Overt jaundice only occurs in about a quarter of cases. Treatment is symptomatic, and in the majority of cases there is complete resolution of all signs and symptoms over the course of a few weeks. Women with significantly impaired liver function may be thrombocytopenic or have abnormal clotting studies. Renal function may also be impaired. In end-stage hepatitis, alteration in mental state may occur as a result of hepatic encephalopathy. There is no evidence that pregnancy affects the course of the disease, nor that hepatitis has any significant effect on pregnancy in the majority of cases. For the small number of pregnant women who develop hepatitis C, it has been suggested that maternal morbidity and mortality is higher than in non-pregnant women. However, this increased risk may be apparent, due to misdiagnosis of conditions such as fatty liver of pregnancy, rather than a genuine risk.

Chronic hepatitis

Chronic persistent hepatitis is usually unaffected by pregnancy. Chronic active hepatitis is associated with impaired fertility; if pregnancy does occur it may be associated with accelerated deterioration in liver function. Treatment includes corticosteroids and antiviral drugs including interferon. The risk of interferon to the fetus is unknown. Lupus antibodies may occur in up to 20% of women with chronic active hepatitis. Chronic active hepatitis may be complicated by arthritis, impaired renal function, myocarditis and neuropathies. Diabetes, hypertension and osteoporosis may also occur as a result of long-term steroid therapy.

Management options

Regional analgesia and anaesthesia are not contraindicated if coagulation studies are normal. If there is chronic impairment of liver function, invasive venous pressure monitoring may assist fluid management, especially if regional anaesthesia is performed. Although fluid overload must be avoided, hypotension will aggravate any reduction in liver blood flow. There may be impaired clearance of lidocaine; dose reduction is advisable.

Patients with severe liver disease often have severely impaired liver function and coagulopathy. Women who have oesophageal varices are at an increased risk of suffering a bleed during pregnancy. Avoidance of pushing during vaginal delivery is recommended, but superimposed obstetric complications (pre-eclampsia, fetal growth restriction) will frequently necessitate operative delivery.

Rapid-sequence induction of general anaesthesia for caesarean section should be used. Suxamethonium can be used safely, despite the greater than normal reduction in plasma cholinesterase levels that is likely to be present. Use of a peripheral nerve stimulator is mandatory, since the action of non-depolarising neuromuscular blockers may be prolonged, and blood glucose levels must be monitored. Opioid analgesia should be used with caution in women with severe hepatic dysfunction.

Standard infection control precautions should be used if women with viral hepatitis are hospitalised.

Key points

- Viral hepatitis is highly contagious.
- Regional analgesia and anaesthesia are not contraindicated, but impaired liver function may be associated with disorders of coagulation.

Further reading

Tran TT. Hepatitis B in pregnancy. *Clin Infect Dis* 2016; **62** (Suppl 4): S314–17.
Westbrook RH, Dusheiko G, Williamson C. Pregnancy and liver disease. *J Hepatol* 2016; **64**: 933–45.

Herpes simplex infection

The herpes simplex virus (HSV) is a common infective agent during both childhood and adult life. Although HSV-1 is traditionally considered to be responsible for orolabial herpes and HSV-2 for genital herpes, there is considerable overlap. HSV is important in pregnancy because of the adverse effects of primary infection on maternal health and premature labour, and also because of the risks of primary neonatal infection, which may be severe.

Problems and special considerations

Primary infection may result in local lesions and viraemia with systemic effects, for example malaise, myalgia, meningitis, encephalitis and hepatitis. Local lesions may reappear weeks to years later, often following emotional or physical stress. Primary infection is associated with a ~40% incidence of neonatal transmission. Secondary infection is not associated with viraemia and the risk of neonatal transmission is under 3%.

Women with severe primary infection may present in premature labour or with acute systemic manifestations, whereas those with active genital lesions may present for caesarean section, performed to reduce neonatal transmission.

It is not known whether epidural or spinal anaesthesia increases the likelihood of central nervous system involvement if there is a history of secondary HSV infection, although there are published series of obstetric regional anaesthesia performed without problems. Epidural morphine is associated with up to 11 times the risk of recurrence of oral lesions compared with parenteral morphine; the mechanism is unclear but may be related to direct activation of the dormant virus in cranial nerve nuclei. Fentanyl has been implicated in a single report. However, there are other confounding factors such as emotional and physical stress that may also account for recurrence.

In primary infection, avoidance of regional anaesthesia is often advised, but less is known about the risks since primary infection at the time of delivery is rare. There are series of successful regional blocks in the presence of primary infection, but numbers are very small.

Management options

Treatment of HSV in pregnancy is by aciclovir, which may be given orally, or intravenously in cases of severe disseminated infection. Caesarean section is the recommended method of delivery when the risk of vertical transmission to the fetus is high, such as in women who have acquired their first infection in the third trimester, or in those with primary active lesions in the last 6 weeks of pregnancy or at the time of delivery. The benefit of caesarean section in the latter group, however, may be reduced if the membranes have been ruptured for longer than 4 hours. Women who present in labour with a recurrent infection, or those who have acquired the primary infection in the first two trimesters of pregnancy and whose labour does not start in the following 6 weeks, may be offered a vaginal delivery.

Mothers should be fully informed of the theoretical risks and benefits of regional anaesthesia, especially before caesarean section when the alternative (i.e. general anaesthesia) is generally perceived as being more hazardous. The neonate born of a mother with HSV should be carefully evaluated for evidence of infection.

Key points

- Primary herpes simplex virus (HSV) infection may cause severe systemic illness and premature labour.
- Neonatal infection may occur if there are active genital lesions.
- The risk of central neural infection following regional anaesthesia in secondary HSV infection is thought to be theoretical only.
- Epidural morphine may cause recurrence of orolabial HSV lesions.

Further reading

Chen YH, Rau RH, Keller JJ, Lin HC. Possible effects of anaesthetic management on the 1 yr followed-up risk of herpes zoster after caesarean deliveries. *Br J Anaesth* 2012; **108**: 278–82.

Corey L, Wald A. Maternal and neonatal herpes simplex virus infections. *N Engl J Med* 2009; **361**: 1376–85.

Foley E, Clarke E, Beckett VA, *et al.*; Royal College of Obstetricians and Gynaecologists. *Management of Genital Herpes in Pregnancy*. London: RCOG, 2014. https://www.rcog.org.uk/gl obalassets/documents/guidelines/management-genital-herpes.pdf (accessed December 2018).

Lee R, Nair M. Diagnosis and treatment of herpes simplex 1 virus infection in pregnancy. *Obstet Med* 2017; **10**: 58–60.

Chapter 142

HIV infection

The prevalence of human immunodeficiency virus (HIV) has been found on population screening to be about 0.15% of pregnant women in England, with the highest prevalence in those born in sub-Saharan Africa (where an estimated ~26 million of the ~37 million people currently living with HIV infection are located). In the UK, the prevalence of the disease in the general population is ~0.16%, compared with 0.4–0.9% in the USA. In parts of central and east Africa, the incidence may reach 20–30% in the larger cities.

The natural course of infection is an acute viral-type illness, followed approximately 3 months later by seroconversion when the patient becomes 'HIV-positive'; progression to the acquired immunodeficiency syndrome (AIDS; characterised by lymphadenopathy and conditions indicating reduced cell-mediated immunity, e.g. chronic opportunistic/invasive infections, chronic diarrhoea, malignancies, neurological involvement) occurs in about two-thirds of cases over the next 10 years, although up to 20% of people who are HIV-positive survive for 20 years without progression to AIDS. Median survival once AIDS is diagnosed is about 3–4 years; in Africa, survival is shorter, with about one-third of infected people progressing to death without developing AIDS itself.

HIV infection has altered the way in which contaminated materials are handled on the labour ward, and the way in which blood and blood products are administered. It is now recommended that all pregnant women undergo routine antenatal HIV testing, as neonatal transmission occurs in 25–30% of cases, with a further 14% infected if the mother breast-feeds; with appropriate medical management of known cases (see below), neonatal transmission can be reduced to under 3%. Since this recommendation by the Department of Health in 1999, the proportion of HIV-infected women diagnosed before delivery in the UK has risen to over 90%.

Human T-cell leukaemia/lymphoma virus (HTLV) types I and II have been found to have a similar prevalence to that of HIV in pregnancy, and screening of blood donations and/or pregnant women is performed in some countries.

Since the target of infection is primarily the lymphocyte, plasma counts of CD4-positive cells (mainly helper T-lymphocytes) have been used to monitor the course of infection and guide treatment. The CD4:CD8 ratio and plasma viral load (amount of viral RNA measurable in the plasma, representing degree of viral replication) are also used.

Problems and special considerations

Problems may be related to the acute viral illness of initial HIV infection.

Problems may also arise from impaired organ function and immunodepression of AIDS. All systems may be affected, either by primary HIV infection or by secondary infection, for example with fungi or other atypical organisms. Co-infection with tuberculosis, hepatitis B or hepatitis C may exist in some patients, and substance abuse is not uncommon. Of particular importance to anaesthetists are neurological manifestations, which may include neuropathy, encephalopathy, meningitis, focal brain lesions, dementia, myelopathy and myopathy, cardiovascular disease such as HIV-associated cardiomyopathy, and haemostatic abnormalities such as thrombocytopenia or platelet function disorders. HIV-positive patients, particularly those with low $CD4^+$ counts, have an increased risk of venous thromboembolism, which may be related to a deficiency in protein C or S or to the use of protease inhibitors.

The effects on organ systems of prophylactic highly active antiretroviral therapy (HAART) must also be considered. These may include blood dyscrasias, gastrointestinal disturbances, neurological and hepatic impairment and increased drug metabolism via hepatic enzyme indication.

There is a risk of transmission of HIV to the neonate. There is also a risk of transmission to medical and midwifery staff, and to other patients.

Management options

All units should offer counselling and testing for at-risk women prenatally or even pre-pregnancy, and this should continue during pregnancy. Many units have protocols in place for joint management of HIV-positive women by obstetricians and HIV specialists.

Acute HIV infection is rarely a known problem on labour ward and in general is managed as for any acute viral illness. For those with acute organ dysfunction, supportive management is directed at the organ system affected. Patients with chronic HIV infection must be assessed carefully before any anaesthetic intervention and managed according to their degree of organ impairment, which in most cases presenting to labour ward will not be severe.

In general, patients with HIV infection are managed as for any obstetric patient, unless specific contraindications exist. Particular care with invasive techniques has been suggested, to reduce the risk of introducing infection, but standard aseptic methods should be adequate if they are followed. The use of epidural or spinal anaesthesia has been questioned for fear of seeding the virus into the cerebrospinal fluid (CSF), thus accelerating the central nervous system (CNS) progression of the infection; because of a theoretical risk of seeding opportunistic infective organisms into the CNS; and because there may be complications related to underlying and undiagnosed CNS pathology. Since CSF involvement occurs very early in HIV infection, however, no further risk is generally felt to exist, and this is supported by clinical experience, albeit limited. Epidural blood patching has also been performed in HIV-positive patients without apparent adverse consequences. There has been no report of secondary CNS infection introduced during administration of regional anaesthesia in the HIV-infected mother, and this risk is generally felt to be theoretical only. Further, if no evidence of CNS involvement exists then most authorities recommend regional anaesthesia as routine. If CNS abnormalities do exist, then management depends on their severity and other considerations such as the presence of other complications.

Most units now treat HIV-positive mothers with antiviral drugs such as zidovudine, which has been shown to reduce transmission to the neonate by up to two-thirds. Combination with elective caesarean section reduces the risk further, to about 1%, although if the mother is well controlled on HAART and the viral load is under 400 copies/ml, vaginal delivery is associated with a similar risk of vertical transmission. There is wide consensus that breastfeeding should be discouraged.

Owing to the implications of testing for HIV, most health authorities advocate the approach of 'universal precautions' to potentially at-risk patients; thus routine management of all women on labour ward should involve the use of protective clothing where appropriate (gloves, goggles, etc., according to individual choice), use of disposable equipment and/or appropriate sterilisation techniques and careful handling and disposal of contaminated sharps. If these practices are routinely followed, the known HIV-positive patient should need no extra measures. Units that have policies such as this have accepted the cost implications of such all-inclusive guidelines, especially given the high cost and high profile of legal proceedings against establishments where cross-infection has occurred.

If an accidental needlestick injury or similar event occurs, local protocols and specialists should be consulted for guidance about prophylactic zidovudine therapy, since this is a controversial area. The risk of seroconversion after needlestick is about 0.3%.

Key points

- HIV-positive mothers may have many systems affected and may be taking several drugs.
- General anaesthetic management is according to standard criteria for indications and contraindications.
- Universal precautions should apply to all patients to reduce contamination of staff.
- Regional anaesthesia is not contraindicated in the HIV-positive parturient.

Further reading

Bull L, Khan AW, Barton S. Management of HIV infection in pregnancy. *Obstet Gynaecol Reprod Med* 2015; **25**: 273–8.

Hignett R, Fernando R. Anesthesia for the pregnant HIV patient. *Anesthesiol Clin* 2008; **26**: 127–43.

de Ruiter A, Taylor GP, Clayden P, *et al.*; British HIV Association. British HIV Association guidelines for the management of HIV in pregnant women. *HIV Med* 2014; **15** (Suppl 4): 1–77.

Malaria in pregnancy

Malaria is a major cause of maternal and fetal morbidity and mortality across the world, especially in tropical and subtropical regions, and though not indigenous to the UK it may present in women who have recently returned from infected areas. Pregnant women are more susceptible to infection (especially if HIV-infected), and are more likely to suffer a recurrence and develop severe complications, with increased risk of death and fetal loss.

Malaria is caused by one of predominantly four *Plasmodium* species: *P. falciparum*, *P. vivax*, *P. ovale* and *P. malariae*. In the UK, malaria is more commonly associated with *P. falciparum* and less so with *P. vivax*. Infection with *P. falciparum* is more insidious and associated with a higher mortality than infection with the other species. In Asia, particularly India, infection with *P. vivax* is more likely, and this can cause a relapsing type of malaria.

The bite of the female *Anopheles* mosquito inoculates *Plasmodium* sporozoites that pass via the bloodstream to the liver and develop into schizonts. The schizonts rupture and release thousands of merozoites into the circulation, which accounts for the typical cyclical nature of symptoms. The merozoites enter red blood cells and once inside can multiply over 2–3 days and infect new red blood cells. In *falciparum* malaria, large numbers of parasites may be sequestered in the placenta, which may be the contributing factor to fetal loss.

Problems and special considerations

Women who are pregnant or planning to become pregnant should be advised not to travel to an endemic area unless necessary. Prevention advice is the same as for the non-pregnant population, though certain antimalarials are relatively contraindicated at certain stages of pregnancy and specialist advice is required.

A high index of suspicion is required, as presentation may be atypical. Clinical features usually develop within 1–3 weeks of infection and may include symptoms of anaemia or fever of unknown origin (which may be very variable or even absent). Splenomegaly may be present. Seizures or coma may be the only presenting symptom of cerebral malaria.

Thick and thin films for malarial parasites should be examined, but parasites may not be visible on peripheral blood films. Rapid diagnostic tests based on malaria antigens are less sensitive; polymerase chain reaction methods may be more accurate.

Haemolytic anaemia may be exacerbated by decreased iron and folate levels, leading to severe anaemia. Thrombocytopenia may occur; when this is associated with haemolysis, it produces a picture that may be confused with HELLP syndrome (see Chapter 85). Disseminated intravascular coagulation may occur in severe malaria. Hypoglycaemia is a common feature and may be aggravated by certain antimalarials. Severe complications such as pulmonary oedema, acute lung injury and cerebral malaria are associated with a high mortality rate.

Fetal mortality associated with malaria is in the region of 15% for *P. vivax* and 30% for *P. falciparum*. Problems for the fetus include prematurity, anaemia, fetal growth restriction and congenital malaria; the last of these may result from transfer of parasites across the placenta and is not always preventable by treatment of the mother. Affected neonates may feed poorly and be pyrexial, irritable or jaundiced (this may be confused with jaundice of the newborn), and may suffer long-term developmental problems such as short stature and metabolic disturbances.

Management options

Severe malaria in a pregnant woman is a medical emergency. The patient with a suspected or proven diagnosis should be managed in a tertiary centre where full facilities and input from specialists in infectious diseases are available. Early admission to the intensive care unit is recommended for all but the mildest disease. Quinine and clindamycin are the standard drugs used for uncomplicated *falciparum* malaria, and chloroquine for the other types; intravenous artesunate or quinine is recommended for severe *falciparum* malaria (see RCOG guidelines for dosage). Close fetal and maternal monitoring is required, and expedited delivery of a late preterm fetus may be necessary. Management of severe complications is largely supportive.

Regional and general anaesthetic techniques have been described in mothers with malaria. If general anaesthesia is used, there are particular considerations: quinine therapy can prolong neuromuscular blockade and the hypoglycaemia induced by its use may be masked under general anaesthesia. Regional anaesthesia may be considered if there is no evidence of cerebral involvement and in the absence of secondary bacterial sepsis.

Key points

- Pregnant women are more susceptible to malaria because of their decreased immunity.
- Malaria may present with atypical symptoms, and mortality is high for both fetus and mother.
- Senior staff should be involved in obstetric and anaesthetic management, and advice should be sought from clinicians experienced in the management of malaria.
- The choice of anaesthetic technique should be based on each individual situation.

Further reading

Lalloo DG, Shingadia D, Bell DJ, *et al.*; PHE Advisory Committee on Malaria Prevention in UK Travellers. UK malaria treatment guidelines. *J Infect* 2016; **72**: 635–49.

Mathew DC, Loveridge R, Solomon AW. Anaesthetic management of caesarean delivery in a parturient with malaria. *Int J Obstet Anesth* 2011; **20**: 341–4.

Royal College of Obstetricians and Gynaecologists. *Malaria in Pregnancy: Prevention*. Green-top Guideline 54A. London: RCOG, 2010 (updated 2017). www.rcog.org.uk/en/guidelines-research-services/guidelines/gtg54a (accessed December 2018).

Royal College of Obstetricians and Gynaecologists. *Malaria in Pregnancy: Diagnosis and Treatment*. Green-top Guideline 54B. London: RCOG, 2010 (updated 2017). www.rcog.org.uk/en/guidelines-research-services/guidelines/gtg54b (accessed December 2018).

Soltanifar D, Carvalho B, Sultan P. Perioperative considerations of the patient with malaria. *Can J Anesth* 2015; **62**: 304–18.

Tarning J. Treatment of malaria in pregnancy. *N Engl J Med* 2016; **374**: 981–2.

Pyrexia during labour

Intrapartum pyrexia is said to occur when maternal temperature is ≥ 38 °C on one reading or ≥ 37.5 °C on two consecutive readings taken at least 1–2 hours apart. Pyrexia in labour may be a marker of infection requiring investigation and antibiotic therapy. However, there are many other medical causes of pyrexia (e.g. inflammatory disease, thyrotoxicosis, pulmonary embolism, malignancy) that should not be forgotten. In addition, epidural analgesia itself may be associated with a gradual increase in maternal (and thus fetal) temperature after about 6–8 hours, of up to 0.5–1 °C, in about 20% of parturients. Most studies, however, are poorly controlled and the phenomenon is controversial (for example, women with predisposing factors for infection are often those who request epidural analgesia).

Suggested mechanisms include alteration of afferent temperature-related neural input to the hypothalamus, impaired thermoregulatory mechanisms in the lower body (such as absent shivering in the legs) and a re-setting of the central 'thermostat'.

The fetal temperature is ~1 °C higher than the maternal core, and follows maternal oral readings more closely than tympanic.

Fetal heart rate may increase as a direct consequence of maternal pyrexia.

Problems and special considerations

The mechanism behind epidural-related fever in labouring women remains controversial; it is thought to be the consequence of a sterile inflammatory reaction. The presence of maternal pyrexia may trigger additional investigations in the mother or neonate or interventions to expedite delivery. It is therefore important that all anaesthetists, obstetricians, midwives and paediatricians are aware that the phenomenon may exist. In protocols and guidelines for the management of pyrexia during labour, provision should be made for the effect of epidurals; separate instructions may be required for mothers with epidurals and those without.

Pyrexia itself has been implicated in causing premature labour and may stress an at-risk fetus. Neonatal encephalopathy is more common if mothers are pyrexial during labour, although whether this is related to the increased temperature itself or to any underlying cause (particularly infection) is uncertain.

Infection causing pyrexia is a potentially serious problem, since severe sepsis may affect both the mother and the fetus. Thus, most protocols call for screening tests and possibly antibiotic therapy if infection is suspected.

Management options

In most cases, mild pyrexia is not in itself troublesome. Fanning, sponging or treatment with paracetamol may be used, although the possibility of masking underlying sepsis should not be forgotten. Pyrexia above 38.5 °C, especially if it occurs within 6 hours of siting the epidural, is unlikely to be related to epidural analgesia. If infection is suspected, screening should include blood cultures, high vaginal swabs and mid-stream urine sampling. Infection may not be accompanied by localising signs, at least initially; in addition, white cell count may increase during normal labour to as high as $30 \times 10^9/l$ (especially if steroids have been given for prematurity).

Mothers who are pyrexial and who request epidural analgesia present a separate dilemma. Local guidelines should be followed, but evidence of infection at the site of injection or sepsis are relative contraindications to neuraxial techniques, since regional blockade may be complicated by localised infection or cardiovascular compromise. For mild localised infection, such as chorioamnionitis (which may be associated with subclinical bacteraemia), regional analgesia is generally felt to be safe if covered with antibiotic therapy.

Set procedures should exist for monitoring of maternal temperature and management of pyrexia, including provision of regional blockade in pyrexial mothers and neonatal screening. A high level of general awareness and education is important, since staff of all disciplines may be unaware of the relationship between epidural analgesia and pyrexia.

Key points
- There are many causes of fever, the most common of which is infection.
- Epidural analgesia exceeding 6–8 hours has been associated with pyrexia.
- Protocols should exist for monitoring of temperature during labour and screening ± treatment of pyrexial mothers.
- Maternal pyrexia does not always contraindicate regional techniques.

Further reading
Riley LE, Celi AC, Onderdonk AB, *et al.* Association of epidural-related fever and noninfectious inflammation in term labor. *Obstet Gynecol* 2011; **117**: 588–95.
Segal S. Labor epidural analgesia and maternal fever. *Anesth Analg* 2010; **111**: 1467–75.
Sultan P, David AL, Fernando R, Ackland GL. Inflammation and epidural-related maternal fever: proposed mechanisms. *Anesth Analg* 2016; **122**: 1546–53.

Migrants and other disadvantaged women

Migration into the European Union (EU) has risen over the last decade, with approximately half of the migrants under 30 years old. It is thought that over a third of live births in the EU occur to mothers who are immigrants. About 500,000–650,000 people have come to live in the UK each year in the last decade, with 300,000–400,000 leaving each year. There is evidence from the Confidential Enquiries into Maternal Deaths, the UK Obstetric Surveillance System (UKOSS) and other national reports that morbidity and mortality are higher in migrant mothers. This is not just limited to international migration; migration from rural to inner-city areas is also increasing, and it is thought that mothers who move in this way have similar risks to those who migrate internationally.

Many of the problems exhibited by migrant parturients are not exclusive to migrants; thus there are other vulnerable and disadvantaged groups of women who should also be considered high-risk, including the homeless, the destitute, drug addicts and sex workers. Many will have mental health issues, and many of these groups overlap (see also Chapter 146, *Psychiatric disease*, and Chapter 147, *Substance abuse*).

Problems and special considerations

The management of pregnancy and safe delivery of the baby in migrant or disadvantaged women provides a challenge to both midwifery and medical staff, for a number of reasons.

Some mothers may present with poor general health, poor nutrition, obesity or coexisting diseases such as tuberculosis, rheumatic heart disease or HIV infection, which may impact on maternal and neonatal outcome. In certain parts of Asia, Africa and the Middle East, female genital mutilation is commonly practised, and this has implications for delivery options.

Migrant mothers may not be entitled to health care, or they may be unaware that they are entitled to it, during pregnancy. They may therefore seek antenatal care late, if at all, and they may be poor attenders of appointments, making it easy for them to be lost to the system. Thus, any pre-existing medical conditions may go untreated or not optimised until late in pregnancy. Similarly, conditions that develop during pregnancy, such as pre-eclampsia or fetal growth restriction, may not be detected.

Language may also pose a barrier to women seeking antenatal care, and this has been identified as a major contributory factor to maternal morbidity.

An accurate past medical history may be difficult or impossible to obtain, and there may be little or no medical records to refer to, either because they do not exist or because they have been lost or even concealed.

Certain cultures or religions may mistrust Western medicine and believe that obstetric intervention (e.g. caesarean section) is linked to death. The mother and/or father may therefore be reluctant to follow the advice of staff when any sort of operative delivery is suggested, leading to delay, poor perinatal outcomes and even fetal or maternal demise.

Previous studies have suggested that the uptake of labour neuraxial analgesia is lower in women from some ethnic groups. This may be related to difficulty in establishing the level of the woman's pain in the presence of a language barrier, the woman's lack of awareness or understanding of the available options for pain relief, her fear of incurring additional costs for the procedure, or cultural reasons. The absence of an in-situ epidural puts these women at an increased risk of receiving general anaesthesia for emergency interventions and the higher morbidity that may be associated with it.

Management options

A multimodal approach is necessary. As in all cases of good obstetric practice, communication is paramount – both within the team (which should include other specialists and social services as appropriate) and with the patient and her partner (and, if necessary, other members of her family).

If a language barrier prevents good communication, then interpreter services must be provided; it is no longer acceptable to use family or staff members to interpret, as they themselves may have limited English skills.

Proper explanation of antenatal care and the plan for delivery is necessary. It may be prudent antenatally to put forward the analgesic options available for labour and, if necessary, a separate appointment may be organised with an anaesthetist and an interpreter. If these are not available, other translation aids may be used. The Obstetric Anaesthetists' Association has leaflets available that may be downloaded, explaining the analgesic options.

Antenatal care should identify any coexisting disease in order that this is optimally managed, and the patient should be advised where to seek help if her symptoms change.

Interpreter services should be available during labour and delivery. Appropriate care and follow-up should also be arranged for the postnatal period.

Key points

- The migrant obstetric population is increasing in number.
- There is a higher morbidity and mortality associated with this group of women, and with other disadvantaged groups.
- Good communication and early antenatal care are paramount in identifying high-risk patients.
- Interpreter services should be available to all women when language is a barrier.

Further reading

Husarova V, Macdarby L, Dicker P, Malone FD, McCaul CL. The use of pain relief during labor among migrant obstetric populations. *Int J Gynaecol Obstet* 2016; **135**: 200–4.

Knight M, Nair M, Tuffnell D, *et al.*; MBRRACE-UK. *Saving Lives, Improving Mothers' Care: Surveillance of maternal deaths in the UK 2012–14 and lessons learned to inform maternity care from the UK and Ireland Confidential Enquiries into Maternal Deaths and Morbidity 2009–14.* Oxford: National Perinatal Epidemiology Unit, University of Oxford, 2016.

Lindquist A, Knight M, Kurinczuk JJ. Variation in severe maternal morbidity according to socioeconomic position: a UK national case–control study. *BMJ Open* 2013; **3**: e002742.

Nair M, Kurinczuk JJ, Knight M. Ethnic variations in severe maternal morbidity in the UK: a case–control study. *PLoS One* 2014; **9**: e95086.

Royal College of Obstetricians and Gynaecologists. *Female Genital Mutilation and its Management.* Green-top Guideline 53. London: RCOG, 2015. www.rcog.org.uk/en/guidelines-research-services/guidelines/gtg53 (accessed December 2018).

Chapter

146

Psychiatric disease

Psychiatric disease has been identified as a risk factor for adverse obstetric and neonatal outcomes, and suicide remains a leading cause of direct maternal death in the reports of the Confidential Enquiries into Maternal Deaths. As well as women with pre-existing psychiatric disease, it is estimated that 10–15% of mothers suffer from postnatal depression, and as many as 60% experience postnatal 'blues'. The risk of admission to hospital with psychosis in the first 3 months after childbirth is more than 300 times greater than at other times.

Much of the challenge in providing effective care to women with psychiatric disease relates to the organisation and funding of services, and the identification of women at risk. Thus there is emphasis on attempting to identify women with a past history of mental illness antenatally, and routine screening questions on booking should include past history and risk factors, including family history. The anaesthetist's involvement is usually restricted to caring for women who present peripartum or who have attempted suicide.

Problems and special considerations

Pre-existing psychiatric disease

Patients may be taking drugs that are affected by pregnancy, that have important maternal or fetal effects, or that affect anaesthesia. Women with bipolar disorder may be maintained on lithium or, less commonly, carbamazepine. Serial monitoring of plasma drug levels is particularly important for these drugs. Lithium may potentiate neuromuscular blockade (with both suxamethonium and non-depolarising neuromuscular blocking drugs). Women with schizophrenia are likely to be taking a variety of antipsychotic drugs, high doses of which can cause sedation and postural hypotension due to α-blockade. The latter is likely to be exacerbated by the physiological changes of pregnancy. Monoamine oxidase inhibitors (MAOIs) have a number of potential interactions, the most important of which concern pethidine and vasopressors. In addition, maternal anticonvulsant therapy may cause neonatal vitamin K deficiency, which may be associated with adverse effects such as haemorrhagic disease of the newborn. Some studies have suggested a link between untreated depression and hypertensive disease of pregnancy, an increased risk of bleeding or need for operative delivery.

Women who have been psychiatrically well and taking maintenance drugs may stop their medication when they become pregnant and present with recurrence of symptoms.

Many of the psychotropic drugs are relatively contraindicated during pregnancy, but a risk–benefit analysis must be made before changing or stopping such medication.

Women with psychiatric disease may lack capacity to give consent to treatment (see below). In acute mental states, they may also refuse treatments, disrupt the care of other patients and not follow feeding policies.

Postnatal psychiatric disease

Women who develop postnatal depression may not have had any warning symptoms or signs. Women with a past history of psychiatric disease or drug dependence may conceal this from obstetricians and midwives because of the perceived stigma of these conditions. Those with a previous history of postnatal depressive psychosis run a 50% risk of recurrence, classically at the same time postnatally as before. It is important for all healthcare professionals to maintain a high level of awareness of such disorders, and to ask all women at booking about previous psychiatric illness.

Substance abuse

Drug abuse is more common in North America than in the UK, but nevertheless it is an important cause of morbidity and mortality in the UK (see Chapter 147, *Substance abuse*). Mothers may conceal their use of recreational drugs, as they may feel that they will be judged, or for fear of being reported to the police or to child protection agencies. Liaison between the general practitioner, social services and maternity services is required.

Management options

Antenatal care

Women with poorly controlled psychiatric disease may default from antenatal care and may thus be at increased risk from undetected complications of pregnancy. They may exhibit hospital phobia and may lack insight into the need for medical care if pregnancy-related problems occur. Continuity of care, which enables a trusting relationship to be developed with one or two healthcare professionals, is vital. A perinatal mental health plan must also be in place and should be accessible to all healthcare professionals who provide care for the woman.

Antenatal discussion about the options for analgesia in labour and the possibility of needing anaesthesia for operative delivery is particularly important, and such discussions should be documented and witnessed by the woman's partner, and a third party if possible. There must be discussion between the psychiatrist, obstetrician, general practitioner and the woman herself about continuing drug therapy throughout pregnancy. Women who are maintained on drug therapy should be monitored regularly to ensure that the pregnancy-related increase in blood and plasma volume does not result in subtherapeutic drug levels.

Labour and delivery

Regional analgesia and anaesthesia are not contraindicated for women with psychiatric disease. Women with untreated or poorly controlled depression may subjectively experience more intense pain in labour and may therefore have an increased need for epidural analgesia.

Women taking an MAOI can receive ephedrine or phenylephrine to correct hypotension caused by regional anaesthesia, but smaller doses than usual should be used, as pressor responses may be exaggerated. Pethidine should be avoided, but fentanyl and morphine have both been used uneventfully.

There is a need for a high level of awareness among all healthcare professionals involved in intrapartum and postnatal care. Symptoms and signs suggestive of depressive illness must be treated promptly. Tri- and tetracyclic antidepressants, the selective serotonin reuptake inhibitor group of antidepressants and MAOIs may all be necessary in the treatment of both non-pregnancy-related and postnatal depression. Electroconvulsive therapy may also be indicated.

Women known to abuse illegal drugs should be treated with particular care. There are numerous interactions with medical drugs, and women frequently abuse multiple drugs.

Consent

A psychiatrist's input may be invaluable in characterising a psychiatric patient's illness and advising on her state of mind, though the decision on whether she has capacity should be made by the treating doctor, after considering such advice (see Chapter 169, *Consent*). The doctrine of necessity allows treatment to be administered without consent if she does not have capacity and this is in the patient's best interests, but it cannot be assumed that what the obstetric team would wish to do always reflects the mother's 'best interests', and a psychiatrist's advice may be useful here too. In the UK, the unborn fetus has no legal status or rights (though it may have moral ones).

If the mother is held in hospital under the Mental Health Act (1983), this only covers treatment of the primary mental condition and does not allow other treatments to be enforced unless they are considered to affect that condition directly.

Patients in whom consent may be problematic require multidisciplinary discussion antenatally in order to formulate a management plan. Often there is extensive discussion but the obstetric anaesthetist is not invited, so that the first contact he/she has may be when analgesia or anaesthesia is required.

Key points

- Psychiatric disease is common in pregnancy.
- A patient's drug therapy requires careful monitoring during and after pregnancy.
- The possibility of substance abuse should always be considered.
- Difficulties with consent should be anticipated and plans made in good time.

Further reading

Cantwell R, Knight M, Oates M, Shakespeare J, on behalf of the MBRRACE-UK mental health chapter writing group. Lessons on maternal mental health. In Knight M, Tuffnell D, Kenyon S, *et al.*; MBRRACE-UK. *Saving Lives, Improving Mothers' Care: Surveillance of maternal deaths in the UK 2011–13 and lessons learned to inform maternity care from the UK and Ireland Confidential Enquiries into Maternal Deaths and Morbidity 2009–13*. Oxford: National Perinatal Epidemiology Unit, University of Oxford, 2015, pp. 22–41.

Gadot Y, Koren G. The use of antidepressants in pregnancy: focus on maternal risks. *J Obstet Gynaecol Can* 2015; **37**: 56–63.

National Institute for Health and Care Excellence. *Antenatal and Postnatal Mental Health: Clinical Management and Service Guidance.* Clinical Guideline 192. London: NICE, 2014 (updated April 2018). www.nice.org.uk/guidance/cg192 (accessed December 2018).

Royal College of Obstetricians and Gynaecologists. Management of women with mental health issues during pregnancy and the postnatal period. *Good Practice* 14. London: RCOG, 2011. www .rcog.org.uk/en/guidelines-research-services/guidelines/good-practice-14 (accessed December 2018).

Substance abuse

The definition of the term 'substance abuse' is difficult, since the use of non-medically indicated substances ranges from socially acceptable activities such as smoking and moderate alcohol intake, to abuse of intravenous drugs. Many types of abuse coexist.

Drug abuse is an increasing problem in inner-city maternity units. Most experience is from the USA, where up to 20% of pregnant women are thought to have abused illicit substances (usually marijuana or cannabis) at some point during their pregnancy.

Problems and special considerations

Problems may be related to the maternal effects of drug use, including acute intoxication, chronic organ impairment and the risk of infection with blood-borne viruses and endocarditis for intravenous drug users; the control of drug use and withdrawal during pregnancy, labour and the postnatal period; and the effects of drug abuse on the fetus and neonate.

Because delivery is seen as a 'normal' process and the mothers may not consider themselves as unwell, they may continue taking the drug(s) up to and through the peripartum period, thus presenting with the acute effects of intoxication, including altered mental state. This may make communication, and especially consent, difficult or impossible. Many addicts present for the first time in labour, with poor antenatal care. There is a greater incidence of sexually transmitted disease in addicts.

Alcohol

Alcohol abuse is a more widespread problem than abuse of many recreational drugs, with well-known manifestations including malnutrition, hepatic disease and cardiac impairment. Acutely intoxicated mothers may have concurrently taken other drugs and may display aggressive behaviour, making regional anaesthesia more challenging. If the stomach is full there may be increased risk of aspiration. Acute withdrawal typically reaches its worst about 24–36 hours after cessation of intake.

A particular feature of alcohol abuse in pregnancy is the fetal alcohol syndrome, which comprises craniofacial, neurological, cardiac, urological and musculoskeletal abnormalities. The upper safe limit of alcohol consumption in pregnancy has not been determined, but recent evidence suggests that even minimal intake may be associated with behavioural difficulties in the child.

Tobacco

Smoking is a common problem worldwide; in the UK its prevalence is about 20% in women of childbearing age. Maternal effects include premature rupture of membranes, placenta praevia, placental abruption and stillbirth. Impaired mucociliary function may increase the incidence of respiratory morbidity associated with general anaesthesia. In the neonate it has long been associated with low birth weight, although the precise mechanism is unclear.

Cocaine

Cocaine, or its water-insoluble derivative crack, causes central and peripheral dopaminergic and adrenergic stimulation resulting in euphoria, increased alertness, vasoconstriction and hypertension. Myocardial ischaemia, malignant arrhythmias or aortic dissection may occur. Cardiotoxicity associated with cocaine use is exaggerated in pregnancy, possibly secondary to increased production of its active metabolite or increased sensitivity of α-adrenergic receptors. Convulsions, intracranial haemorrhages and renal, hepatic and haematological impairment (including thrombocytopenia) have been reported. Cocaine abuse has been associated with increased incidence of spontaneous abortion, placental abruption, premature labour and fetal morbidity and mortality. Prolonged action of suxamethonium has also been reported.

Diagnosis may be difficult since its use is often denied, and the presentation may resemble that of pre-eclampsia and phaeochromocytoma. Urine remains positive for cocaine metabolites up to 3 days after use, and testing has been suggested in all at-risk groups (e.g. known users of other drugs, unbooked pregnancies).

Opioids

Opioid abuse is associated with hepatic, renal, pulmonary and cardiovascular impairment. Gastric emptying is delayed. The incidence of pre-eclampsia is reportedly increased. Addicts may require central venous cannulation because of their poor peripheral veins. Apart from these considerations, opioid withdrawal may complicate labour and delivery, and postoperative analgesia may be difficult to provide. Withdrawal typically occurs 8–16 hours after cessation of intake and may present with tachycardia, hypertension, myalgia and agitation that worsen over 1–3 days. Opioid antagonists may precipitate acute withdrawal (including neonatal). Neonatal withdrawal may occur several days postpartum. Other neonatal effects of opioid addiction include increased fetal loss and fetal growth restriction.

Cannabis (marijuana)

Cannabis is a potent psychoactive drug that has been associated with increased incidence of arrest of labour and fetal morbidity. Cardiac arrhythmias including tachycardia or bradycardia, hypotension and myocardial depression have also been reported, especially if large doses are taken.

Amphetamines

Although less commonly abused than the above drugs, amphetamines acutely cause similar effects to cocaine including hypertension, arrhythmias, agitation, fever and confusion. Fetal effects include fetal growth restriction, premature labour and placental abruption. Acute ingestion may increase the requirement for anaesthetic drugs, whereas chronic abuse may result in central depression and depletion of catecholamine stores. Both regional and general anaesthesia may be accompanied by severe hypotension in chronically abusing patients.

Others

Experience with methylenedioxymethylamphetamine (MDMA; 'ecstasy') and solvent abuse in obstetrics is limited, but the same maternal manifestations may occur as are seen in non-pregnant subjects. Barbiturate abuse is less common now; its main problems are acute intoxication and chronic addiction/withdrawal.

Management options

Substance abuse may be difficult to identify in pregnant women but should always be considered in the differential diagnosis of any atypical case, for example when a woman presents with unexplained collapse or acute confusion. The timing of the most recent intake in relation to labour and delivery should be established. General management is directed at any specific organ impairment (including central nervous system depression) and providing appropriate nutrition, psychological support and counselling.

Management of acute alcohol withdrawal includes oral chlormethiazole or benzodiaze-pines. Alcohol infusion may also be used (10–150 ml/h of a 5–10% solution) although it may suppress uterine contractions.

If abusers of cocaine require general anaesthesia, pre-treatment with antihypertensive drugs should be considered, since severe hypertension and arrhythmias may follow tracheal intubation. Labetalol has been suggested as the drug of choice, as pure β-blockade may precipitate severe hypertension and coronary vasoconstriction via unopposed α-stimulation. Glyceryl trinitrate has also been used. Benzodiazepines have been recommended to reduce sympathetic activity. Drugs causing sympathetic stimulation (e.g. ketamine) should be avoided. During regional anaesthesia, haemodynamic instability may be greater than normal and resistance to ephedrine has been reported, possibly related to noradrenaline depletion (directly acting vasopressors such as phenylephrine may be preferable). Increased requirement for analgesic supplementation during caesarean section has also been described.

Management of opioid addicts is often simplified if opioids are avoided altogether and local anaesthetic alone is used for regional analgesia and anaesthesia.

Key points

- Problems of substance abuse in pregnancy/labour include the maternal effects of chronic abuse, acute effects on presentation and fetal/neonatal effects.
- A high index of suspicion is required in all atypical cases on the labour ward.

Further reading

Jones HE, Deppen K, Hudak ML, et al. Clinical care for opioid-using pregnant and postpartum women: the role of obstetric providers. Am J Obstet Gynecol 2014; 210: 302–10.

Louw KA. Substance use in pregnancy: the medical challenge. Obstet Med 2018; 11: 54–66.

Scott K, Lust K. Illicit substance use in pregnancy. Obstet Med 2010; 3: 94–100.

Wong S, Ordean A, Kahan M; Society of Obstetricians and Gynecologists of Canada. SOGC clinical practice guidelines: Substance use in pregnancy, no. 256. Int J Gynaecol Obstet 2011; 114: 190–202.

Young JL, Lockhart EM, Baysinger CL. Anesthetic and obstetric management of the opioid-dependent parturient. Int Anesthesiol Clin 2014; 52: 67–85.

Chapter 148

Obesity

The World Health Organization (WHO) has classified obesity according to body mass index (BMI) (Table 148.1). In the UK, around one in five pregnant women is obese by the WHO definitions. Obesity in pregnancy has been defined as weight > 91 kg, or > 110–120% of ideal body weight, or BMI $\geq$ 30 kg/m^2 at the first antenatal consultation. The obese mother presents significant challenges to the obstetric anaesthetist, and obesity has been highlighted as an important factor contributing to maternal mortality.

Problems and special considerations

The physiological changes that occur in pregnancy already put the parturient at risk, and obesity puts further stress on the limited physiological reserve of the pregnant mother.

The risks of diabetes, hypertension, coronary artery disease and obesity-related cardiomyopathy are all increased. Airway closure may occur within tidal volume, especially in supine and semi-supine positions. A small number of morbidly obese women may develop secondary pulmonary hypertension and chronic right ventricular failure.

Antenatal assessment, including accurate estimation of gestation, may be difficult.

Airway-related morbidity and mortality is increased in obese parturients, who have a high incidence of symptomatic reflux and are at greater risk of gastric aspiration, and of difficult or failed intubation.

Aortocaval compression will occur in all but the full upright and full lateral positions, owing to the large pannus.

Fetal growth restriction is possible, as well as the more commonly occurring macrosomic fetus. Malpositions are common, and there is a higher incidence of birth defects and

Table 148.1 World Health Organization classification of obesity

		Body mass index
Underweight		< 18.5 kg/m^2
Normal		18.5–24.9 kg/m^2
Overweight		25.0–29.9 kg/m^2
Obese	class 1	30.0–34.9 kg/m^2
	class 2	35.0–39.9 kg/m^2
	class 3	> 40.0 kg/m^2

stillbirth. Furthermore, monitoring the fetus ante- and intrapartum is more difficult in the obese patient.

The obese mother has an increased likelihood of developing pre-eclampsia, of requiring operative delivery (a risk of caesarean section of 30–50% has been reported) and of postpartum haemorrhage. Thromboembolic disease and infective postoperative complications are also more common.

The massively obese woman may not fit on a standard operating table, and she may exceed the weight limit of a standard hospital lift.

Intravenous access and non-invasive monitoring of the mother may be difficult. The use of invasive arterial monitoring has been suggested where it is thought that the blood pressure cuff may not give accurate blood pressure measurements.

Regional anaesthesia may be difficult, and there is an increased risk of epidural failure and dislodgement of the epidural catheter in obese patients.

Management options

Thromboprophylaxis should be used, preferably with low-dose heparin (in increased doses; Table 148.2), and graduated compression stockings should be worn for the entire hospital admission – this alone needs special consideration, since it may be difficult or even impossible to find stockings that fit effectively. Specialised equipment such as a bariatric operating table or hoist must be made available as required. H_2-antagonists and antacids should be used throughout labour.

Difficulty in securing intravenous access should be anticipated, as should difficult tracheal intubation. For labour, the benefits of regional analgesia usually outweigh the risks of epidural haematoma resulting from heparin prophylaxis. Early use of epidural analgesia should be recommended, since the risk of obstetric intervention is greater. Although identification of landmarks is difficult, standard-length needles can be used for the majority of women. The use of ultrasound may help to identify the midline and the need for a longer needle. The lowest effective concentrations of local anaesthetic combined with an opioid should be used; combined spinal–epidural (CSE) analgesia offers a suitable alternative. The aim should be to minimise any motor blockade while providing effective analgesia. There is some anecdotal evidence suggesting that the incidence and severity of postdural puncture headache is reduced in obesity, perhaps because of increased intra-

Table 148.2 CMACE/RCOG recommended daily doses of low-molecular-weight heparin in obese parturients

Weight	Enoxaparin	Dalteparin	Tinzaparin
91–130 kg	60 mg [a]	7500 units	7000 units [a]
131–170 kg	80 mg [a]	10,000 units	9000 units [a]
> 170 kg	0.6 mg/kg [a]	75 units/kg	75 units/kg [a]

[a] May be given in two divided doses.
Reproduced with permission from Royal College of Obstetricians and Gynaecologists. *Reducing the Risk of Thromboembolism During Pregnancy and the Puerperium.* Green-top Guideline 37a. London: RCOG, 2015. www.rcog.org.uk/en/guidelines-research-services/guidelines/gtg37a.

abdominal pressure. Once an epidural has been sited, these patients should be reviewed regularly during labour, and there should be a low threshold to re-site a non-functioning epidural early.

For caesarean section, regional anaesthesia is usually recommended in preference to general, and an existing epidural can usually be extended for emergency delivery. Where a de novo block is required, CSE anaesthesia may be preferable to single-shot spinal anaesthesia, because it allows better control over the final height of the block and surgical difficulty may lead to prolonged operating time. It is important to pay meticulous attention to avoidance of aortocaval compression.

If general anaesthesia is necessary, the risks of hypoxia and regurgitation of gastric contents should be assumed to be higher than in the non-obese pregnant woman. Adequate preoxygenation is essential, and tipping the operating table head-up may help to increase the functional residual capacity (FRC) and improve the efficiency of preoxygenation.

Difficulty with tracheal intubation should be anticipated and suitable aids should be readily available (see Chapter 38, *Failed and difficult intubation*). Often, extra pillows are required under the patient's shoulders and neck to position the mother optimally. The so-called 'ramped' position (external auditory meatus and sternal notch in the same horizontal plane) has been advocated in obese patients as this is thought to be associated with the optimal position for intubation as well as improving the FRC; it may be achieved using ordinary pillows and/or blankets or specific wedge-shaped pillows, possibly also altering the configuration of the operating table.

Trained and experienced anaesthetic assistance is essential, and the presence of a second anaesthetist is desirable.

In order to ensure good oxygenation, higher tidal volumes, the use of positive end-expiratory pressure (PEEP) and a higher inspired oxygen concentration have been recommended. Residual neuromuscular blockade has been implicated in maternal death and is a particular hazard in the obese woman. A peripheral nerve stimulator should be used to confirm reversal of neuromuscular blockade, and the trachea should be extubated with the patient in a slightly head-up position. Recovery from general anaesthesia should take place in a well-lit recovery area under the supervision of trained recovery staff.

Good postoperative analgesia, for example with epidural or spinal opioids, is important to allow early mobilisation. Abdominal wall blocks performed intraoperatively and intravenous patient-controlled opioid analgesia in the postoperative period are recommended for women in whom the central neuraxial route is unavailable. Postoperative physiotherapy should be provided, and high-dependency midwifery care should also be available.

Key points
- The obese mother has an increased risk of obstetric and anaesthetic complications.
- Early regional analgesia for labour should be encouraged.
- Difficulty with tracheal intubation should be anticipated.
- Thromboprophylaxis should be used in appropriate dosage.

Further reading

Centre for Maternal and Child Enquiries;
Royal College of Obstetricians and Gynaecologists. *Management of Women with Obesity in Pregnancy*. London: CMACE/RCOG, 2010. www. rcog.org.uk/womens-health/clinical-guidance/management-women-obesity-pregnancy (accessed December 2018).

Ellinas EH. Labor analgesia for the obese parturient. *Anesth Analg* 2012; **115**: 899–903.

Lim CC, Mahmood T. Obesity in pregnancy. *Best Pract Res Clin Obstet Gynaecol* 2015; **29**: 309–19.

Mace HS, Paech MJ, McDonnell NJ. Obesity and obstetric anaesthesia. *Anaesth Intensive Care* 2011; **39**: 559–70.

Uzoma A, Keriakos R. Pregnancy management following bariatric surgery. *J Obstet Gynaecol* 2013; **33**: 109–14.

Chapter

149

Kidney disease

Women with chronic kidney disease (CKD) may present in pregnancy. Some women, including those with no known pre-existing renal dysfunction, may develop acute kidney injury (AKI) in pregnancy or the puerperium, perhaps as a complication of a pregnancy-related problem. Either way, it has implications for the obstetric anaesthetist.

Although pregnancy was uncommon in patients with CKD in the past, improvements in the care of patients requiring renal replacement mean that women on dialysis programmes or having received renal transplants are increasingly likely to present to the maternity department. Conversely, pregnancy-related AKI related to an obstetric complication should be becoming less common as care of the sick mother (in both the maternity suite and the intensive care unit) improves, although there are few data relating to this.

It should be remembered that the normal physiological changes of pregnancy result in an increased glomerular filtration rate and a lowering of the 'normal' blood indices of renal function. Thus, the usual blood urea concentration in pregnancy is 3.0–4.0 mmol/l and the creatinine concentration 55–65 mmol/l. In contrast to non-pregnant subjects, a moderate increase in blood urea concentration in a pregnant woman may thus represent significant renal impairment.

Problems and special considerations

Pre-existing disease

In terms of general anaesthetic management, the problems of pre-existing renal disease are the same as in the non-pregnant population. These include the underlying cause of renal impairment, systemic manifestations of renal failure (in particular hypertension and ischaemic heart disease, thrombocytopenia and anaemia), the patient's medication, altered handling of drugs and fluid management, including the nature and timing of dialysis.

Obstetric management may be influenced by the above factors and any history of previous abdominal surgery, including the presence of a transplanted kidney. There is an increased risk of pre-eclampsia in mothers with renal impairment. The fetus may also be at risk, either from the underlying disease that caused renal impairment or from the above complications.

Pregnancy-related acute kidney injury

Typically, pregnancy-related AKI is especially associated with pre-eclampsia, HELLP syndrome, septic abortion and massive haemorrhage (traditionally caused by placental abruption, although any cause of hypovolaemia may be followed by AKI). Other important causes include pyelonephritis, drug reactions (especially non-steroidal anti-inflammatory drugs,

NSAIDs), acute fatty liver, incompatible blood transfusion and thrombotic microangiopathies. In most cases, AKI is caused by acute tubular necrosis, although cortical necrosis has been seen after abruption and pre-eclampsia. Problems are those of AKI generally, especially related to fluid balance and the apparently increased susceptibility of pregnant women to developing pulmonary oedema.

Management options

Parturients with pre-existing kidney disease should have their renal function closely monitored and blood pressure optimised during pregnancy. Severe anaemia may need to be corrected. Discussion with renal physicians and obstetricians is required regarding the timing of dialysis and method of delivery. Any arteriovenous shunt should be noted and steps taken to protect it during labour and/or delivery. Standard anaesthetic and analgesic techniques are suitable, given the above considerations, although regional anaesthesia may not be appropriate in some patients with coagulopathy or in those who have had recent haemodialysis. Drugs excreted renally should be used with caution, and those known to impair renal blood flow or function (especially NSAIDs) should be avoided. The management of women with previous renal transplant is discussed in Chapter 154, *Transplantation*).

Management of AKI in pregnancy is along standard lines. Preventive management aims at the identification of risk factors and early intervention, for example correction of hypovolaemia. Careful fluid balance is especially important, given the propensity of obstetric patients to pulmonary oedema, and invasive haemodynamic monitoring may be required in some women. Serum electrolytes must be monitored, particularly in women receiving magnesium therapy. Renal replacement therapy may occasionally be needed. Most mothers regain normal renal function, depending on the underlying cause, although a degree of renal impairment may persist postpartum.

Key points

- Mothers with chronic kidney disease require careful monitoring and an interdisciplinary approach.
- Obstetric anaesthetic management uses standard techniques, taking into account the underlying cause and systemic effects of renal dysfunction, use of drugs and problems relating to fluid management.
- Acute kidney injury may develop during or after obstetric catastrophes; management is along standard lines, and recovery of function is usual.

Further reading

Acharya A. Management of acute kidney injury in pregnancy for the obstetrician. *Obstet Gynecol Clin North Am* 2016; **43**: 747–65.
Chinnappa V, Ankichetty S, Angle P, Halpern SH. Chronic kidney disease in pregnancy. *Int J Obstet Anesth* 2013; **22**: 223–30.
Galvagno SM, Camann W. Sepsis and acute renal failure in pregnancy. *Anesth Analg* 2009; **108**: 572–5.
Liu Y, Ma X, Zheng J, Liu X, Yan T. Pregnancy outcomes in patients with acute kidney injury during pregnancy: a systematic review and meta-analysis. *BMC Pregnancy Childbirth* 2017; **17**: 235.
Webster P, Lightstone L, McKay DB, Josephson MA. Pregnancy in chronic kidney disease and kidney transplantation. *Kidney Int* 2017; **91**: 1047–56.

Steroid therapy

In pregnancy, steroids are used for the same inflammatory conditions as in the non-pregnant state, such as sarcoidosis and rheumatoid arthritis. They may also be used for obstetric medical conditions, for example recurrent miscarriages or antiphospholipid syndrome. Finally, maternal administration of glucocorticoids (usually dexamethasone or betamethasone) has been shown to reduce the incidence of respiratory distress syndrome and related complications in premature babies; the drugs are usually given as two doses 12–24 hours apart. The benefit is greatest at 30–32 weeks' gestation and when delivery occurs within 1–7 days after the administration of steroids.

Problems and special considerations

Anaesthetic concerns are related to the underlying reason for steroid therapy, the presence of side effects of steroids and the requirement for supplementary steroids to cover the stress of delivery.

Side effects

These are well known and no different in the pregnant state to those in the non-pregnant state, and they may be of relevance to the anaesthetist (e.g. electrolyte disturbance, osteoporosis). In general, hydrocortisone and prednisolone are about 90% metabolised by the placenta and therefore little reaches the fetus. However, maternal dosage above 10 mg prednisolone per day has been associated with neonatal adrenal suppression, and similar effects are theoretically possible in breastfed neonates, although reported measured concentrations of steroids in breast milk have been extremely low. There are unlikely to be adverse maternal effects of short-term administration of steroids given for premature delivery, although a raised white cell count is common and this may potentially complicate the diagnosis if infection is suspected. Transient reductions in fetal heart rate variability have been reported.

Steroid supplementation

Severe hypotension characterises the acute adrenocortical insufficiency of Addison's disease, and hypotension may also occur following surgery or trauma in chronic takers of steroids who do not receive supplementation, presumably as a result of suppression of the adrenals' ability to mount a stress response. This has led to the recommendation that all patients on steroid therapy should receive supplementation perioperatively. However, the population at risk is uncertain, although most authorities would include all those with more than a week's steroid therapy within the last 3–6 months. If too much supplementary steroid is given, there is at least a theoretical risk of increased susceptibility to infection; in addition, many patients dislike taking increased doses because depression and other mood changes may be apparent even after a short time, although other side effects typically take longer to occur. Finally, the amount of steroid reaching the neonate through breast milk, even though it is small, should be kept to a minimum.

Management options

In general, the management plan for these women should be made in collaboration with an endocrinologist, and adapted according to the particular circumstances of the case.

For general surgery, a more logical approach than the traditional '200 mg hydrocortisone 6-hourly' is to consider the normal endogenous response to surgery and to ensure that the equivalent amount of steroid is provided: for example, 25–50 mg hydrocortisone for minor surgery, 75–100 mg for intermediate surgery and 100–150 mg for major surgery (note that 1 mg prednisolone is equivalent to 4 mg hydrocortisone). This daily amount is required for 1–3 days depending on the extent of surgery and should include any therapy the patient is already taking, such as a maintenance dose.

Labour and delivery (including caesarean section) should generally be considered major surgical stress, although the stress of a prolonged and difficult labour is likely to be greater than that of a simple and rapid one. If the patient is already taking adequate steroid to cover the daily requirement, no extra steroid should be required so long as the usual dose can be taken orally. If supplementation is necessary, it can be given as intravenous hydrocortisone or oral prednisolone, each tapered after the required period. It is recommended that parturients with Addison's disease be commenced on hydrocortisone at the start of active labour or before a planned caesarean section, at a dose of 50–100 mg 6–8-hourly or on a continuous infusion of 200–300 mg per 24 hours, until delivery. This dose should be doubled post-delivery then tailed off to the pre-pregnancy dose after 24–48 hours, as clinically appropriate.

Key points

- Steroids may be given for medical or obstetric purposes.
- Side effects may be important to the anaesthetist just as in the general population, although they are usually not a problem after administration for premature delivery.
- Steroid cover should be given according to the particular circumstances of the case, but most patients require less than is traditionally given.

Further reading

Kemp MW, Newnham JP, Challis JG, Jobe AH, Stock SJ. The clinical use of corticosteroids in pregnancy. *Hum Reprod Update* 2016; **22**: 240–59.
Lebbe M, Arlt W. What is the best diagnostic and therapeutic management strategy for an Addison patient during pregnancy? *Clin Endocrinol* 2013; **78**: 497–502.
McDonald SD. Antenatal corticosteroids for women at risk of preterm delivery. *BMJ* 2017; **356**: j1467.

Trauma in pregnancy

Trauma during pregnancy may be coincidental or related to instability and difficulty moving, especially in the third trimester. It is a consistent cause of maternal death, usually associated with road traffic accidents but also including other forms such as violence, suicide and falls. One per cent of women of childbearing age who suffer major trauma in the UK are pregnant, and pregnant trauma patients tend to have a worse outcome. Fetal mortality rate is up to 50% in major trauma. Although the general principles are the same as in non-pregnant women, the physiological effects of pregnancy and the presence of the fetus impose particular conditions upon the presentation, assessment and management of injured mothers.

Problems and special considerations

The increased metabolic demands of pregnancy make the mother less tolerant of hypotension, poor organ perfusion and hypoxaemia. Assessment of circulating volume status may be complicated by the increased cardiac output, pulse rate and blood volume of pregnancy and the potential for aortocaval compression. Injury to the abdomen and/or pelvis may result in fetal injury, maternal urinary tract injury or severe haemorrhage from the increased vascularity.

Obstetric complications include premature rupture of membranes, premature labour, uterine rupture and placental abruption; the last may occur even with minor trauma and is an especially common cause of fetal death. Fetomaternal haemorrhage may occur, with maternal sensitisation to fetal blood antigens if susceptible.

The fetus is susceptible to the effects of drugs given to the mother.

Management options

General resuscitation is as for any injured patient, following the principles of advanced trauma life support, with the risk of aortocaval compression and gastric aspiration borne in mind. Hypotensive resuscitation is often recommended in trauma patients; however, there is no evidence to support its use in the pregnant patient, and its effects on uteroplacental perfusion will be detrimental to the fetus. Intravenous access should be secured above the diaphragm, where venous return is not compromised by the uterus. If chest drainage is indicated, landmarks may be changed in the presence of a gravid uterus, and drains may need to be inserted at a higher intercostal space. The choice of drugs administered to the mother will be influenced by the stage of the pregnancy. In the early stages, teratogenicity should be considered, and in the second and third trimesters the effect of the drugs on fetal growth and uterine function must be taken into account.

In the management of acute head injury, the normal blood gas values for pregnancy (arterial partial pressure of carbon dioxide approximately 4 kPa) must be remembered, especially if artificial ventilation is required. The risk of acid aspiration should be considered when airway reflexes are obtunded, and early intubation and ventilation may need to be considered.

Many of these women will require diagnostic radiological investigations, especially for head or spinal cord injury. Computerised tomography (CT) requires that the fetus is screened from the ionising radiation. Magnetic resonance imaging (MRI) requires an immobile patient, which may necessitate general anaesthesia with all its attendant risks. Aortocaval compression must be avoided at all times. Access to the MRI scanner may not be possible in an advanced state of pregnancy.

The fetus should be monitored for several hours at least, since placental abruption or fetomaternal haemorrhage may be delayed. In addition, the fetus may have suffered direct injury itself (risk increases with increasing gestational age) or be stressed by any concomitant hypotension, hypoxaemia or maternal therapeutic drugs or manoeuvres (e.g. inotropes, mannitol, furosemide, hyperventilation for control of intracranial pressure).

Caesarean delivery should be for obstetric reasons. Epidural analgesia can be an integral part of the management of labour or operative delivery.

Once the patient is stabilised, definitive surgical management of trauma injuries should follow the principles of non-obstetric surgery in pregnancy (see Chapter 8, *Incidental surgery in the pregnant patient*).

Key points

- The general principles of managing trauma in pregnancy are as for non-pregnant patients.
- Pregnant women are more susceptible to the effects of hypotension and hypoxaemia.
- Aortocaval compression must be avoided at all times.
- Assessment may be complicated by the physiological changes of pregnancy.
- Placental abruption and fetomaternal haemorrhage are particular risks. The former may be a cause of concealed haemorrhage and unexplained cardiovascular instability.

Further reading

Battaloglu E, Porter K. Management of pregnancy and obstetric complications in prehospital trauma care: faculty of prehospital care consensus guidelines. *Emerg Med J* 2017; **34**: 318–25.

Huls CK, Detlefs C. Trauma in pregnancy. *Semin Perinatol* 2018; **42**: 13–20.

Mendez-Figueroa H, Dahlke JD, Vrees RA, Rouse DJ. Trauma in pregnancy: an updated systematic review. *Am J Obstet Gynecol* 2013; **209**: 1–10.

Chapter 152

Jehovah's witnesses

There are 8.5 million Jehovah's Witnesses worldwide, meaning that encountering a Jehovah's Witness in the medical workplace is not uncommon. The combination of the potential for major haemorrhage and the limitation of blood product administration makes the pregnant Jehovah's Witness a challenge for the anaesthetist. Observational study suggests that the pregnant Jehovah's Witness has a greatly increased risk of morbidity and death.

Problems and special considerations

Understanding the motivation and conviction behind blood product refusal is important when providing care to a Jehovah's Witness. This primarily stems from a literal interpretation of the Bible, for example:

> For the life of every creature is its blood: its blood is its life. Therefore I have said to the people of Israel, You shall not eat the blood of any creature, for the life of every creature is its blood. Whoever eats it shall be cut off. Leviticus 17:14

This has been interpreted by Jehovah's Witnesses to mean that the acceptance of blood products will result in the loss of their faith and place in their community; the alternative option is preferable to many.

Secondly, Jehovah's Witness information sources cite the medical benefits of refusal of blood products such as avoiding exposure to blood-borne diseases, immune-system reactions and human errors; alternatives such as bloodless surgery and blood conservation techniques are recommended. While the benefits of avoiding blood transfusion are clearly supported by an evidence base, depending on the clinical context, this is often not transferable to the acute major haemorrhage that may be seen in obstetrics.

Management options

The pregnant Jehovah's Witness should be seen in both obstetric and anaesthetic antenatal clinics. This gives the opportunity for optimisation and planning before delivery. Anaemia must be treated; if oral iron is inadequate, intravenous iron should be offered. Supplemental folate and vitamin C can be added. Erythropoietin may be offered to those refractory to iron, and may be acceptable.

The antenatal review also gives the opportunity to explore which blood products or synthetic products (if any) are acceptable, and which techniques, such as cell salvage, may be used (Table 152.1). There may be significant variation between what different Jehovah's Witnesses find acceptable; the individual patient's wishes should be clearly documented,

Table 152.1 Usual range of acceptability to Jehovah's Witnesses of blood and blood-related products (note that individual patients may have very specific views, and these must be sought and documented in each case)

Usually acceptable	Sometimes acceptable	Usually not acceptable
Iron, folate	Albumin	Whole blood
Tranexamic acid	Clotting factors	Packed red cells
Desmopressin	Immunoglobulins	White cells
	Cryoprecipitate	Platelets
	Recombinant erythropoietin	Plasma
	Prothrombin complex concentrate	
	Factor VIIa concentrate	
	Cell salvage	
	Cardiopulmonary bypass	
	Haemofiltration	

and she must be reassured as to the confidentiality of her decision. If the woman has an advance directive, a copy should be prominently displayed in her notes. A frank discussion regarding the individual's risk of haemorrhagic complications of pregnancy and labour, and the potential consequences (including death), should occur to ensure that decisions are informed, and this discussion should be recorded in the clinical notes. It must be made clear that there are currently no blood substitutes with the ability to carry oxygen that are licensed for use in the UK, a misunderstanding that is sometimes encountered. Most hospitals and trusts will have a pro forma for patients who might refuse blood and related products.

Jehovah's Witnesses may be subject to coercion by family members or others (e.g. religious leaders), such that they may state their refusal of blood products if others are present, but agree to certain treatments when the options are discussed in private. Staff must be aware of this risk and be certain that the views recorded reflect those of the woman herself, free of coercion.

Of those who will accept cell salvage, some may request a continuous circuit to be used, such that there is no 'break' in the continuity of blood leaving and entering the body. This has also been requested when performing epidural blood patches, the mechanics of which have been detailed in case reports.

Senior experienced clinicians should lead care in the peripartum period. During delivery, prompt use of uterotonics is recommended. Mechanical techniques to control haemorrhage, including hysterectomy, may be considered sooner than in non-Jehovah's Witnesses in the event of major haemorrhage. This should have been discussed during the antenatal visits.

Alternative intraoperative techniques to counter blood loss and its effects, such as permissive hypotension and normovolaemic haemodilution, need careful consideration in the obstetric setting. Case reports have described the use of peripartum hyperbaric oxygen therapy in the critically anaemic Jehovah's Witness, to maximise oxygen delivery.

In emergency clinical situations, where the patient does not have the capacity to make informed decisions, advice should be sought from the hospital legal team. In general, the patient's views must be respected, even if this results in her death. However, if there is any doubt as to the mother's wish not to receive blood products under any circumstances (e.g. if this is not clearly documented in the notes or in a signed advance directive), then the default position would be to preserve life.

Key points

- Advance communication and preparation and multidisciplinary team work are essential when caring for the pregnant Jehovah's Witness.
- The views of Jehovah's Witnesses vary regarding receipt of blood and blood-related products, and these must be sought and clearly documented for each individual patient, including all circumstances in which such treatments would or would not be acceptable.
- The risk of coercion by family members and others must be considered, and the true wishes of each patient ascertained.
- Certain treatments (e.g. cell salvage and epidural blood patch) may be acceptable if a continuous circuit of blood is maintained.

Further reading

Jehovah's Witnesses. Official website. www.jw.org/en (accessed December 2018).
Lawson T, Ralph C. Perioperative Jehovah's Witnesses: a review. *Br J Anaesth* 2015; **115**: 676–87.
Mason CL, Tran CK. Caring for the Jehovah's Witness parturient. *Anesth Analg* 2015; **121**: 1564–9.

Malignant disease

There have been continuing improvements in the treatment of malignancies affecting children and young adults, and in the management of the reduced fertility that commonly follows such treatment. Thus, there are increasing numbers of women with treated (but not necessarily cured) malignant disease who become pregnant. In addition, malignant disease may occasionally present for the first time during pregnancy, and it may also be related to the pregnancy itself. Cancer prevalence rates in pregnancy are increasing (approximately 1 per 1000 pregnancies), primarily owing to older maternal age and the use of detection modalities that are now considered safe in pregnancy. The most common cancers seen are breast cancer, cervical cancer, haematological malignancies and melanoma.

Problems and special considerations

General problems of malignancy

These may be local (compression effects, local invasion, scarring, etc.), metastatic (liver involvement, etc.) or general (malaise, anaemia, endocrine effects, weight loss and cachexia). There may also be problems relating to treatment, such as side effects of cytotoxic drugs and steroids, and fibrotic effects of radiotherapy. There may be coagulation abnormalities or increased risk of deep-vein thrombosis necessitating anticoagulant therapy. Electrolyte disturbances (e.g. hypercalcaemia) may be a feature of the malignancy or its treatment.

Problems during pregnancy

Malignancies may be affected by the changing hormonal profile of pregnancy and its effects on the tissues; this may make certain tumours more aggressive (e.g. breast cancer, melanoma). Diagnoses may be delayed because of the overlap of symptoms with those of the pregnancy. Some maternal malignancies may metastasise to the fetus or placenta (e.g. melanoma), although in general this is rare. Women who have had childhood cancer may be at increased risk of complications in pregnancy, including gestational diabetes, hypertensive disorders and anaemia; an increased level of antenatal input may therefore be warranted.

The risks and benefits to the mother, the fetus and future fertility of administering or withholding treatment need careful consideration. The patient's medication may need altering, especially in early pregnancy, since many cytotoxic drugs are harmful to the fetus; systemic chemotherapy is associated with prematurity, congenital malformations, neurocognitive dysfunction, cancer and fertility problems in the fetus. There will be concerns about the use of radiotherapy to treat malignancy during pregnancy; the rapidly growing fetus is particularly radio-sensitive, and effects will depend on gestational age and the exposure dose. Concerns related to surgical intervention are the same as those for other surgical procedures in pregnancy (see Chapter 8, *Incidental surgery in the pregnant patient*).

In addition, the normal psychological stresses of pregnancy and delivery are especially intense if the mother has (or has had) cancer. The physiological demands of normal pregnancy may stress the more susceptible systems in the mother with malignant disease; for example, anaemia may become more pronounced, and mild cytotoxic-induced cardio-myopathy may become more severe. Finally, there may be direct effects of the malignancy or its treatment on the uterus and birth canal, such as scarring from cervical or perineal surgery, or abdominal adhesions.

A particular form of malignant disease affecting pregnancy is that arising from the placenta itself (gestational trophoblastic neoplasia), comprising hydatidiform mole, invasive mole, choriocarcinoma and placental site trophoblastic tumour. The incidence is 1 in 714 live births, and it is more common at the extremes of reproductive age, in east and southeast Asia, and if previous pregnancies have been affected. The pregnancy itself is non-viable, and concerns about the fetus do not apply. These tumours generally respond well to chemotherapy, even if metastatic spread has occurred, with a mortality below 1%. Molar pregnancy may be associated with hyperemesis, hypertensive disease, anaemia, ovarian cysts and, rarely, hyperthyroidism. Surgical evacuation may be associated with excessive bleeding, and may be followed by pulmonary oedema or acute lung injury, possibly related to trophoblastic pulmonary embolism.

Management options

General care is directed towards the particular organs or systems affected by the malignancy itself and its treatment. Thus all mothers who have or have had a malignancy require careful antenatal assessment, paying particular attention to haematological and major organ function, with decisions concerning anaesthetic management made accordingly. Some mothers may knowingly have put their lives at risk in order to give the fetus the best chance of survival, and this must be respected when managing their analgesia and anaesthesia.

In trophoblastic neoplastic disease, uterine evacuation may be adequate surgical management, but hysterectomy may be required in more invasive disease, especially in older women. Surgery may also be required for torsion of, or haemorrhage into, ovarian cysts. Chemotherapy may be required if human chorionic gonadotrophin levels remain elevated or in metastatic disease.

In terms of anaesthetic management, the above considerations should be taken into account and appropriate measures taken regarding investigation (including liver and thyroid function blood tests and chest radiography), monitoring and management. General anaesthesia is usually recommended, since uterine bleeding may be rapid and severe, and blood should be cross-matched and ready before surgery.

Key points

- Malignancies may be present before pregnancy, may develop or be diagnosed during pregnancy, or may arise from the pregnancy itself.
- Problems may be related to general effects of malignancies or those related to the interaction between malignancy, its treatment and pregnancy.
- Gestational trophoblastic neoplasia represents a particular form of malignancy.

Further reading

Basta P, Bak A, Roszkowski K. Cancer treatment in pregnant women. *Contemp Oncol (Pozn)* 2015; **19**: 354–60.

Morice P, Uzan C, Gouy S. Gynaecological cancers in pregnancy. *Lancet* 2012; **379**: 558–69.

Salani R, Billingsley C, Crafton SM. Cancer and pregnancy: an overview for obstetricians and gynecologists. *Am J Obstet Gynecol* 2014; **211**: 7–14.

Chapter 154

Transplantation

Advances in transplant surgery and immunosuppressive drug treatment have led to increasing numbers of women with transplanted organs choosing to embark on pregnancy. Pregnancy following renal transplantation is now almost commonplace, and successful pregnancy following liver, heart and heart–lung transplantation has been reported. The major considerations for the medical staff caring for the pregnant transplant recipient are the effects of immunosuppressive therapy, the alteration in physiological function of the transplanted organ and the impact of the physiological changes of pregnancy.

Problems and special considerations

Immunosuppressive therapy

All transplant patients are at risk of organ rejection and therefore require long-term immunosuppressive therapy. There is no evidence that pregnancy itself increases the risk of rejection, which, in the case of renal transplants, is about 10% in the first year and up to 40% after 5 years.

Infections, both bacterial and viral, are more common because of the immunosuppressed state, with urinary tract infections (already more common during pregnancy) the most frequent infectious complication. The immunosuppressed patient is at risk of infection with uncommon pathogens, and it is therefore important to take appropriate cultures before beginning treatment.

Immunosuppressive drugs include cyclosporin, azathioprine and corticosteroids. Frequent monitoring of drug levels is required because of the changing blood volume during pregnancy, weight gain and altered drug metabolism, although in some cases the dose requirement may be reduced rather than increased.

Cyclosporin is associated with systemic hypertension (caused by activation of the sympathetic nervous system), and women with transplanted organs also have an increased risk of developing pre-eclampsia – an incidence of 30% has been reported. Pre-eclampsia may be difficult to diagnose because of the pre-existing hypertension and proteinuria. There have also been reports of thrombotic complications occurring in patients receiving cyclosporin, leading to recommendations that prophylactic heparin should be considered during pregnancy.

Azathioprine is associated with abnormal liver function tests and thrombocytopenia.

The problems associated with long-term corticosteroid therapy are well known (see Chapter 150, *Steroid therapy*); of specific concern during pregnancy are hypertension and glucose intolerance. There is an increased incidence of hypertension and gestational diabetes post-transplantation, regardless of medication.

Immunosuppressive drugs are associated with a relatively low rate of fetal abnormality (cyclosporin is less teratogenic than azathioprine) but an increased rate of preterm delivery and fetal growth restriction.

Kidney transplant

Pre-pregnancy factors associated with a deterioration in renal function in renal transplant recipients are hypertension requiring medication, a raised serum creatinine level and proteinuria. In the absence of these factors, there is no evidence that pregnancy has an impact on graft outcome. It is important to monitor renal function closely throughout pregnancy; as with hypertension, there may be difficulty with differential diagnosis if pre-eclampsia develops.

Liver transplant

Alkaline phosphatase and serum transaminase levels increase during pregnancy; bilirubin and prothrombin time do not change and can be used to assess liver function during pregnancy. Liver function usually resolves quickly after transplantation, and concern about drug metabolism is usually not necessary in a well-functioning graft. The rate of caesarean delivery after liver transplant is about 50%; reasons suggested for this include the increased incidence of gestational diabetes and hypertensive disorders, and an increased tendency towards fetal distress.

Heart and heart–lung transplant

The transplanted heart is denervated, and thus there are no vagal influences acting upon it. Adequate cardiac output is dependent on maintenance of adequate preload. Heart rate can increase in response to hypovolaemia or vasodilatation, but this response is delayed compared with that of the normal pregnant woman; a high block may be particularly poorly tolerated. There is considerable controversy regarding the response of the denervated heart to adrenergic agonists, with reports of both extreme hypersensitivity and blunted response. Likewise there have been reports of bradycardia and even sinus arrest following administration of neostigmine, despite theoretical grounds for believing that the drug should not alter the rate of the denervated heart.

Afferent denervation of the heart prevents the patient from experiencing angina, but the anaesthetist and obstetrician should be aware that the woman with a cardiac transplant is at increased risk of coronary artery disease (20% by 1 year post-transplant and up to 50% by 5 years), which can only be reliably detected by cardiac catheterisation. Assessment of graft function includes pulmonary function tests, chest radiograph, arterial blood gas analysis, ECG, echocardiogram and cardiac catheterisation. There is some limited evidence from case series to suggest that graft failure may be higher in heart–lung transplantation than in other solid organ transplants after pregnancy.

Obstetric outcomes

Apart from the increased incidence of pre-eclampsia with cyclosporin, parturients who are recipients of transplanted organs have an increased risk of premature delivery, fetal growth restriction and the need for operative delivery. Surgery may be complicated by the previous transplant, and the risk of postoperative infection is also increased. There is also a risk of transplant rejection during pregnancy, possibly related to the physiological changes in pregnancy and alterations in drug metabolism.

Management options

Fertility is reduced in women with end-stage organ failure, because of hypothalamic-pituitary–gonadal dysfunction, but fertility tends to improve after 6 months with a well-functioning graft. Most women are advised not to become pregnant for 1–2 years after transplantation, in order to allow organ function and immunosuppressive therapy to stabilise. Pregnancy after organ transplantation may be considered high-risk and should be managed by a multidisciplinary team.

There are reports of successful vaginal delivery following kidney, heart, heart–lung and liver transplants. As a general rule, caesarean section is only indicated for obstetric complications, although each case must be considered individually. Anaesthetic priorities are to maintain adequate perfusion to the graft organ, but this should not differ from routine obstetric anaesthesia. A recent platelet count should be checked before neuraxial techniques, as it may be affected by pre-eclampsia, liver or kidney dysfunction, or immunosuppressive agents.

The woman with a well-functioning liver or kidney transplant can be treated as normal and may receive epidural analgesia and either regional or general anaesthesia. For renal patients, particular attention should be paid to venous access, keeping cannulae as peripheral as possible and preserving any sites for shunts and fistulae. Nephrotoxic agents are probably best avoided.

Epidural analgesia has been used for heart transplant recipients in labour, and regional anaesthesia (both epidural and spinal) has been used successfully for operative delivery; a combined spinal–epidural with a small spinal dose may be preferable to avoid a sudden and severe drop in blood pressure. Adrenaline is probably best avoided as an epidural additive, as an exaggerated tachycardia may be seen. If general anaesthesia is required, care should be taken with tracheal intubation in the presence of a tracheal–bronchial suture line. Airways may be more reactive after lung transplant, and agents that cause bronchospasm are best avoided. It is important to avoid dehydration and to use adequate preloading, but the risks of catheter-related sepsis probably outweigh the benefits of central venous pressure monitoring in these patients. Ephedrine has been used in normal doses, but it is wise to use small increments because of the risk of exaggerated response to the drug. If ineffective, a directly acting vasopressor such as noradrenaline or phenylephrine can be used; these drugs will cause vasoconstriction without a reflex bradycardia.

Infectious complications remain one of the major risks for all transplant recipients, and scrupulous attention to aseptic technique is therefore vital. There is an increased risk of red blood cell antibodies arising from transplanted organs; early discussion with the blood bank is advised to mitigate problems. Thromboembolism risk should be documented, as there is an increased incidence of thromboembolic disease.

An augmented dose of corticosteroids during delivery has been recommended to reduce the risk of graft rejection; this should be discussed with the transplant physician.

Key points

- Immunosuppressive drugs are used by all transplant recipients.
- Cyclosporin is associated with systemic hypertension and proteinuria.
- Transplanted hearts are denervated and cardiac output is primarily dependent on preload.
- Successful vaginal delivery with epidural analgesia has been reported following organ transplantation.

Further reading

Bramham K, Nelson-Piercy C, Gao H, *et al.* Pregnancy in renal transplant recipients: a UK national cohort study. *Clin J Am Soc Nephrol* 2013; **8**: 290–8.

Chittka D, Hutchinson J. Pregnancy after renal transplantation. *Transplantation* 2017; **101**: 675–8.

Moaveni DM, Cohn JH, Hoctor, KG, Longman RE, Ranasinghe JS. Anesthetic considerations for the parturient after solid organ transplantation. *Anesth Analg* 2016; **123**: 402–10.

Mohamed-Ahmed O, Nelson-Piercy C, Bramham K, *et al.* Pregnancy outcomes in liver and cardiothoracic transplant recipients: a UK national cohort study. *PLoS One* 2014; **9** (2): e89151.

Vos R, Ruttens D, Verleden SE, *et al.* Pregnancy after heart and lung transplantation. *Best Pract Res Clin Obstet Gynaecol* 2014; **28**: 1146–62.

Chapter 155

Critical care in pregnancy

The importance of critical care provision in pregnancy is increasingly being recognised. In 2013, a study by the Intensive Care National Audit and Research Centre (ICNARC) and the Obstetric Anaesthetists' Association (OAA) examined a large dataset of obstetric admissions to the intensive care unit (ICU). Women were more likely to be admitted to ICU in the postpartum period than while pregnant, and haemorrhage was the commonest cause in this group, followed by hypertensive disorders. Antenatal admissions were more heterogeneous but pneumonia, respiratory failure and sepsis predominated.

Most series give an overall ICU admission rate of 0.2–9 per 1000 deliveries, although there is much variation between countries and even units as a result of differences in patient population and selection. Most patients stay in the ICU for less than 3–4 days. Mortality rates are difficult to estimate for the above reasons but are generally low overall (in the order of 3–4% in reported UK series), although they range from 0% to 20% in published series worldwide. Objective prediction of mortality is hampered by the relative inability of standard scoring systems (e.g. APACHE) to allow for the physiological changes of pregnancy or the particular spectrum of conditions seen in pregnancy (e.g. platelet count has greater importance in obstetric patients than in the non-pregnant population).

However, such data only provide information on women who were admitted to ICU, and not those who were managed on the ward. The Confidential Enquiries into Maternal Deaths (CEMD) focus on deaths and therefore do not give a complete picture of critical illness and pregnancy, although recent reports have included sections about ICU management and selected causes of morbidity, in order to extract lessons to be learned. The need for adequate provision of ICU or high-dependency beds, especially in smaller delivery units, is repeatedly stressed. Some units have the facilities to provide high-dependency care on the labour ward; if not, clinicians will have a lower threshold for transfer to a general ICU. More recently, emphasis has been on providing 'intensive care' to the sick mother within the maternity unit – i.e. before she is actually admitted to the ICU; critical care outreach teams can provide valuable support.

Problems and special considerations

A modification of the Department of Health's 2000 classification of critical care has been suggested for obstetrics (Table 155.1).

General ICU care is as for non-obstetric patients. Particular points to note include:

- The risks to the fetus and the need for fetal monitoring (if antepartum)

Table 155.1 Classification of critical care, modified for obstetrics

Level 0	Normal ward care of low-risk mother
Level 1	Additional monitoring or intervention, or step down from higher level of care (e.g. risk of haemorrhage, neuraxial analgesia, oxytocin infusion, mild pre-eclampsia, medical condition such as congenital heart disease or diabetes)
Level 2	Single organ support
	• Respiratory (e.g. requiring continuous oxygen, continuous positive airway pressure, bi-level positive airway pressure)
	• Cardiovascular (e.g. pre-eclampsia requiring intravenous antihypertensives, arterial or central venous lines, cardiac output monitoring, intravenous antiarrhythmic/antihypertensive/vasoactive drugs)
	• Neurological (e.g. magnesium to control seizures, intracranial pressure monitoring)
	• Hepatic (e.g. acute fulminant hepatic failure with consideration of transplantation)
Level 3	Advanced respiratory support or two other organ systems support

- The requirements of the patient's partner and family
- The midwifery care required in the puerperium (if postpartum)
- The need for attention to drug safety if breastfeeding
- The physiological changes of pregnancy, including especially:
  - Increased risk of aspiration and higher incidence of a difficult airway
  - Increased oxygen demands and changes in respiratory function
  - Apparently increased propensity of critically ill obstetric patients to develop acute lung injury
  - Susceptibility to aortocaval compression
  - Increased cardiac output and other cardiovascular changes
  - Haematological changes including anaemia, increased risk of deep-vein thrombosis (DVT) and susceptibility to disseminated intravascular coagulation

These effects of pregnancy may be overlooked by staff unfamiliar with managing pregnant women. This problem may increase with the separation of anaesthesia and intensive care medicine training in the UK, as non-anaesthetic intensivists are less likely to have spent time on the labour ward during their training.

Finally, there may be psychological problems in the mother who is, or has been, critically ill, both before and after delivery. The fetus is likely to have been affected by her illness, increasing the stress upon her. The ICU environment is a far from ideal place to deliver or care for a baby.

Management options

The CEMD reports emphasise prompt recognition of the deteriorating parturient, early involvement of senior clinical staff and multidisciplinary team working.

Routine ICU support includes prophylaxis against DVT and stress ulcers. Management of any associated organ failure is along standard lines. In severe respiratory failure in pregnancy, early referral to a specialist unit able to provide extracorporeal membrane oxygenation (ECMO) is advised. Premature labour is always a risk of severe maternal illness; however, the use of tocolytic drugs may be considered too risky for the mother. Aortocaval compression must be avoided at all times.

Caesarean section may be required in order to improve the mother's condition, for example in severe cardiac or respiratory disease or hypertensive disorders. A perimortem caesarean delivery may be required in the event of maternal cardiac arrest; critical care staff should be alerted to this possibility, and appropriate equipment should be readily available.

Postpartum haemorrhage may be severe if a coagulopathy is present. Breast milk may be collected postpartum but may be unsuitable for use because of maternally administered drugs. If breast milk is not collected for neonatal feeding or to maintain lactation until the mother is well enough to nurse, lactation can be suppressed with bromocriptine, although this is not recommended routinely (especially in pre-eclampsia) since hypertension, stroke and myocardial infarction have followed its use.

Regular obstetric review should occur on the ICU, and neonatal support must be accessible. Management specific to the obstetric population must be clearly communicated – for example fluid therapy in pre-eclampsia. Good communication between all the involved clinicians (obstetricians, intensivists, etc.) and between the midwife and ICU nursing staff is vital to ensure that continuity of care is achieved with regard to treatment decisions and information given to relatives. Once discharged from hospital, outpatient obstetric and critical care follow-up should be offered to discuss events and monitor recovery from critical illness.

Key points

- Worldwide, between 0.2 and 9 obstetric patients per 1000 are admitted to the intensive care unit.
- Hypertensive disorders and haemorrhage are the most common causes of admission.
- Basic principles apply, but the special needs of the fetus and the neonate, the mother and her family, and the physiological effects of pregnancy, must be remembered.
- Overall mortality of obstetric ICU admissions in UK series is 3–4%.

Further reading

American College of Obstetricians and Gynecologists. Practice Bulletin No. 158: Critical care in pregnancy. *Obstet Gynecol* 2016; **127**: e21–8.

Gaffney A. Critical care in pregnancy: is it different? *Semin Perinatol* 2014; **38**: 329–40.

Guntupalli KK, Hall N, Karnad DR, *et al.* Critical illness in pregnancy: part I: an approach to a pregnant patient in the ICU and common obstetric disorders. *Chest* 2015; **148**: 1093–104.

Guntupalli KK, Karnad DR, Bandi V, *et al.* Critical illness in pregnancy: part II: common medical conditions complicating pregnancy and puerperium. *Chest* 2015; **148**: 1333–45.

Intensive Care National Audit and Research Centre. Female admissions (aged 16–50 years) to adult, general critical care units in England, Wales and Northern Ireland, reported as 'currently pregnant' or 'recently pregnant', 1 January 2009 – 31 December 2012. London: ICNARC, 2013. www .icnarc.org/Our-Audit/Audits/Cmp/Our-National-Analyses/Obstetrics (accessed December 2018).

Plaat F, Wray S. Role of the anaesthetist in obstetric critical care. *Best Pract Res Clin Obstet Gynaecol* 2008; **22**: 917–35.

Royal College of Anaesthetists, Royal College of Obstetricians and Gynaecologists, Royal College of Midwives, *et al. Care of the Critically Ill Woman in Childbirth: Enhanced Maternal Care.* London: RCoA, 2018. www.rcoa.ac.uk/document-store/enhanced-maternal-care-2018 (accessed December 2018).

Modified early obstetric warning scores

Chapter 156

Improving the care of the critically unwell obstetric patient is repeatedly mentioned in the Confidential Enquiries into Maternal Deaths (CEMD) reports, with early recognition of deterioration highlighted as a key aim; when clinical deterioration occurs it can be rapid in the parturient.

Use of an early warning score has been recommended since the 2003–2005 Enquiry; such a score can be used to identify patients with observations that are outside a predefined range, to trigger a graded response. It is thought that by using a scoring system, smaller changes in clinical condition will be detected earlier than by waiting for an obvious picture of deterioration to emerge. Their utility depends upon partial physiological decompensation that is recognised and acted upon during a window of opportunity before full decompensation.

A 2014 survey of practice indicated that use of an obstetric early warning score was universal across the UK hospitals surveyed, a dramatic improvement over the previous 10 years.

Problems and special considerations

The standardised National Early Warning Score (NEWS) chart cannot be applied to the obstetric population, given the altered physiology of pregnancy, so modified early obstetric warning scores (MEOWS) have been developed to identify women with observations outside the expected norm. A MEOWS chart would usually be used from 20 weeks' gestation until 6 weeks postpartum.

Parameters looked at may include systolic and diastolic blood pressure, respiratory rate, heart rate, fractional inspired oxygen required to maintain an oxygen saturation of at least 96%, temperature, and level of consciousness (Figure 156.1). Of all the variables recorded, a change in respiratory rate is the most sensitive, but is often the parameter that is poorly measured or not recorded. The parameters recorded take into account the altered physiology of pregnancy, for example a higher heart rate and respiratory rate.

MEOWS charts are colour-coded as a visual cue to the severity of abnormal parameters. The National Institute for Health and Care Excellence (NICE) has recommended that early warning scores trigger three grades of response: a low-score group that results in increased frequency of observations and alerting of the nurse in charge; a medium-score group, resulting in an urgent call to the medical team caring for the patient; and a high-score group resulting in an emergency call to a team with critical care competencies. The actual response is subject to local policy and dependent on local skill mix and staff.

Date/Time															
Systolic blood pressure															
< 80 mmHg	3														
80–89 mmHg	2														
90–139 mmHg	0														
140–149 mmHg	1														
150–159 mmHg	2														
> 160 mmHg	3														
Diastolic blood pressure															
< 90 mmHg	0														
90–99 mmHg	1														
100–109 mmHg	2														
> 110 mmHg	3														
Respiratory rate (breaths per minute – bpm)															
< 10 bpm	3														
11–17 bpm	0														
18–24 bpm	1														
25–29 bpm	2														
> 30 bpm	3														
Heart rate (beats per minute – bpm)															
< 60 bpm	3														
60–110 bpm	0														
111–149 bpm	2														
> 150 bpm	3														
Oxygen to maintain saturations > 96%															
Room air	0														
24–39%	1														
> 40%	3														
Temperature															
< 34 °C	3														
34–35 °C	1														
35.1–37.9 °C	0														
38–38.9 °C	1														
> 39 °C	3														
Conscious level															
Alert	0														
Not alert	3														

Figure 156.1 Example MEOWS chart. Many units have added additional lines, e.g. for recording neurological status, pain, nausea, state of liquor/lochia, etc. Each variable is scored according to the values present, and specific actions (e.g. whom to refer/escalate to) are triggered by set thresholds.

Management options

A standardised MEOWS chart has been recommended in the CEMD reports, but a national evidence-based standard has not emerged. There are many variations in existence and some have not been validated; many scores have been designed through clinical consensus rather than through research or statistical analysis. Studies have suggested that MEOWS charts can over-detect severe sepsis, and that simpler tools are more sensitive. A scoring system based on an example MEOWS in the 2003–2005 CEMD report was validated for use at detecting maternal morbidity using data from a single centre. A scoring system has been developed through clinical and statistical analysis using the UK's Intensive Care National Audit and Research Centre (ICNARC) Case Mix Programme database, which has demonstrated excellent discrimination between survivors and non-survivors; its applicability to morbidity on the labour ward, however, has not been validated.

More recently, multidisciplinary work suggests that only six parameters should contribute to the score: respiratory rate, oxygen saturation, heart rate, systolic blood pressure, diastolic blood pressure, and temperature. Any other observations that may be useful in obstetric patients, such as urine output or lochia, should be recorded separately, so as not to confuse documentation. It has also been pointed out that altered level of consciousness is not an early warning sign.

An important feature of MEOWS charts is that they need to be applied to *all* women in the unit, not just to those considered at high risk, since experience has shown that identifying the latter group is unreliable unless a systematic scoring system is used.

Key points

- Use of a modified early obstetric warning score (MEOWS) can help to identify the deteriorating parturient. However, once identified, appropriate action must be triggered by present scores.
- For a screening tool to be effective it must be safe, cost-effective and validated.

Further reading

Carle C, Alexander P, Columb M, Johal J. Design and internal validation of an obstetric early warning score: secondary analysis of the Intensive Care National Audit and Research Centre Case Mix Programme database. *Anaesthesia* 2013; **68**: 354–67.

Isaacs RA, Wee MY, Bick DE, *et al.*; Modified Obstetric Early Warning Systems Research Group. A national survey of obstetric early warning systems in the United Kingdom: five years on. *Anaesthesia* 2014; **69**: 687–92.

McGlennan AP, Sherratt K. Charting change on the labour ward. *Anaesthesia* 2013; **68**: 338–42.

Quinn AC, Meek T, Waldmann C. Obstetric early warning systems to prevent bad outcome. *Curr Opin Anaesthesiol* 2016; **29**: 268–72.

Singh S, McGlennan A, England A, Simons R. A validation study of the CEMACH recommended modified early obstetric warning system (MEOWS). *Anaesthesia* 2012; **67**: 12–18.

Invasive monitoring

The increase in the number of pregnant women with significant coexisting medical disease has led to a need for high-dependency facilities during labour, delivery and the puerperium. In addition, women with complications of pregnancy such as pre-eclampsia may require high-dependency care. In these situations, an understanding of the pathophysiological changes that are taking place may be improved by the use of invasive monitoring.

Successive reports of the Confidential Enquiries into Maternal Deaths (CEMD) have recommended the more frequent and earlier use of invasive monitoring in the management of obstetric haemorrhage.

Problems and special considerations

Midwives are not intensive care nurses, and invasive monitoring may only aid management if the data obtained are reliable and correctly interpreted. All invasive cardiovascular monitoring has significant morbidity associated with its use, such as line sepsis, accidental arterial puncture, pneumothorax and even death. Insertion of pulmonary artery catheters is associated with a particularly high morbidity, and their use is rarely indicated nowadays.

The relative risks and benefits of invasive monitoring need to be assessed carefully – the difficulties of conducting labour and delivery on an intensive care unit may, in some circumstances, outweigh the potential benefits of such monitoring. The implications of the CEMD recommendations are that all obstetric units should be able to care for women with central venous pressure (CVP) monitoring, and that if it is not possible to do so, these women should be transferred to an intensive care unit.

Management options

Direct arterial pressure monitoring

Intra-arterial monitoring provides valuable information in conditions where even brief periods of hypotension or hypertension might cause significant morbidity or mortality. Women with severe cardiac disease resulting in a fixed cardiac output require continuous blood pressure monitoring if epidural analgesia is used in labour, and before induction of either general or regional anaesthesia for operative delivery.

Direct arterial pressure monitoring is desirable in women with severe pre-eclampsia, or those receiving intravenous infusions of antihypertensive agents.

On rare occasions, an intra-arterial cannula may be inserted to facilitate frequent arterial blood gas analysis in women with severe respiratory pathology.

Most midwives are not used to managing arterial lines, and it is therefore vital to ensure that the line is clearly labelled to minimise the risk of its being confused with an intravenous line. The insertion site must be readily accessible and kept visible at all times. It is sensible to explain the purpose of the line to the mother and to involve her in responsibility for its care.

Central venous pressure monitoring

Insertion of a central venous catheter to measure right atrial pressure may give valuable information in women with coexisting cardiac disease. Most protocols for managing women with severe pre-eclampsia also suggest insertion of a CVP line to aid in fluid management, although it is important to realise that the information obtained (right atrial pressure) may not accurately reflect pulmonary artery or left atrial pressure (see Chapter 86, *Hypertension, pre-eclampsia and eclampsia*).

The least invasive technique is recommended for women who are undelivered, i.e. use of a long line inserted from a peripheral vein (usually in the antecubital fossa). It may be technically difficult to cannulate the subclavian or internal jugular vein in the neck of a pregnant woman. She will be intolerant of the head-down position, and the need to adopt lateral tilt or the supine wedged position may distort the usual anatomical landmarks. The apprehension caused by attempting insertion of a neck line may provoke hypertension or arrhythmias caused by increased circulating catecholamines. In addition, the pre-eclamptic woman may have considerable soft tissue oedema of the face and neck and may also be thrombocytopenic.

A clear right atrial pressure waveform on a directly transduced trace may provide confirmation of correct placement of the line without the need for radiological confirmation, although the decision about whether to perform radiography should follow consideration of the relative risks and benefits. Chest radiography should be performed regardless of whether the woman is delivered if there is any anxiety about correct placement or complications of insertion.

Midwives should be able to look after women with CVP lines, and there should be continued education led by the anaesthetic team to ensure that new and existing staff are familiar with this aspect of care of high-risk patients.

Pulmonary artery catheterisation

Though the traditional gold standard for measurement of cardiac output, pulmonary artery catheterisation is becoming less common generally, since its use has been linked to increased mortality in some studies (although patient selection may be a confounding factor). In obstetrics, many authorities would reserve its use for extreme cases of impaired global cardiac function such as cardiomyopathy, or for severe pre-eclampsia with impaired left ventricular function. The risks are those of CVP monitoring plus the potential for pulmonary artery rupture and infarction, as well as technical problems such as knotting of the catheter. Recent studies have suggested that non-invasive measurements of cardiac output such as transthoracic echocardiography may give comparable results without the risk of such complications (see below).

Other cardiac output monitoring techniques

Cardiac output correlates better with uteroplacental perfusion than heart rate and blood pressure, so cardiac output monitoring may be a useful adjunct in obstetric care. The choice of cardiac output monitor depends on whether accuracy (demonstrated by validation studies) or trend measurements are required. The degree of invasiveness and whether the woman is conscious must also be considered. The information obtained should be clinically useful within the correct time frame and impact positively on clinical care.

Non-invasive methods of cardiac output monitoring, such as transthoracic or trans-oesophageal echocardiography, suprasternal Doppler ultrasound and electrical bioimpedance, have been used in the obstetric setting. These techniques have inter-observer variation but may be useful in specific cases (e.g. with severe cardiac disease) or as research tools. Point-of-care echocardiography is gaining popularity, particularly within the obstetric critical care setting; basic echocardiography skills can help distinguish between causes of hypotension and help guide fluid therapy. Arterial waveform analysis techniques have been suggested as alternatives in obstetric practice; these include the LiDCOplus (LiDCO, Cambridge, United Kingdom) and PiCCOplus (Pulsion Medical Systems, Munich, Germany), and the uncalibrated Vigileo monitor (Edwards Lifesciences, Irvine, California). These devices provide beat-to-beat data and are generally precise and reliable in terms of cardiac output measurement, and can thus monitor the patient's responsiveness to fluids and vasopressors. They are therefore thought to be more useful than the measurement of filling pressures.

Key points

- High-dependency care of women with coexisting medical disease or obstetric complications of pregnancy may require invasive monitoring.
- If appropriate monitoring cannot be provided in the maternity unit in which the woman is intending to deliver, arrangements should be made to transfer her care to another unit.

Further reading

Armstrong S, Fernando R, Columb M. Minimally- and non-invasive assessment of maternal cardiac output: go with the flow! *Int J Obstet Anesth* 2011; **20**: 330–40.

Dennis AT, Dyer RA. Cardiac output monitoring in obstetric anaesthesia. *Int J Obstet Anesth* 2014; **23**: 1–3.

Fujitani S, Baldisseri MR. Hemodynamic assessment in a pregnant and peripartum patient. *Crit Care Med* 2005; **33** (10 Suppl): S354–61.

Paech M, James M. Maternal hemodynamic monitoring in obstetric anesthesia. *Anesthesiology* 2008; **109**: 765–7.

Chapter

Neonatal assessment

Formal assessment of the newborn baby is important: to allow documentation of the neonate's general state of wellbeing; as a prognostic exercise, to identify neonates at risk and focus medical attention on them; possibly as a means of following progress over time; and as a research tool for determining the effects of various interventions or conditions on neonatal outcome (e.g. drug therapy, anaesthetic techniques, epidemiological factors). Various methods have been described; as far as obstetric anaesthesia is concerned, the important ones are those that focus on the neonate's gross physiological status at or shortly after birth, and those that assess its neurobehaviour.

Problems and special considerations

The easier the system for assessment (and therefore the more attractive it is to busy clinicians), the less its ability to discern subtle differences, and thus the less useful it is as a tool, especially when the effects being studied are likely to be small (e.g. a possible difference in the effects of two similar drugs in labour). Conversely, tiny differences revealed by very sensitive measurements may be of uncertain significance clinically. In addition, factors that might ordinarily be prognostic may be susceptible to the actions of anaesthetic agents – for example, ketamine may be associated with falsely high scores when using systems that rely heavily on muscle tone.

Methods of assessment

Measures of overall physiological status

- **Time to sustained respiration (TSR).** The time between delivery and sustained spontaneous ventilation is a very crude indicator of neonatal wellbeing, but it does indicate babies that need special attention and attempts to quantify the degree of impairment. It does not distinguish between babies who are slow to breathe unsupported for different reasons (e.g. drugs, congenital defects), and is best suited to birth asphyxia. It is rarely performed routinely.
- **Apgar score.** Described by the American anaesthesiologist Virginia Apgar in 1953, the system comprises five variables, each scoring 0–2 (Table 158.1). The Apgar score is now a standard tool and is recorded routinely after virtually all deliveries. It is usually performed at 1 and 5 minutes after birth, although it may be repeated thereafter. A modified system, 'Apgar minus colour' (maximum of 8), has been suggested but is rarely used.
- **Umbilical cord blood gas analysis** at delivery is a reflection of the metabolic status of the fetus and the adequacy of fetal oxygenation in the immediate peripartum period.

459

Table 158.1 Apgar scoring system

	0	1	2
Heart rate	Absent	< 100	> 100
Respiratory effort	Nil	Weak cry	Strong cry
Muscle tone	Limp	Poor tone	Good tone
Reflex irritability	Nil	Some movement	Strong withdrawal
Colour	Blue/pale	Pink body/blue extremities	Pink

The Royal College of Obstetricians and Gynaecologists (RCOG) recommends the measurement of cord blood gases in all neonates delivered by caesarean section or by instrumental delivery for fetal distress, or where there have been concerns over fetal wellbeing during labour.

Tests of neurobehavioural status

The following tests are sometimes referred to eponymously:

- **Neurobehavioural assessment score (NBAS).** Developed in 1973 by the American paediatrician Brazelton, the NBAS is the most commonly used of the detailed neurobehavioural assessment systems. It takes 45–60 minutes and requires trained staff to perform it.
- **Early neonatal neurobehavioural scale (ENNS).** Developed in 1974 by the American anaesthetist Scanlon, the ENNS is less complicated than the NBAS and therefore quicker to perform (about 5–10 minutes). It examines wakefulness, tone and the response to various stimuli, including the presence or absence of neonatal reflexes.
- **Neurological and adaptive capacity score (NACS).** Developed in 1982 by the paediatrician Amiel-Tison and anaesthetic colleagues in San Francisco, the NACS takes about 5 minutes to perform and is a relatively crude measure, mainly examining neonatal tone. It has been claimed that the NACS can distinguish between the effects of asphyxia and those of drugs, although this has been challenged. It has, however, been widely used in obstetric anaesthetic studies because of its ease of use.

Effects of anaesthetic drugs

In general, the more gross an effect, the easier it is to show it; thus, for example, maternal pethidine can readily be demonstrated to suppress neonatal condition at birth and affect neurobehaviour and feeding for 1–2 days postpartum, by using relatively crude scoring systems. However, more subtle tools such as the NBAS are required to investigate smaller effects, and their significance may be disputed. Finally, the difficulty in conducting randomised studies, and the inadequate size of most studies that have looked at measures of neonatal assessment in depth, mean that no clear conclusions can be drawn in many cases. However, the overall effects of maternal anaesthetic and analgesic drugs on the neonate can be summarised:

- **Systemic drugs.** Impairment is seen depending on the dosage and the test used: the more sensitive the assessment system, the greater the effect. Thus effects on alertness and responsiveness may be detected by using the NBAS and ENNS before respiratory depression is seen. Some effects of pethidine are apparent 24–48 hours postpartum, and subtle differences, for example in feeding, may persist for up to 6 weeks.
- **Regional anaesthesia.** Lidocaine was suspected of impairing the ENNS in the 1970s (the 'alert but floppy baby') but this was not substantiated subsequently. There is no hard evidence of impairment after regional anaesthesia or analgesia for labour or caesarean section with various local anaesthetics or opioids. Although some studies have claimed to find differences, the difficulty of using adequate controls and conflicting results from other studies make these uncertain.
  Hypotension lasting less than 2–3 minutes has not been associated with demonstrable effects, although Apgar score, acid–base profiles and crude neurobehavioural scores have been found to be affected if hypotension is prolonged. The place of regional anaesthesia when the fetus is compromised is still debated by anaesthetists and others, most anaesthetists supporting its use.
- **General anaesthesia.** The effects of general anaesthesia have been greater than those of regional anaesthetic techniques in most studies. Low concentrations of volatile agents are thought to have little effect.

Key points

- The more complex the method used to assess the neonate's state, the more subtle the changes found.
- Anaesthetic and analgesic drugs have all been implicated in affecting neurobehaviour to some degree; this is generally agreed for systemic opioids and general anaesthesia but less certain for regional anaesthetic techniques, as long as hypotension is mild and limited.
- In terms of neonatal neurobehaviour, regional anaesthesia for delivery of the severely compromised fetus is thought by most anaesthetists to have advantages over general anaesthesia, but this is still disputed.

Further reading

Littleford J. Effects on the fetus and newborn of maternal analgesia and anesthesia: a review. *Can J Anesth* 2004; **51**: 586–609.
Reynolds F. Labour analgesia and the baby: good news is no news. *Int J Obstet Anesth* 2011; **20**: 38–50.

Neonatal physiology and pharmacology

The physiology of the neonate is best considered in relation to the various body systems. Some of these are considered elsewhere in this book, but a brief summary of the main points follows. Physiological factors that result in specific differences in drug handling by the neonate are also considered here. It should be remembered that functioning of the neonate's organ systems is closely related to the gestation at which it is born. Finally, factors that are important in the fetus may be equally important after birth; thus many of the following points refer to both the fetus and the neonate.

Circulatory system

In the fetus, oxygenated blood returning from the placenta is directed through the foramen ovale via the left atrium into the left ventricle, and thence preferentially to the brain. Deoxygenated blood from the brain passes via the right atrium and ventricle into the pulmonary artery; since the pulmonary vascular resistance is high, the blood passes through the ductus arteriosus into the aorta and thence via the two umbilical arteries (arising from the internal iliac arteries) to the placenta (Figure 159.1).

At birth, the systemic vascular resistance increases as the umbilical arteries close, whereas the pulmonary vascular resistance decreases as air is drawn into the lungs. Thus, the circulation takes up the adult pattern, although the circulation remains transitional for

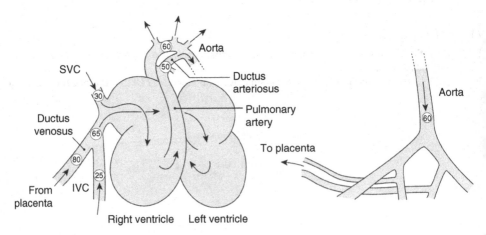

Figure 159.1 Diagram of fetal circulation. IVC, inferior vena cava; SVC, superior vena cava. Arrows denote flow of blood. Figures refer to the approximate oxygen saturation.

about 2 weeks in term neonates, and fetal circulation may persist if pulmonary vascular resistance remains high (e.g. caused by hypoxaemia, acidosis, hypovolaemia or hypothermia). The neonate relies mainly on heart rate for maintenance of cardiac output, the stroke volume being relatively fixed.

Respiratory system

Two-thirds of the pulmonary fluid is expelled from the chest by compression during delivery (reduced in caesarean section and if the neonate is small) and the remaining fluid is rapidly absorbed. Lung inflation is important to assist transition from the fetal to the adult circulation and to promote pulmonary surfactant production. Surfactant is required to enable alveolar expansion and is present in only small amounts up until about 34 weeks' gestation, although its production can be stimulated by maternal steroid therapy.

Fetal haemoglobin (containing α and γ chains) comprises about 80% of the circulating haemoglobin in the fetus. Its oxyhaemoglobin dissociation curve is shifted to the left compared with that of adult haemoglobin; thus transfer of oxygen from maternal to fetal blood is encouraged. Fetal haemoglobin normally persists for about 2–3 months after delivery, but this may be extended if there is a haemoglobinopathy affecting adult haemoglobin.

The response of the neonate to hypoxia is discussed in Chapter 160, *Neonatal resuscitation*.

Neurological system

The blood–brain barrier is generally accepted to be less complete in the neonate than in the adult, making the neonate more susceptible to depressant drugs such as opioids, and its function may be compromised further in the presence of hypoxia or acidosis. In premature babies, the fragile periventricular vessels are susceptible to fluctuations in arterial blood pressure and hypoxia, resulting in intraventricular haemorrhage.

Other systems

Heat production in the neonate is achieved by oxidation of brown fat, which results in increased oxygen requirements. It may be inadequate if there has been fetal growth restriction. Thus, a warm environment for delivery is especially important.

Pharmacology

Uptake of drugs by the fetus is considered in Chapter 16, *Placental transfer of drugs*. The low plasma protein-binding capacity of the fetus and neonate results in a greater amount of free drug in the plasma compared with that in the adult. Lipid-soluble drugs (e.g. anaesthetics) are extensively bound to fetal and neonatal tissues, offsetting this effect. Finally, fetal acidosis may result in the 'trapping' of drugs, which may persist postpartum if the neonate remains acidotic. The relative immaturity of both target organs (e.g. brain) and organs involved in metabolism (e.g. liver) makes the neonate more susceptible to many drugs administered to the mother before delivery or directly to the neonate after delivery.

Key points

- Major circulatory and respiratory changes occur at birth.
- The neonate may exhibit the effects of intrapartum insults, and remains susceptible to insults occurring postpartum

Further reading

Morton S, Brodsky D. Fetal physiology and the transition to extrauterine life. *Clin Perinatol* 2016; **43**: 395–407.

Neonatal resuscitation

Published studies have reported some degree of resuscitation being required in up to 5–14% of neonates overall, although this may be higher in selected cases. Most neonates require assisted ventilation only. The need for resuscitation may often be predicted from the events and course of the pregnancy and labour (including the presence of meconium, the fetal heart rate and pH during labour and the mother's condition), although up to a third of cases occur after apparently normal labours.

There has been a trend in recent years for paediatricians not to attend uncomplicated elective caesarean sections, since surveys have suggested that the requirement for neonatal resuscitation is low in such cases, especially when the indication for caesarean section is previous operative delivery, and when regional anaesthesia is used. In such situations, anaesthetists should not take on the responsibility of resuscitating the neonate, since their primary responsibility is to care for the mother. However, all personnel in the delivery suite (including obstetric anaesthetists) should be competent at basic neonatal resuscitation.

Problems and special considerations

Cardiovascular

The change from fetal to adult circulation normally accompanies delivery and the inspiration of air into the lungs. If there is poor lung inflation, high inflation pressures, hypercapnia, hypothermia or acidosis, the circulation (which remains transitional for about 2 weeks after birth in term neonates) may return to the fetal configuration.

The neonate relies on a fast heart rate for cardiac output since stroke volume is relatively fixed. The neonatal heart responds to hypoxaemia with bradycardia, which in turn worsens oxygen delivery. The initial treatment is oxygenation.

Respiratory

The squeezing of the chest during vaginal delivery helps to expel the fluid contained within the lungs in babies born this way. In babies born by caesarean section, this effect is absent and respiratory support is more likely to be required, especially superimposed on the underlying reason for emergency operative delivery. Uterine contractions themselves help to expel fluid, and even a short labour may be beneficial.

The first breath needs to overcome the forces tending to keep the alveoli collapsed, and thus requires greater effort.

If meconium is present, its dispersal throughout the lungs during resuscitation may result in the meconium aspiration syndrome.

Hypoxaemia typically leads to vigorous respiratory efforts followed by a period of primary apnoea (accompanied by bradycardia), during which stimulation may provoke respiration. After a few gasps a period of terminal apnoea ensues, during which active resuscitation is required. It is possible for both stages to occur in utero if the fetus is hypoxic.

Evidence of tissue damage (including brain tissue) caused by hyperoxia, especially after a period of asphyxia, has led to the avoidance of high concentrations of oxygen for neonatal resuscitation, with air being the gas recommended initially.

Management options

Appropriate equipment includes an oxygen source, funnel, bag and facepiece, suction, laryngoscopes, tracheal tubes (sizes 2.5–3.5 mm, non-shouldered) and a radiant heater. The laryngeal mask airway has been used for neonatal resuscitation and has been suggested as being faster, more reliable and thus safer than tracheal tubes, although its use is not yet widespread.

The basic principles of the 'ABC' of resuscitation apply in neonatal resuscitation, with a focus on ventilation over drug administration. The latest Resuscitation Council (UK) algorithm is shown in Figure 160.1.

Vigorous oropharyngeal suction may cause apnoea. If meconium aspiration is suspected, direct laryngoscopy and pharyngeal or laryngeal suction under direct vision is preferred, with tracheal intubation if meconium is seen below the cords. Gentle suction and removal of meconium should take place before lung inflation unless the heart rate is under 60 beats/minute.

It is recommended that the pulse oximetry sensor be positioned on the right hand to provide an accurate measurement of oxygen saturation in the preductal circulation.

If controlled ventilation is required, the first breath should be held for 2–3 seconds to help expand the alveoli, with subsequent breaths lasting for 0.5–1.0 seconds. A maximum of 30–35 cmH$_2$O should be administered (20–25 cmH$_2$O if preterm). If heart rate does not increase or oxygenation (as indicated guided by oximetry) remains unacceptable despite effective ventilation, oxygen should be considered instead of air.

Cardiac massage is performed either by encircling the baby's chest with the hands and compressing the sternum with the thumbs, or by using the index and middle fingers. The sternum should be depressed 1–2 cm. Compressions should occur at 120/minute, at a ratio of 3:1 with breaths. ECG monitoring may aid the accurate assessment of neonatal heart rate.

Intravenous access is usually obtained most easily with an umbilical venous catheter – the single umbilical vein is accompanied by two umbilical arteries, which aids its identification. Drugs are rarely required; doses are given in Table 160.1. The cannula should be flushed with saline after each drug is administered. The intraosseous route has also been used.

The neonate should be kept warm and dry throughout resuscitation, with the body temperature maintained between 36.5 and 37.5 °C.

Therapeutic hypothermia should be considered for babies at term or near-term with evolving moderate or severe hypoxic–ischaemic encephalopathy.

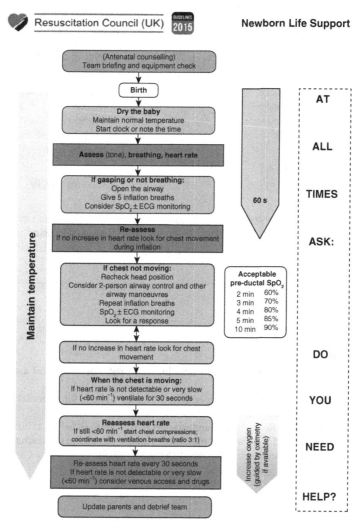

Figure 160.1 Algorithm for neonatal resuscitation. Reproduced with permission from Resuscitation Council (UK). Resuscitation and support of transition of babies at birth, 2015. www.resus.org.uk/resuscitation-guidelines/resuscitation-and-support-of-transition-of-babies-at-birth.

Key points

- Some degree of neonatal resuscitation is required in up to 5–14% of deliveries overall, but the incidence is higher in selected cases.
- The anaesthetist's first duty is to the mother.
- Before delivery, it should be possible to predict two-thirds of cases in which neonatal resuscitation will be required.
- Basic principles are similar to those of adult resuscitation, but with more emphasis on lung inflation and less on drugs.

Table 160.1 Drugs used in neonatal resuscitation

Drug	Dose	Notes
Naloxone	100 µg/kg IM	Should be considered if maternal opioids given
Adrenaline	10 µg/kg IV (0.1 ml/kg of a 1:10,000 solution) initially; 10–30 µg/kg IV if ineffective	If no significant cardiac output despite effective significant lung inflation and chest compression 50–100 µg/kg intratracheally is roughly equivalent to 10 µg/kg IV
Volume expansion	10–20 ml/kg	0.9% saline initially
Sodium bicarbonate 4.2%	1–2 mmol/kg IV (2–4) ml/kg	High concentrations of bicarbonate have been associated with intraventricular haemorrhages

IM, intramuscular; IV, intravenous.

Further reading

Berger TM. Neonatal resuscitation: foetal physiology and pathophysiological aspects. *Eur J Anaesthesiol* 2012; **2**: 362–70.

Guay J, Lachapelle J. No evidence for superiority of air or oxygen for neonatal resuscitation: a meta-analysis. *Can J Anesth* 2011; **58**: 1075–82.

Resuscitation Council (UK). Resuscitation and support of transition of babies at birth. London: Resuscitation Council, 2015, www.resus.org.uk/resuscitation-guidelines/resuscitation-and-support-of-transition-of-babies-at-birth (accessed December 2018).

Perinatal mortality

Perinatal mortality rate (PMR) is defined as the number of stillbirths plus the number of neonatal deaths within the first completed week of life, per 1000 total live births. It was proposed by the World Health Organization in 1975 as an international definition of late fetal and early neonatal loss and is a measure of antepartum care and wellbeing, care during delivery and immediate care postpartum. Perinatal mortality is thus generally accepted as a good indicator of general health and healthcare provision across different countries.

In developed countries, PMR is about 6–12 per 1000 births, whereas in developing countries rates of up to 60 per 1000 births are reported, although many countries are unable to provide data. In England and Wales it has fallen from 32.8 per 1000 in 1961 to 6.6 per 1000 in 2016.

In some countries, infant mortality rate (IMR; the number of deaths in the first completed year after delivery per 1000 total live births) is used as the standard indicator, and it is generally about 3–8 in developed countries. In the UK, it was 3.8 in 2016, compared to 4.6 in 2009.

Problems and special considerations

Apart from difficulties collecting data, the figures are susceptible to variations in other definitions used; for example in the UK, an upward 'blip' in PMR was caused in 1991 when the definition of a live birth was changed from 28 weeks' to 24 weeks' gestation.

Perinatal mortality has been found to increase with lower birth weight, lower gestational age, lower social class, maternal age < 20 or > 40, parity < 1 or > 5, body mass index > 30 kg/m^2, presence of medical conditions, method of delivery (e.g. forceps) and poor management of labour. It has been estimated that application of what is already known about good and poor practice would achieve a greater reduction in perinatal mortality than any other single measure.

For many years, the annual Confidential Enquiry into Stillbirths and Deaths in Infancy (CESDI) reported on causes of perinatal death and areas of suboptimal care, joining with the Confidential Enquiries into Maternal Deaths (CEMD) in 2003. From 2012, the programme has been commissioned by the Healthcare Quality Improvement Partnership (HQIP). Recommendations from the enquiries include establishing strategies and protocols for improving communication, training and peripartum clinical practice, appropriate involvement of senior medical staff and improvements in neonatal resuscitation.

Key points

- Perinatal mortality rate (PMR) equals the number of stillbirths and neonatal deaths within the first completed week of life, per 1000 total live births.
- PMR is generally accepted as a measure of the quality of provision of general health care for a particular country, as well as specific maternity and neonatal care.
- In the UK, PMR was 6.6 in 2016.

Further reading

Draper ES, Gallimore ID, Kurinczuk JJ, *et al.*; MBRRACE-UK Collaboration. *MBRRACE-UK Perinatal Mortality Surveillance Report, UK Perinatal Deaths for Births from January to December 2016.* Leicester: Infant Mortality and Morbidity Studies, Department of Health Sciences, University of Leicester, 2018.

Chapter

162

Drugs and breastfeeding

Mothers often ask their anaesthetist for information about breastfeeding after anaesthetic and surgical interventions. The majority of drugs administered to the mother enter her breast milk, but many are present in pharmacologically insignificant amounts and do not therefore pose a risk to the baby. The amount of drug that a breastfed baby receives depends on the concentration of drug in the milk and the volume of milk taken by the baby. In the first few days following delivery, the baby receives colostrum and then very small volumes of milk, so that any drug exposure is likely to be minimal. It is, however, common sense to administer drugs to the breastfeeding mother only if they are considered essential.

The British National Formulary (BNF) contains a comprehensive list of drugs that are known to be present in breast milk following maternal administration, but also points out that in many cases there are insufficient data to enable accurate information to be provided.

Breastfeeding and anaesthesia

Production of breast milk is dependent on adequate maternal hydration and regular stimulation (either by the baby feeding or by the mother expressing her milk). A mother scheduled for anaesthesia and surgery should be encouraged to feed her baby as near as possible to the planned time of surgery and also as soon as she feels able to postoperatively. In some cases it may be more appropriate for her to express milk preoperatively if the procedure or recovery period is expected to be long.

There is some evidence to suggest that following a caesarean section under regional anaesthesia compared with general anaesthesia, mothers are able to breastfeed more quickly; this is presumed to be due to the maternal and neonatal effects of general anaesthesia, but more research is required in this area. It has been proposed that babies born to mothers receiving epidural analgesia in labour are more likely to have delayed breastfeeding, but the evidence for this is extremely weak.

Intravenous and inhalational agents

Both thiopental and propofol are found in breast milk in insignificant amounts following maternal administration, and current data suggest that a mother can breastfeed as soon as she has adequately recovered from a general anaesthetic. Levels of volatile agent excreted into breast milk are also negligible (most information relates to halothane, but extrapolation of data based on pharmacokinetic information suggests that isoflurane, sevoflurane and desflurane would be present in breast milk in even lower concentrations). Neuromuscular blocking agents are large, water-soluble, ionised quaternary ammonium compounds and therefore are not excreted into breast milk in any measurable quantity.

Analgesics

Transfer of non-steroidal anti-inflammatory drugs and paracetamol into breast milk has been extensively studied, and neither type of analgesic is present in clinically important quantities.

Therapeutic doses of morphine and diamorphine given for postoperative analgesia (following either caesarean section or other surgical intervention) can be given to the mother as required, though the lowest effective dose for shortest duration should be administered. For those who require opioid analgesia for a longer period, it would be sensible to monitor the neonate for signs of opioid side effects. Longer-acting opioids given more than an hour before delivery may inhibit the neonatal suckling reflex. Codeine is no longer recommended for use in breastfeeding mothers because of the possibility of the mother or neonate being a rapid metaboliser, leading to supratherapeutic levels of morphine. The Medicines and Healthcare products Regulatory Agency (MHRA) currently recommends the prescription of tramadol or dihydrocodeine (at the lowest effective dose) instead, though evidence for their use remains limited. Maintenance on a methadone programme is not considered incompatible with breastfeeding, and there are no longer any restrictions on the maximum dose considered safe, although the lowest dose possible is generally recommended.

Antiemetics

All the commonly used antiemetics carry a manufacturers' warning to 'use with caution' or 'use only if essential'.

Benzodiazepines

Prolonged administration of benzodiazepines should be avoided because of the risk of neonatal toxicity and withdrawal symptoms. Diazepam is found in clinically significant quantities in breast milk and may cause hypotonia and impaired suckling in the baby. However, use of a single dose of temazepam or lorazepam as a premedicant drug is not contraindicated. Similarly, use of midazolam for intravenous sedation or during general anaesthesia is considered safe.

Other drugs

Anticoagulants

Warfarin and low-molecular-weight heparins are considered to be safe in breastfeeding mothers.

Antidepressants and anticonvulsants

The reports of the Confidential Enquiries into Maternal Deaths have highlighted the risk of postnatal depression and its potential to lead to postnatal psychosis and suicide. There are numerous case reports offering conflicting advice about the use of psychotropic and anticonvulsant drugs in lactating women. Since the recommendations vary with each individual drug, specialist advice should be sought.

Antihypertensives

It is common for pre-eclamptic women to receive β-blocking drugs for several weeks following delivery. Atenolol is excreted in breast milk in measurable amounts, and there is some evidence that it may cause neonatal bradycardia, hypotension or cyanosis; the World Health Organization advises using an alternative agent, particularly when the infant is less than 1 month old, given the immature renal function.

Key points

- Most drugs are excreted into breast milk, but information about the effects on the neonate is scarce.
- Commonly used anaesthetic and analgesic drugs can be safely used in breastfeeding mothers.

Follow-up

Follow-up of mothers after obstetric analgesia and anaesthesia is important for the woman, the individual anaesthetist and the hospital – and for obstetric anaesthesia as a whole. In an ideal world, all anaesthetists would aim to follow up their own patients. This ideal is often not practical; therefore follow-up has to become part of the routine of an obstetric anaesthetic service. At local, national and international levels, data collection enables anaesthetists to assess risk and monitor standards of care.

Problems and special considerations

The purpose of routine follow-up is to provide feedback on the anaesthetic care received, and to identify complications. Follow-up of women who have had analgesia or anaesthesia administered by the anaesthetist should ideally be carried out within 24 hours. However, it may be difficult to see all women before they are discharged from hospital. This early discharge to the community means that anaesthetists must rely on midwifery, obstetric and general practitioner colleagues to refer back any problems. Areas that anaesthetists might wish to follow up can be divided into anaesthetic interventions perceived to be uncomplicated, and those where there was a problem.

Management options

After an uncomplicated intervention

Follow-up of this group is important, to ensure that women are satisfied with their treatment and, if not, why not. The follow-up interview gives the woman a chance to voice her opinion of the treatment she received. The anaesthetist should be responsive to criticisms of the service as a whole, since many women make their comments in order to help improve the service to others.

Questions to be asked at follow-up could include the following:

- **Relating to analgesia in labour** – Were you satisfied with the pain relief you received for the first and second stages of your labour? Were you able to mobilise during labour where appropriate? Has your sensation returned to normal? Have you a headache? Have you any comments about the care that you received?
- **Relating to regional anaesthesia** – Were you satisfied with the anaesthesia that you received? Did you feel any discomfort or pain at any time during the caesarean section? Have you had good postoperative pain relief? Are you mobile? Are you able to pass urine? Has your sensation returned to normal? Have you a headache? Have you any comments about the treatment that you received?

- **Relating to general anaesthesia** – Did you have a good sleep? Do you remember going to sleep? Do you remember waking up? Do you remember dreaming or waking up during the operation? Do you have a sore throat, sore muscles or headache? Were you in pain when you woke up? Has the postoperative pain relief been adequate (at rest and on movement)? Have you had nausea or vomiting? Have you any comments about your treatment?

After a problem with anaesthesia or analgesia

The most common problems associated with an anaesthetic intervention are:
- Difficulty in siting a regional analgesic
- Accidental dural puncture
- Paraesthesia during insertion of a spinal or epidural, and/or neurological symptoms afterwards
- Poor analgesia in labour (especially in the second stage if the epidural was inadequately topped up)
- Pain during caesarean section or operative delivery

Patients with the above problems should always be followed up, ideally by a consultant obstetric anaesthetist. Continuity of care is important for these patients, and involvement of other specialists, where appropriate, should occur at an early stage. For example, neurological consultation should be sought when there is any doubt as to the cause of a headache or neurological deficit. Early involvement of a clinical psychologist with a special interest in post-traumatic stress disorder following childbirth (if one is available) may be useful when there has been a painful experience during delivery.

Communication with the women, their partners and the midwifery and obstetric staff is essential to ensure that any problems, however small, are dealt with quickly and comprehensively. All women who have had a problem should have the opportunity to see the consultant obstetric anaesthetist after discharge from hospital. A follow-up visit at around 6–8 weeks post-delivery is useful for both the women and the obstetric anaesthetist. This consultation allows the lines of communication to remain open and offers the opportunity for a frank and open dialogue about any problems.

Key points
- Follow-up is important in both straightforward and complicated cases.
- Follow-up does not end when the woman leaves hospital.
- Consultant anaesthetic involvement is important.
- Communication is vital between all the professional groups involved.

Further reading

Cook TM, Counsell D, Wildsmith JA; Royal College of Anaesthetists Third National Audit Project. Major complications of central neuraxial block: report on the 3rd National Audit Project of the Royal College of Anaesthetists. *Br J Anaesth* 2009; **102**: 179–90.

Jenkins JG. Some immediate serious complications of obstetric epidural analgesia and anaesthesia: a prospective study of 145,550 epidurals. *Int J Obstet Anesth* 2005; **14**: 37–42.

Nguyen T, Slater P, Cyna AM. Open vs specific questioning during anaesthetic follow-up after Caesarean section. *Anaesthesia* 2009; **64**: 156–60.

Maternal satisfaction

Maternal satisfaction has become a major outcome measure, mentioned in several important documents and strategies concerned with childbirth; it is used to reflect the quality of maternity service provision. Anaesthetists have an important role to play in maternal satisfaction, since for many women aspects of their analgesia and anaesthesia can have an enormous effect on how they view their overall experience, in some cases irrespective of what happened in other areas of their care. Conversely, mothers' rating of their satisfaction with analgesia or anaesthesia in general, and different techniques in particular, may be affected by several factors unrelated to the anaesthetic itself. Despite this, studies comparing different techniques often quote measures of global satisfaction as evidence that one technique is superior to another. Similarly, obstetric anaesthetists are encouraged to assess and audit maternal satisfaction with the obstetric anaesthetic service as a marker of quality of performance, and patient feedback has been proposed as an important component in the process of consultants' revalidation.

Problems and special considerations

Apart from the confounding effects of various unrelated factors, as described above, another difficulty relates to the measuring tool used to assess satisfaction. Methods used have varied from simple 'satisfaction scales', such as a visual analogue scale or verbal rating scale, to complex evaluations of different modalities that combine to produce a positive experience of childbirth such as fulfilment (e.g. happiness), lack of distress (e.g. pleasure) and physical wellbeing (e.g. lack of pain). The simpler systems will always be more attractive to busy clinicians such as anaesthetists than the more complex and time-consuming ones, even though simple questions such as 'Are you satisfied?' or 'Rate your satisfaction on a scale of 1–10' are not very useful as objective outcome measures. The Royal College of Anaesthetists currently recommends that satisfaction with labour epidural analgesia should be verbally rated, as excellent, satisfactory, unsatisfactory or no benefit.

Studies suggest that factors associated with dissatisfaction include being excluded from one's care and decisions relating to it, poor communication and lack of information, bad outcome (although there may be strong satisfaction with the medical care if this is perceived to have been good) and being led to expect a particular event and then not experiencing it (e.g. receiving assurance that an epidural will be available but not receiving it because the anaesthetist is unavailable).

Despite initial assumptions that effective analgesia in labour automatically guarantees maternal satisfaction, this is not necessarily the case, and factors such as control and involvement in decision making may be more important. It is often suggested that satisfaction is increased when motor block is minimised by using low-dose epidural techniques or patient-controlled epidural analgesia.

Management options

Until more work is done on the interplay between specific factors that contribute to maternal satisfaction, obstetric anaesthetists have to fall back on the use of vague and non-specific methods of assessing it. It is probably more important to assess dissatisfaction, which may indicate deficiencies in service and facilitate quality improvement, but any single measure of satisfaction is only as good as the methods used to obtain it. It is also important to ensure that if a mother has had a bad experience in childbirth but the anaesthetic care has been good and appropriate, her adverse opinion should not extend to include the anaesthetist, although achieving this may be difficult.

Attention meanwhile should be paid to those factors that have been shown to be important in promoting maternal satisfaction, such as involving the mother in decisions, keeping her informed, being prompt and courteous and other desirable general professional attitudes. Similarly, any expression of dissatisfaction should be taken seriously and an attempt made (and recorded in the notes) to discuss the particulars of the case, perhaps by offering an appointment at a later date. Medicolegal experience supports this approach as one of the most important factors in preventing subsequent legal action.

Key points

- Maternal satisfaction is an increasingly recognised but poorly defined measure of quality of care.
- Involving women in their care, good communication and honesty are important factors in increasing maternal satisfaction.
- Women expressing dissatisfaction should be identified and offered the opportunity to discuss their care further with a senior member of staff.

Further reading

Dickinson JE, Paech MJ, McDonald SJ, Evans SF. Maternal satisfaction with childbirth and intrapartum analgesia in nulliparous labour. *Aust N Z J Obstet Gynaecol* 2003; **43**: 463–8.

Dualé C, Nicolas-Courbon A, Gerbaud L, *et al.* Maternal satisfaction as an outcome criterion in research on labor analgesia: data analysis from the recent literature. *Clin J Pain* 2015; **31**: 235–46.

Hodnett ED. Pain and women's satisfaction with the experience of childbirth: a systematic review. *Am J Obstet Gynecol* 2002; **186**: S160–72.

Robinson PN, Salmon P, Yentis SM. Maternal satisfaction. *Int J Obstet Anesth* 1998; **7**: 32–7.

Antenatal education

Women preparing for childbirth make use of many sources of information. These will typically include discussion with other women, magazine articles, books and classes. Classes may be run by the general practice or the maternity unit, or by external bodies such as the National Childbirth Trust (NCT). Antenatal education is beneficial, since it has been shown that the well-informed mother will cope better with labour, but it is important that the information provided should be accurate, well balanced and relevant to local services.

Problems and special considerations

Retention of information

The middle of a painful labour is the wrong time to attempt to provide quite complex information about regional analgesia. In addition to the pain itself and the inevitable tension, the mother may well be under the influence of powerful sedative or analgesic drugs. Theoretically, the antenatal period is the ideal time to educate mothers about pain relief and anaesthesia for caesarean section. Unfortunately, many studies have shown that the ability of patients to recall details of explanations is poor, and that such information tends to be retained for the short term only. This problem is exacerbated by the fact that many primigravidae who have epidural analgesia in labour were not originally planning to use it; these women would be especially unlikely to recall information given in the antenatal period.

Written information

Poor recall of verbal explanations implies that antenatal classes should be supplemented with written information that women can take home and read at leisure; audiotapes and videos can also be very helpful. When preparing these sources, it is important to target them at a relatively low level of comprehension; it is all too easy to slip into medical jargon and unnecessarily complicated language. Studies have shown that written information for patients should be set at a reading age of about 12 years. The needs of mothers whose first language is not English should also be considered, and the Obstetric Anaesthetists' Association (OAA) has several translations of its information for mothers available on its website, including in smartphone/tablet format.

Content

Mothers need balanced information to enable them to make rational decisions; this is an essential element of the principle of consent. Talks, leaflets, videos and other information sources all need to present an unbiased view of the benefits and risks of the available alternatives, and they should be based on the best available evidence. Inevitably, material that is designed to inform a large number of women will be too complex for some and have insufficient detail for others; it is therefore essential that mothers should be able to discuss their concerns individually with an anaesthetist if necessary, and antenatal education should not be seen as a substitute for this facility.

Management options

Providing a regular antenatal class is a major (and almost certainly unpaid) commitment, often involving regular evening lectures. Equally, not every anaesthetist is suited to giving informal talks to large groups of mothers and fathers. In some circumstances, it is better to enlist the help of parentcraft teachers, who may be willing to put across the anaesthetist's message themselves. If this is to be done successfully, however, it is essential that the teachers fully understand and agree with the content and emphasis of the information. The anaesthetist should still attend the classes on a regular basis, and must be available (not necessarily on the same day) to deal with any queries outside the teacher's experience. Audiovisual aids are useful, particularly as a prompt if the talk is delegated to someone else, but slides must be kept simple, jargon-free and not gory.

The use of written or video material is worthwhile, but preparation to an acceptable standard is more difficult than might be imagined. Many hospitals have departments dedicated to providing patient information, and their help should be sought at an early stage. Presentation in an attractive format is also important, and this will almost certainly require professional input. Production of high-quality leaflets is not cheap, and it is tempting to seek sponsorship from a company with a commercial interest in pregnancy or labour; however, many midwives are reluctant to distribute information that appears to endorse products, and their views should be sought before embarking on such a course. In general, the cooperation of midwifery staff is important in ensuring that the target audience is reached, and they should therefore be involved at the preparation stage.

It is important to remember that antenatal education often misses the most socially deprived – and hence high-risk – mothers. The extent of this problem may be assessed by discussion with local community midwives, who may be willing to establish 'outreach' clinics for this vulnerable group.

Several national organisations, including the OAA, have produced leaflets, videos and smartphone applications about pain relief in labour. These provide an attractive way of informing mothers in the antenatal period, but care should be taken if using such material to ensure that the information given reflects local practice and experience.

Key points

- Antenatal education allows explanation of key facts in a low-stress environment.
- Retention of information given in the antenatal period is poor.
- Information should be accurate, locally relevant and carefully targeted.
- Leaflets and videos are useful supplements, but may be difficult to prepare.

Further reading

Bethune L, Harper N, Lucas DN, *et al.* Complications of obstetric regional analgesia: how much information is enough? *Int J Obstet Anesth* 2004; **13**: 30–4.

Broaddus BM, Chandrasekhar S. Informed consent in obstetric anesthesia. *Anesth Analg* 2011; **112**: 912–15.

Fortescue C, Wee MY, Malhotra S, Yentis SM, Holdcroft A. Is preparation for emergency obstetric anaesthesia adequate? A maternal questionnaire survey. *Int J Obstet Anesth* 2007; **16**: 336–40.

Obstetric Anaesthetists' Association. [Information for mothers.] www.labourpains.com (accessed December 2018).

Audit

Medical audit is a process by which certain aspects of practice are assessed and compared with predefined standards. If those standards are not met, then the reasons for not meeting them are analysed and addressed; subsequent audits can be used to confirm that the situation has improved (thus completing the audit 'loop'). Audit should be distinguished from research, which seeks to determine what the standards should be, resulting in 'generalisable knowledge'. Research, for example, might suggest that drug A is best for uterine relaxation in premature labour, whereas audit might determine whether drug A is in fact being used appropriately in a particular unit, and show that the right intervention might improve this. In practice, many projects do not fit into either category precisely: for instance, the first step of an audit may produce 'generalisable knowledge' that might be applicable in other units.

Audit is widely supported as a means of encouraging evidence-based medicine and improving standards of care.

National audit

The best-known and oldest obstetric audit is the annual report of the Confidential Enquiries into Maternal Deaths, in which obstetric deaths are analysed, their causes determined and management compared against 'best practice', and recommendations made about standards of care in maternity units (see Chapter 89, *Maternal bortality*). Anaesthetic and critical care aspects are considered by specific anaesthetic and intensivist assessors, respectively. Other than this, there is no comprehensive national obstetric anaesthetic audit system, although most units have a system for collecting some measure of activity and outcomes. This causes problems with estimating true incidences of adverse outcomes, since the denominators are rarely known (e.g. the number of general anaesthetic caesarean sections in the UK), although there have been recent attempts by the Royal College of Obstetricians and Gynaecologists (and more recently by anaesthetic organisations, particularly the Obstetric Anaesthetists' Association) to collect these basic data.

The National Audit Projects of the Royal College of Anaesthetists provided national data on complications related to neuraxial analgesic and anaesthetic techniques (NAP3), complications related to airway management (NAP4), awareness under general anaesthesia (NAP5) and perioperative anaphylaxis (NAP6); all these reports included information from obstetric cases.

Local audit

At unit level, rates of epidurals in labour, accidental dural punctures, anaesthesia for caesarean section and complications are commonly recorded. Whether this information is used for 'true' audit as defined above is uncertain. In addition, definitions of these various terms may not be uniform among units – for example, should 'epidural rate' include spinals and combined spinal–epidurals, and should the denominator be the number of women delivering, the number of women in labour, or the number of babies delivered? Finally, the real impact of sometimes expensive audit on actual outcome of care has been repeatedly questioned.

It is important to perform audit with specific aims, rather than simply to collect data for its own sake. Simple audit can easily be performed for particular aspects of care, such as to assess whether antacid prophylaxis is being given to all patients before elective caesarean section or to labouring mothers in high-risk groups, or whether appropriate investigations are being performed in pre-eclamptic patients before regional analgesia. Administrative aspects can also be audited, for example response times of anaesthetists on call or provision of adequate teaching on the labour ward. The value of an audit is increased by concentrating on objective data: for instance, satisfaction is commonly measured following obstetric anaesthesia, but data derived from vague satisfaction scales may be a poor reflection of quality of service.

In recent years, the concept of quality improvement (QI) has been proposed as a better means of monitoring and improving service delivery than audit, since the latter is a static process in which improvements are made in steps, after each audit cycle. In QI, a continuous cycle of monitoring and intervention allows a more dynamic process of improvement.

Finally, if the data are unreliable any project is worthless; thus each audit should be planned carefully to ensure that high-quality data are collected. During each cycle, the audit can itself be audited by sampling the data collected and checking them for accuracy and completeness.

Key points

- Audit comprises:
  1. Assessment of practice
  2. Comparison against 'best practice'
  3. Analysis of any shortcomings
  4. Correction of deficient practice
  5. Repeating the assessment

Further reading

Holdcroft A, Verma R, Chapple J, et al. Towards effective obstetric anaesthetic audit in the UK. Int J Obstet Anesth 1999; 8: 37–42.

Knight M, Bunch K, Tuffnell D, et al.; MBRRACE-UK. Saving Lives, Improving Mothers' Care: Lessons learned to inform maternity care from the UK and Ireland Confidential Enquiries into Maternal Deaths and Morbidity 2014–16. Oxford: National Perinatal Epidemiology Unit, University of Oxford, 2018.

National Institute of Academic Anaesthesia. National Audit Projects. https://www.nationalauditprojects.org.uk/National_Audit_Projects (accessed December 2018).

Paech M, Sinha A. Obstetric audit and its implications for obstetric anaesthesia. Best Pract Res Clin Obstet Gynaecol 2010; 24: 413–25.

Wagstaff DT, Bedford J, Moonesinghe SR. Improvement science in anaesthesia. Curr Anesthesiol Rep 2017; 7: 432–9.

Labour ward organisation

Chapter 167

Unplanned situations and emergencies inevitably arise in the best-managed obstetric units, but good organisation should be able to reduce these to a minimum. Anaesthetists are present in most labour wards for a majority of the working week, are involved in the care of the complex cases that test the organisational structure, and are accustomed to communicating with other medical and non-medical staff. They are therefore ideally suited to help in the planning of the various aspects of labour ward organisation.

Problems and special considerations

The labour ward is a potential hotbed of organisational problems. Workload may vary suddenly and dramatically, and the urgent nature of many admissions makes forward planning very difficult. A variety of specialists are intimately involved with the care of the patients, and conflicts, although regrettable, are inevitable. Priorities are often difficult to establish, and prolonged periods of routine work may be suddenly interrupted by an extreme emergency. All of this makes careful organisation essential but very difficult.

Maternity care is by far the largest source of medicolegal litigation in Europe and the USA, and analysis of claims commonly implicates communication and other organisational factors – for example, failure to notify the anaesthetist of an impending caesarean section until the last minute, resulting in inappropriate anaesthetic decisions or excessive delay.

In many labour wards in the UK and elsewhere, mothers identified as low-risk are frequently cared for solely by a midwife. This situation, although not hazardous in itself, calls for careful guidelines to ensure early communication of potential problems to relevant medical staff. The problem can be exacerbated if independent practitioners are allowed to admit their clients to the labour ward.

Although the role of the anaesthetist is more widely appreciated by midwives and obstetricians than in the past, there is still a tendency in some units to regard him/her as an 'outsider', only to be summoned when required. This attitude fosters poor communication and should be discouraged.

Management options

There should be a consultant anaesthetist responsible for the provision of the obstetric anaesthetic service. A labour ward working party or equivalent, meeting on a regular basis, is an ideal forum in which to raise concerns and maintain communication, and there must be an anaesthetist on this body.

Guidelines and protocols should be drawn up to cover both routine care and the management of difficult cases and emergencies, and must be agreed by all parties involved. These guidelines should be updated frequently, be readily available on the labour ward and be distributed to all new staff, who should undergo a formal familiarisation programme before being allowed 'on call'. Standards laid down in guidelines should be the subject of regular audit. Independent practitioners who require admitting rights must also agree to abide by the unit guidelines.

A formal scheme for reporting all critical incidents and 'near-misses' must be in place, and a blame-free culture established to encourage staff to utilise the system. Regular multidisciplinary morbidity meetings are useful to identify potential organisational problems. Information from these should pass to a risk management committee (also multidisciplinary), responsible for ensuring good practice and minimising risk to patients.

Good communication is the most important factor in a well-managed labour ward. A system should be in place to ensure that potentially difficult cases are referred to an anaesthetist early in the antenatal period, and that the anaesthetist is also notified when they are admitted. Management plans and other relevant clinical information should be easily accessible to the care team at all times. The anaesthetist should be familiar with all the patients on labour ward, and this is best achieved by participating in joint ward rounds with the obstetricians and midwives. The duty anaesthetist must be rapidly contactable at all times; 'bleep' systems should not be relied upon as a sole means of contact. The names and methods of contacting consultant staff should be visible at the central desk. In general, anaesthetists should ensure that they are regarded as part of the 'team', rather than as someone to be called when the situation is desperate.

Extreme emergencies such as cardiorespiratory arrest are very uncommon on the labour ward, but a successful outcome depends on a rapid, efficient response – and this can be threatened by the very rarity of such events. National guidelines on the management of common emergencies such as anaphylaxis should be posted in a visible place. The whereabouts of resuscitation equipment and drugs must, of course, be known to all staff, and regular 'drills' for emergencies such as maternal collapse and massive antepartum haemorrhage should be carried out to ensure that the system works smoothly. Robust systems for data collection should be in place to enable the conduct of clinical audit, the identification and follow-up of complications, and the assessment of outcomes.

Detailed guidelines covering the above points, and more, have been published by the Obstetric Anaesthetists' Association, the Association of Anaesthetists of Great Britain and Ireland, and the Royal Colleges of Midwives and of Obstetricians and Gynaecologists. These documents serve as useful reminders of the various aspects of labour ward organisation that need attention, and also serve as tools for ongoing audit.

Key points

- Poor organisation results in unnecessarily hasty, and sometimes incorrect, decision making.
- Anaesthetists should be involved in labour ward management.
- Good, early communication will help prevent many disasters.

Further reading

Obstetric Anaesthetists' Association, Association of Anaesthetists of Great Britain and Ireland. *OAA/ AAGBI Guidelines for Obstetric Anaesthetic Services*, 3rd edn. London: AAGBI, 2013. www .aagbi.org/sites/default/files/obstetric_anaesthetic_services_2013.pdf (accessed December 2018).
Royal College of Anaesthetists, Royal College of Midwives, Royal College of Obstetricians and Gynaecologists, Royal College of Paediatrics and Child Health. *Safer Childbirth: Minimum Standards for the Organisation and Delivery of Care in Labour*. London: RCOG Press, 2007. www.rcog.org.uk/globalassets/documents/guidelines/wprsaferchildbirthreport2007.pdf (accessed December 2018).

Midwifery training

Obstetric anaesthetists are part of the delivery suite team. This involves working closely with midwives, who are often the lead professionals caring for the pregnant woman. It is therefore important to understand the training that midwives have received, and for senior anaesthetists to take responsibility for teaching obstetric analgesia and anaesthesia and the management of critically ill obstetric patients to midwives.

Training and regulation of midwives was formally established following passage of the Midwives Act in 1902, with the establishment of the Central Midwives Board (CMB). In 1983, the CMB was replaced by the United Kingdom Central Council for Nursing, Midwifery and Health Visiting (UKCC), whose functions were taken over by the Nursing and Midwifery Council (NMC) in 2002. The NMC register currently has ~618,000 nurses, ~33,000 midwives and ~8000 dual-qualified nurse-midwives.

Special considerations

Midwives working in the NHS have completed either a degree course in midwifery (usually 3 years) or a midwifery short programme (at least a year and a half) if they already have a nursing qualification. The structure of the courses varies considerably, as does the obstetric anaesthetic involvement.

Midwifery training usually requires the following topics to be covered:

- Biological sciences, applied sociology and psychology, and aspects of professional practice
- Pain in labour, the pain pathways involved, and pain relief (including both non-pharmacological and pharmacological methods)
- Anaesthesia, including both regional and general anaesthesia in pregnancy

These modules do not have to be taught by obstetric anaesthetists, although in most training schools there is a good relationship between the midwifery tutors and obstetric anaesthetists, who may as a result be involved in many hours of teaching. This relationship has led to increasing awareness that anaesthetists are involved with the sick maternity patient and that they should be involved in teaching both high-dependency care and the recognition of clinical risk factors. Teaching of these skills is particularly important for direct-entry midwives and has led to the following topics often being taught by obstetric anaesthetists:

- Postoperative and recovery skills, including basic airway management manoeuvres and monitoring of recovery from neuraxial blockade
- Risk factors associated with women who have medical problems
- Care of the critically ill woman, e.g. high-dependency care for women who have pre-eclampsia, sepsis or haemorrhage

This extension of the teaching role of the obstetric anaesthetist may require around 18 hours of teaching to be given to each group of students. The students who have general nursing qualifications will require less time than the direct-entry students.

In order to practise, midwives must be registered with the NMC. To remain registered, they must maintain a professional portfolio as evidence of their keeping up to date, and notify the NMC annually of their intention to practise. Part of midwives' continuing professional development and training will include the practical management of epidural analgesia. The ability to administer epidural top-ups requires additional in-service teaching, which is usually done on the delivery suite. A certificate is issued to the midwife on completing the training satisfactorily. The exact requirements of the training differ depending on local practice and may require an update of resuscitation skills.

Anaesthetists are often involved in other areas of professional development, for example intravenous cannulation, resuscitation (adult and neonatal) and specific high-dependency and simulation training.

Key points

- It is important that obstetric anaesthetists are involved in midwifery training.
- Midwives require instruction during their midwifery training, as well as continuous education and maintenance of skills once qualified.

Consent

Consent for treatment comprises a number of components:

- Provision of adequate information to, and its understanding by, the patient
- The ability of the individual to retain and assimilate this information, weigh up the alternatives and consequences, and come to and communicate a decision (in ethical and legal parlance, often referred to as 'capacity' and 'competence', respectively)
- Allowing adequate time for the process
- Voluntariness, i.e. no coercion by others

Consent may be implied or expressed. Implied consent is usually assumed when a patient cooperates in allowing a minor procedure, such as venepuncture, to take place. For a more major procedure such as epidural anaesthesia, the maintenance of a suitable posture might be taken to imply consent to continue, but it would be unwise to rely on this in the absence of a full discussion.

There is no legal difference between written and verbal consent. The only advantage of the former is that it provides concrete evidence that a discussion took place if a dispute arises.

Failure to obtain consent before performing a procedure could lead to an action against the anaesthetist for battery – the unlawful touching of another person. In practice, this is rarely, if ever, an issue in claims against doctors. Far more likely is the claim that a lack of informed consent resulted in a complication (if the patient had only been told of the risk, she would not have undergone the procedure), which amounts to a claim of negligence. (A 2005 House of Lords judgment means that a doctor may now be found negligent with respect to the provision of adequate information to the patient even if this failure had no effect on the patient's decision to undergo treatment.)

The amount of information that a doctor must impart to a patient to aid her in making a decision has traditionally been based on the 'Bolam principle' from 1957, which holds that an action – in this case the failure to mention a complication – is not negligent if it can be shown that the doctor has acted in accordance with a 'responsible body of medical persons skilled in that particular art'. However, this principle, which essentially allows the profession to set its own standards, has increasingly been challenged, particularly by the 'Bolitho principle' from 1997, by which the views or practice of a body of medical opinion can only be considered as 'reasonable' or 'responsible' if it holds up against 'logical analysis'. Thus, for example, an anaesthetist who did not explain the risk of nerve injury after an epidural might claim that many other anaesthetists would also not explain this (a defence based on Bolam) – but the courts might decide that this is unacceptable practice nonetheless (Bolitho).

These principles have been superseded by the landmark Montgomery case of 2015, which ruled that doctors have a duty to disclose risks if 'a reasonable person in the patient's position would be likely to attach significance to the risk, or the doctor is or should reasonably be aware that the particular patient would be likely to attach significance to it'. The law thus requires that each patient should be given the information that a reasonable patient might want *and* that she herself would want, not what the treating doctor thinks she needs. Further, she should be informed of the alternatives to the treatment being discussed. So, for instance, a woman undergoing caesarean section should be told the risks and benefits of regional anaesthesia *and* those of general anaesthesia, even though the former is being proposed as the best and safest option for her.

Problems and special considerations

The principles of consent to treatment in obstetric anaesthesia are essentially no different from those in any other field, the main distinction being that, in the often fraught circumstances that surround labour and delivery, they may be more difficult to apply.

Prior information about epidural analgesia – e.g. in the antenatal clinic – is generally accepted as improving the consenting process, but it should be borne in mind that up to half of primigravidae who end up with an epidural were not intending to have one beforehand.

Questions may arise over the issue of capacity when the mother is in the full throes of labour, especially when she is exhausted and/or has received powerful analgesic drugs. The practitioner treating the patient (in this case, the anaesthetist) is the person who must make the decision of whether or not the mother does have the capacity to understand what is being explained or proposed to her. If yes, then she is able to consent to (or refuse) treatment as in any other situation, even if this goes against a previous statement in the form of a birth plan – i.e. a woman with capacity is able to change her mind. If no, then the anaesthetist is obliged to treat her in her 'best interests' – which may not necessarily mean siting an epidural. In such a situation, the anaesthetist must attempt to determine what her best interests are, for example based on her birth plan and, where possible, discussions with her partner and midwife about her prior views and strength of feeling. Trainee anaesthetists would be well advised to consult with senior staff should such a situation occur. It is important in such circumstances to explain the difficulties of the situation to the woman's partner, to record the discussions in the patient's notes, and to visit her postpartum to explain events to her.

Consent is ultimately a matter between the anaesthetist and the patient. However, the partner's views should not be dismissed summarily; they are important participants in the birth process and should be encouraged to listen to the anaesthetist's explanation and accept the woman's decision. As outlined above, the partner can also be a key provider of evidence as to what a woman's 'best interests' might be if she lacks capacity to give consent.

The presence of the fetus does not interfere with the patient's right to make an autonomous decision about her own care, even if the decision taken will compromise the wellbeing of her unborn child. It is, of course, still very important that the risks and benefits to the fetus are also explained to the mother when seeking consent to a particular course of action. An emergency court order to authorise treatment may be requested in such circumstances, but will only be granted if the court concludes that the woman lacks the relevant decision-making capacity and that the treatment is in her best interests.

Patients whose first language is not English are as entitled as any others to an adequate explanation in their own language. The partner may act as translator in an emergency, but this is a very poor substitute for using an official interpreter. In hospitals where a substantial proportion of patients are from ethnic minorities, suitable interpreters should be made available (e.g. via telephone) at all times.

In difficult cases, it is wise to make sure that a witness (usually the midwife) is present, that all present agree on what has been said and decided, and that appropriate notes are made in the medical records, detailing the discussion and the decision.

Management options

Good antenatal education about pain relief and anaesthesia, supported by booklets and/or videos, is an important part of the obstetric anaesthetist's job, and it is best not delegated to midwives unless the information that they disseminate is scrupulously checked. Every obstetric unit, in conjunction with the anaesthetic team, must provide advice in early pregnancy about pain relief during labour.

Signed consent for epidural analgesia in labour is not currently considered necessary, and in most units only verbal consent is taken. What is important is to give an adequate explanation of the risks and benefits that are applicable to each particular woman making a decision in the prevailing circumstances. This will obviously vary according to the situation, but a note should always be made listing the matters discussed and identifying reasons why an explanation was brief or curtailed. If the procedure is difficult or prolonged, then verbal permission to continue must be sought at regular intervals.

For regional techniques, most obstetric anaesthetists would now consider, as a minimum, explanation of the risk of partial or complete failure of the technique, dural puncture and headache, motor block, a fall in blood pressure, neurological complications, sensation during caesarean section and the possibility of conversion to general anaesthesia. An explanation of the risks of regional anaesthesia for caesarean section should always include the possibility of discomfort, pain and conversion to general anaesthesia. Failure to do this has resulted in many negligence claims against anaesthetists and trusts.

When offering anaesthetic options for elective caesarean section, it is perfectly reasonable to stress the maternal advantages of regional block, but there is no argument at present for insisting on this when there are no contraindications to general anaesthesia. A patient undergoing emergency caesarean section with a functioning epidural in situ is a different proposition entirely, and every effort should be made to encourage an epidural top-up, with refusal being carefully recorded in the notes.

Key points

- It is difficult to provide complex information to a woman in painful labour. Antenatal education makes this task much easier.
- Women with capacity are able to change their mind at any time; those without capacity should be treated in their 'best interests'.
- The risks and benefits discussed with the patient should always be recorded.
- A pregnant woman's autonomy is not affected by the fact that she is carrying a fetus.

Further reading

Broaddus BM, Chandrasekhar S. Informed consent in obstetric anesthesia. *Anesth Analg* 2011; **112**: 912–15.

Chan SW, Tulloch E, Cooper ES, *et al.* Montgomery and informed consent: where are we now? *BMJ* 2017; **357**: j2224.

McCombe K, Bogod DG. Paternalism and consent: has the law finally caught up with the profession? *Anaesthesia* 2015, **70**: 1016–19.

Wheat K. Progress of the prudent patient: consent after Chester v Afshar. *Anaesthesia* 2005; **60**: 217–19.

Yentis SM, Hartle AJ, Barker IR, *et al.* AAGBI: consent for anaesthesia 2017. *Anaesthesia* 2017; **72**: 93–105.

Medicolegal issues

Obstetric anaesthetists may be involved in medicolegal issues in a number of different contexts, all of which have relevance or potential relevance to obstetric care. These may concern consent and capacity (see Chapter 169, *Consent*); various statutes such as the Mental Capacity Act, Mental Health Act, Data Protection Act, Human Tissue Act and Human Rights Act; involvement in coroners' courts; the risk of being accused of assault and/or battery; and claims of negligence. It is the last, however, that is by far the most likely reason for an obstetric anaesthetist to encounter the legal system.

Claims within the NHS are handled by NHS Resolution (which was formerly known as the NHS Litigation Authority, NHSLA), although the named NHS body itself is the defendant so that negligence claims are made against (and defended by) the trust and not the individual employees involved in the case. However, staff working outside the NHS may be personally named in negligence claims.

There is a general trend in the UK towards patients seeking redress in the courts when they think that they have been harmed as a result of a negligent act on the part of their medical attendants. In 2017–18, the NHS made payments in excess of £1.63 billion in respect of negligence claims, a 33% increase over the previous year. Since the Clinical Negligence Scheme for Trusts (CNST) started in 1995, surgery (39%), medicine (19%) and obstetrics and gynaecology (18%; obstetrics 10%) have been the most commonly involved specialties, with anaesthesia accounting for 2%. However, obstetrics and gynaecology accounts for 51% of the costs, and within anaesthetic claims, regional and obstetric anaesthesia accounts for ~40% of the costs of claims. Before it became NHS Resolution in 2017, the NHSLA developed a 5-year strategy to help address the escalating costs of claims; one area of focus is obstetric claims, and in 2017 the Early Notification Scheme of potential cases of brain damage at birth was launched, which aims to assist with record keeping, duty of candour, mediation and peer support.

For a negligence claim to succeed, the patient has to demonstrate: (1) that the doctor had a duty of care towards her (normally not a matter for contention); (2) that there was a failure of that duty of care (the standard applied here is that of the ordinary doctor professing skill in anaesthesia); and (3) that she has suffered harm as a result. The test for causation is that were it not for the failure of care, the harm would not have occurred. However, a judgment in 2005 in the House of Lords relating to consent has established that, even were this not to apply, the doctor may still be found negligent.

Problems and special considerations

Consent

Consent is equally valid whether written or verbal, the only difference being that a record of the former is retained in the hospital notes as confirmation if a case comes to court after some years. Consent is only valid if it is informed, which means that the patient has been presented with enough information about the risks and benefits of the procedure to make a sensible choice. This can obviously be difficult in practice if a patient is in severe pain and under the influence of Entonox or opioids, as is often the case when epidural analgesia is needed in labour. It is generally agreed that provision of information in the antenatal period is best, although many women may not consider it applicable to them at this time (see Chapter 169, *Consent*).

Regional analgesia and anaesthesia

The extent of information required when seeking consent for regional analgesia or anaesthesia is controversial, although most surveys suggest that some women would wish to know most, if not all, complications. Most obstetric anaesthetists would now consider, as a minimum, explanation of the risk of partial or complete failure of the technique, dural puncture and headache, motor block, a fall in blood pressure, neurological complications, sensation during caesarean section and the possibility of conversion to general anaesthesia. Signed, written consent is not generally considered necessary currently, although the pertinent aspects of the discussion should be recorded, and a note made if the patient's condition does not allow for a full explanation. Antenatal access to an anaesthetist should be available for women who have particular concerns.

Pain during caesarean section

Pain felt during caesarean delivery under spinal or epidural anaesthesia is thought to be the most common source of successful litigation against UK obstetric anaesthetists, accounting for 31% of obstetric claims related to regional anaesthesia. In practice, a pain-free procedure cannot be guaranteed, and the anaesthetist must mention this possibility when obtaining consent. The level of block must be carefully checked before starting the operation, and recorded, along with the sensory modality used. Any complaint of pain should be taken seriously, documented and treated.

Headache

Headache following accidental dural puncture is a common source of complaint. The occurrence of a dural tap is not, in itself, enough to demonstrate negligence, as long as the epidural technique was acceptable and the headache was correctly managed. This means that good analgesia should be established for labour and the patient followed up daily while in hospital. Any complaint of headache, neck pain or visual disturbances should be documented, and definitive treatment, in the form of epidural blood patch, should be offered early. Any mother who has suffered a dural tap or postdural puncture headache should be encouraged to contact the hospital if there is a recurrence or worsening of symptoms. These patients should be routinely followed up at 6–10 weeks postpartum.

Backache

Claims are often made for backache after epidural analgesia, but few, if any, succeed. Prospective studies have shown that new long-term backache is common following childbirth but is not related to whether or not regional analgesia has been used.

Management options

It is far easier to minimise the risk of litigation than to deal with it once it arises. Sensible guidelines for the management of common obstetric anaesthetic situations are essential. Good communication with patients and relatives, and keeping them informed, will ensure them of one's good intentions – very few patients institute proceedings against doctors who have communicated well. Most hospitals now have an efficient risk-management procedure that includes rapid response to complaints, with the result that patients, most of whom only want an explanation of what went wrong and an apology, will often be content without needing to take more formal action. Complaints from mothers or their partners, however informal, must be handled at a senior level.

If, despite these precautions, legal action ensues, then good record keeping will help the anaesthetist to recall what happened long after the case has faded from memory. Even if it was always an individual anaesthetist's routine practice to give a test dose after siting an epidural, for example, it will be difficult to convince a judge of this fact without documentary evidence relating to the particular case. The same applies to the explanations given when obtaining consent for a procedure. A case of negligence will often come down to the anaesthetist's recollection versus that of the patient – needless to say, she will remember the whole incident perfectly, while the anaesthetist may have performed many similar procedures since. Equally, it is well documented that the patient's recollection of the consent process is poor, so documentation of the consent discussion is essential. The need for accurate records is particularly important when the complaint is of a subjective nature, such as pain or awareness during caesarean section. (See also Chapter 171, *Record keeping*.)

An accusation of negligence is a very painful and traumatic experience for a doctor, and it is important to seek support from peers and seniors, especially those who have experience of medicolegal practice.

Key points

- Negligence claims against obstetric anaesthetists continue to increase.
- Good relations should be maintained with patients and their relatives.
- Any complaint should be dealt with promptly.
- Full records are the best defence and should include details of explanations given before consent.

Further reading

Cook TM, Bland L, Mihai R, Scott S. Litigation related to anaesthesia: an analysis of claims against the NHS in England 1995–2007. *Anaesthesia* 2009; **64**: 706–18.

McCombe K, Bogod DG. Learning from the law: a review of 21 years of litigation for pain during caesarean section. *Anaesthesia* 2018; **73**: 223–30.

NHS Litigation Authority. Claims (including factsheets). Available via https://resolution.nhs.uk (accessed December 2018).

Szypula K, Ashpole KJ, Bogod D, *et al.* Litigation related to regional anaesthesia: an analysis of claims against the NHS in England 1995–2007. *Anaesthesia* 2010; **65**: 443–52.

Yentis SM, Hartle AJ, Barker IR, *et al.* AAGBI: consent for anaesthesia 2017. *Anaesthesia* 2017; **72**: 93–105.

Record keeping

Chapter 171

The increase in negligence litigation against doctors in general, and obstetric anaesthetists in particular, has led to increased concerns about the standard of record keeping in hospitals. Many hospitals now have clinical risk managers, and one of the main tasks of these individuals is to ensure that records are clear, complete and retrievable. Many practitioners criticise the current medicolegal climate as leading to the practice of 'defensive medicine', but in the area of record keeping at least, the benefits for practitioner and patient alike are clear. There is no doubt that record keeping has often been poor in the past, and that this has led to delays, unnecessary repetition of investigations and breakdowns in communication.

Increasingly, certain aspects of medical record keeping are being done electronically (e.g. prescribing, recording of intraoperative observation) but the unpredictable nature of obstetric analgesia and anaesthesia makes such systems difficult to design and implement in the maternity setting.

Special considerations

Legibility

Although it is not always easy to maintain good legibility in the emergency situation, every effort should be made to ensure that entries in the notes, and particularly signatures, can be read. While most doctors can read their own handwriting, this is not always true 20 years later, and it should be borne in mind that the interpretation will often be made by someone other than the writer. Each signature in the notes should be followed by the author's name in capital letters.

Hospitals rarely release original notes, and solicitors usually receive a photocopied bundle of records, often prepared in haste by the most junior office assistant. Therefore, black ink (it photocopies better) should be used, and notes should not be written in the extremes of the margin (often missed in the photocopying process).

Contemporaneity

The courts appreciate that it is often impossible to keep good, contemporaneous records in the midst of dealing with a crisis. It is perfectly in order, for example, to copy a series of blood pressure results from the monitor 'trends' screen into the record after an operation. Similarly, it is quite reasonable to sit down after a dangerous situation has been stabilised and make a retrospective record of what happened – in this instance, however, the time at which the record was written should be included in the entry. It is even acceptable to go back and alter or add notes some time after the event – as long as the alterations are honest – but it must be made very clear in the notes that these are later additions. In general, complex notes should be made as soon as possible after the event, while the memory is fresh.

Completeness

While it may be one's standard practice to warn of the risk of headache before siting an epidural or to assess the level of block after instituting spinal anaesthesia for caesarean section, it is prudent to note that this has been done in each individual case – and ideally, this record should include the incidence quoted. An anaesthetist's actions may be queried many years after the event, by which time he/she will have no recollection of the individual case; the patient, on the contrary, will remember it as if it were yesterday. In this situation, the defence that something must have been done, because it was one's routine practice always to do so, does not carry much weight if there is no mention of it in the notes.

Reasons for making clinical decisions – such as withholding a blood patch for a postdural puncture headache because it seems to be improving – should always be carefully noted, especially when the decision deviates from standard guidelines. Finally, all entries should be dated, timed and signed legibly.

The maintenance of complete records can be encouraged by developing forms with prompts for commonly omitted data, such as level of block and mode of testing after regional anaesthesia. Good record keeping can also be encouraged by stressing its value in departmental guidelines. One of the most effective methods for ensuring standards is to incorporate a review of clinical records into the audit programme.

Retrievability

The best records in the world will be of no help if they cannot be found. Anaesthetic notes, especially epidural forms, are often made on sheets that do not form part of the main record. There must be a system in place for incorporating these into the bound folder, preferably not by just inserting them into a pocket in the back.

Obstetric litigation may arise up to 21 years after the birth of the child. Maternity records must be kept for at least this long, and this often causes considerable logistic problems, as does the difficulty in tracing the practitioners involved after such a long period.

Key points

- Notes should be written clearly and legibly in black ink.
- The date, time and the author's name should be included.
- Even if a practice is routine, details should be noted.

Further reading

McCombe K, Bogod DG. Learning from the law: a review of 21 years of litigation for pain during caesarean section. *Anaesthesia* 2018; **73**: 223–30.

Chapter 172

Minimum standards, guidelines and protocols

Recent years have seen a proliferation of documents aimed at standardising and improving medical care. These are variously known as standards, guidelines and protocols and are developed at local, national and even international level. There are no firm, accepted definitions of these terms, and in practice they are often used interchangeably. However, the term 'minimum standards' tends to be used for establishing general standards of services and care to which practitioners and units should aspire, while 'protocols' tends to refer to specific management of a particular condition or group of conditions. 'Guidelines' is commonly used in both contexts.

Such documents are increasingly used throughout medicine. They are seen as an efficient way of maintaining good practice, although they may have some disadvantages (Table 172.1). They are generally seen as an important part of risk management.

Current national standards and guidelines

In the UK, the Association of Anaesthetists of Great Britain and Ireland (AAGBI) has produced a series of standards and guidelines over the past 20 years. In the field of obstetric anaesthesia, the Obstetric Anaesthetists' Association (OAA) produced its *Recommended Minimum Standards for Obstetric Anaesthesia Services* in 1994. In 1998, both organisations jointly produced *Guidelines for Obstetric Anaesthesia Services*, which was most recently updated in 2013. This important document specifies recommendations for staffing levels; acceptable response times; monitoring during regional analgesia and caesarean section; theatre, recovery, high-dependency and intensive care unit facilities; availability of blood; consent; support services; assistance and departmental guidelines. In addition, it has a section on professional relationships with midwives and obstetricians.

The Royal College of Anaesthetists (RCoA) produces an online document, *Guidelines for the Provision of Anaesthetic Services* (GPAS), which has a chapter dedicated to obstetric service provision. This covers staffing requirements, equipment and support services, training, governance, organisation and areas of special requirement such as the acutely unwell or obese parturient. The RCoA has also produced an audit recipe book (with an obstetric section) that details standards of care for trusts to measure themselves against, as a method of maintaining and improving quality of service.

In 1999, the Royal Colleges of Midwives and Obstetricians and Gynaecologists published *Towards Safer Childbirth – Minimum Standards for the Organisation of Labour Wards*, setting out recommendations for organisational aspects of maternity services and risk management, which was updated in 2007.

Table 172.1 Advantages and disadvantages of minimum standards, guidelines and protocols

Advantages	Can support local departments/units in their argument for adequate resources/facilities
	Encourage practitioners/units to examine their own practice and establish good risk-management procedures
	Represent an overview from established authorities
	Increase uniformity of practice, especially where there is a large turnover of staff
	Allow better adherence to evidence-based practice
	Improve management of rare but serious conditions, e.g. anaphylaxis, major haemorrhage
	Can be used for teaching and training of staff
	May reduce the risk of medicolegal claims
	Required by most accreditation/assessment authorities as an indicator of good risk management
Disadvantages	Require continuous updating and removal when obsolete
	Lay the organisation or individuals open to potential criticism if not adhered to or if badly written
	May be ignored if the targets set are seen as unrealistic
	May restrict clinical freedom
	May result in blind adherence to a set management path, even though it may be inappropriate in certain circumstances
	May remove the incentive to 'think for oneself'
	Rely on consensus; if opinions vary widely the resultant protocol may be too loose to be useful

The National Institute for Health and Care Excellence (NICE) aims to produce evidence-based guidance on best practice, and it has an extensive section on obstetric care that covers topics such as midwifery staffing, use of intraoperative cell salvage and maternal request for caesarean section.

In the USA, the American Society of Anesthesiologists (ASA) produced its *Guidelines for Regional Anesthesia in Obstetrics* in 1988 and amended them in 1991. *Practice Guidelines for Obstetrical Anesthesia*, the report by the ASA's Task Force on Obstetrical Anesthesia, was produced in 1999 and most recently updated in 2016; it aims to be evidence-based, covering most aspects of obstetric anaesthetic practice. The ASA's *Guidelines for Regional Anesthesia in Obstetrics* and *Optimal Goals for Anesthesia Care in Obstetrics* (the latter produced jointly with the American College of Obstetricians and Gynecologists, ACOG) were published in 2000, and were subsequently replaced by a new document published in 2009 by ACOG and ASA entitled *Optimal Goals for Anesthesia Care in Obstetrics*.

Local protocols and guidelines

It is important that these are written clearly and unambiguously. Once a protocol has been written, it becomes an important legal document (e.g. in future claims that negligence occurred) even if it has not yet been formally introduced, since merely by existing it demonstrates that any other management is suboptimal. This potential exposure to criticism and possibly legal action has deterred some clinicians from utilising protocols more widely.

Each version of a protocol should be dated and previous ones removed in order to maintain consistency throughout the unit. Obsolete ones should be stored, since subsequent legal actions may refer to guidelines that were in force at the time of the supposed mismanagement.

Although there have been calls for national protocols that can be used by all units, most prefer to alter basic schemes to suit the local circumstances.

Writing a protocol requires the clinical problem or procedure to be carefully defined at the start. It is important that protocols are written by multidisciplinary groups and that all individuals involved are consulted before their introduction, since the protocols must be willingly followed by all clinicians unless specific exclusion criteria are met. Management of cases meeting exclusion criteria should also be covered. It is equally important that adherence to the protocol is audited to ensure consistency of management.

Medicolegal considerations

As a method of protecting the practitioner from legal actions for negligence, documents of this type are obviously a double-edged sword, since they could be a useful weapon for lawyers when the stated standards have not been achieved.

In practice, however, standards and guidelines have not been afforded a great deal of weight in courts of law in the UK or USA. This is partly because, although they may reflect the views of a group of senior and respected practitioners, they are rarely firmly based on good scientific evidence, and there is often an equally respectable opinion that would support a different course of action or standard of care. Furthermore, since such documents and their authors cannot be cross-examined in court, greater weight is often attached to the evidence given directly by expert witnesses. Finally, guidelines and protocols cannot cover every clinical scenario, and expert clinical judgement must be applied to determine the most appropriate management of individual patients.

Key points

- Minimum standard documents provide a useful reference when developing local protocols and are an impetus to improving and maintaining the quality of medical care.
- Local protocols and guidelines can improve clinical management and form an important part of risk management.
- Many potential problems can be avoided by careful writing and achieving consensus.
- Each copy should be dated, and obsolete versions removed from all clinical sites and kept for future reference.

Further reading

ACOG Committee on Obstetric Practice. ACOG Committee Opinion No. 433: optimal goals for anesthesia care in obstetrics. *Obstet Gynecol* 2009; **113**: 1197–9.

American Society of Anesthesiologists. Practice guidelines for obstetric anesthesia: an updated report by the American Society of Anesthesiologists Task Force on Obstetric Anesthesia and the Society for Obstetric Anesthesia and Perinatology. *Anesthesiology* 2016; **124**: 270–300.

McGarrity L, O'Connor R, Young S. A national survey of obstetric anaesthesia guidelines in the UK. *Int J Obstet Anesth* 2008; **17**: 322–8.

National Institute for Health and Care Excellence. Fertility, pregnancy and childbirth. NICE guidance. www.nice.org.uk/guidance/conditions-and-diseases/fertility-pregnancy-and-childbirth (accessed December 2018).

Obstetric Anaesthetists' Association, Association of Anaesthetists of Great Britain and Ireland. *OAA/ AAGBI Guidelines for Obstetric Anaesthetic Services*, 3rd edn. London: AAGBI, 2013. www .aagbi.org/sites/default/files/obstetric_anaesthetic_services_2013.pdf (accessed December 2018).

Royal College of Anaesthetists, Royal College of Midwives, Royal College of Obstetricians and Gynaecologists, Royal College of Paediatrics and Child Health. *Safer Childbirth: Minimum Standards for the Organisation and Delivery of Care in Labour*. London: RCOG Press, 2007. www.rcog.org.uk/globalassets/documents/guidelines/wprsaferchildbirthreport2007.pdf (accessed December 2018).

Royal College of Anaesthetists. *Guidelines for the Provision of Anaesthesia Services for an Obstetric Population 2018*. GPAS, Chapter 9. London: RCoA, 2018. www.rcoa.ac.uk/system/files/GPAS-20 18-09-OBSTETRICS.pdf (accessed December 2018).

Royal College of Anaesthetists. *Raising the Standard: a Compendium of Audit Recipes*, 3rd edn. London: RCoA, 2012. www.rcoa.ac.uk/ARB2012 (accessed December 2018).

Risk management

Risk management is a process by which adverse outcomes are minimised by analysing their causes and instituting preventive steps, thus reducing both the chance of an adverse event occurring and its cost (both clinical and financial), should it occur. Although it may involve audit or quality improvement projects, the emphasis is more on the analysis of individual real or potential adverse events rather than assessment of standards of practice generally. This approach is widely used throughout (and outside) health care to reduce risk and also liability.

Problems and special considerations

Traditionally, anaesthetic risk has been seen as individual-based (e.g. arising from human error), but recent emphasis has focused on risk being operating-room-based (arising from the interaction between anaesthetists and their working environment, in this case labour ward), and most recently system-based (human actions superimposed on inherent flaws in a system or process).

Examples of system-based errors might be seen in the case of a patient with pre-eclampsia who presents unbooked late in pregnancy, requires emergency caesarean section but is not given antacid prophylaxis because her drug chart is missing, and is then anaesthetised by a junior trainee, aspirates on induction and is transferred to another hospital because of a shortage of intensive care beds.

Management options

Important steps in the development of a risk-management programme include:

- Analysis of risks (e.g. morbidity and mortality meetings, critical incident reporting schemes)
- Prevention of risks associated with routine activities (e.g. proper training and supervision, provision of trained anaesthetic assistants)
- Avoidance of particularly high-risk practices (e.g. general anaesthesia for caesarean section)
- Minimising the severity of adverse events should they occur (e.g. having an antacid prophylaxis protocol in place)
- Risk financing (e.g. indemnity)
- Having a system in place for dealing with disasters and complaints: this may reduce both psychological sequelae and legal proceedings

Such a programme has implications for training, purchase and upkeep of equipment and other potentially costly processes but should ultimately reduce costs related to legal actions.

Relatively simple measures can be taken to reduce the risks attached to specific activities, such as analysing a single procedure (e.g. caesarean section) at all its stages or focusing on a specific complication (e.g. dural tap) and working back. A climate in which mistakes and critical incidents can be openly discussed without fear of retribution is important. More formal analytical techniques (e.g. root cause analysis) can be used to reveal underlying weaknesses in systems; such methods may have a role in helping to predict incidents but are usually employed to analyse incidents once they happen.

Once a risk-management programme is instituted, specific audits can then be performed to highlight areas where inadequacies still exist. Protocols are generally seen as a way of reducing risk if they are widely circulated and followed (itself a worthy subject of audit). Wider use of critical incident reporting schemes has been suggested as a more effective means of improving service than traditional reliance on outcome studies (e.g. looking at mortality), firstly because serious adverse outcomes are rare, and secondly because a proactive approach is inherently more attractive than a reactive one.

The organisation that handles claims against NHS bodies is called NHS Resolution (previously the NHS Litigation Authority; see Chapter 170, *Medicolegal issues*). Through its Clinical Negligence Scheme for Trusts (CNST), NHS bodies are encouraged to improve their structure and processes through financial incentives. The costs of the scheme are met by the bodies themselves according to whether they meet required CNST standards of organisational structure, routine and high-risk clinical care, and communication. Trusts may meet none (level 0), some (levels 1 or 2) or all (level 3) standards, and their contributions are adjusted accordingly.

Key points

- Risk may involve human actions and/or an underlying flawed system.
- Management includes:
  - Analysis
  - Reduction of risk attached to routine activities
  - Avoidance of high-risk activities
  - Damage limitation
  - Risk financing

Further reading

Boothman RC, Blackwell AC. Integrating risk management activities into a patient safety program. *Clin Obstet Gynecol* 2010; **53**: 576–85.

Pettker CM. Systematic approaches to adverse events in obstetrics, Part I. Event identification and classification. *Semin Perinatol* 2017; **41**: 151–5.

Pettker CM. Systematic approaches to adverse events in obstetrics, Part II. Event analysis and response. *Semin Perinatol* 2017; **41**: 156–60.

Smith R. Clinical risk management in obstetric practice. *Obstet Gynecol Reprod Med* 2017; **27**: 277–84.

Post-crisis management

Obstetric anaesthesia is a particularly stressful subspecialty of anaesthesia. It is important that all staff are aware that there are times when colleagues may need someone to talk to, and they may need support in communicating with the patient and other colleagues. It is also clear that proper debriefing after catastrophes is an important part of risk management.

A crisis may be precipitated by a variety of factors, some obvious and others less obvious (Table 174.1).

Problems and special considerations

Obstetric anaesthesia is a particularly stressful subspecialty, for several reasons:

- The anaesthetist is looking after two people – the mother and the baby – during an important life event. There is therefore much at stake should things go wrong.

Table 174.1 Causes of major stress when support and counselling of colleagues may be required

Serious adverse outcome	Maternal death or severe impairment
	Fetal death or severe impairment
Unexpected crisis	Anaphylaxis
	Failed or difficult tracheal intubation
	Shoulder dystocia
	Sudden severe maternal haemorrhage
	Maternal cardiac arrest
Complication of technique	Accidental dural puncture
	Neurological deficit following regional analgesia and anaesthesia
Failure of technique	Awareness during general anaesthesia for caesarean section
	Pain during regional anaesthesia for caesarean section
	Failed regional anaesthesia for labour
Human error	Giving the wrong drug or blood
	Not checking a blood result
	Wrong route of injection of drugs
Other	Letter of complaint from patient or solicitor
	Formal complaint from other hospital staff
	Violence from patient or relative/partner
	Coincidental professional or personal crisis

- Both mother and fetus may be physiologically stressed and thus have less reserve than healthy patients. When adverse events occur, they often do so rapidly and without warning, with little time to treat them before irreparable damage occurs. Obstetrics thus represents a truly 'high-risk' area of medical practice.
- Pregnancy is perceived as a normal physiological function in which the outcome should be safe and happy. The public expectations are very high, and it is inevitable that these high expectations may sometimes not be met.
- It is obvious that a maternal death will be a very traumatic event, but less obvious that a junior anaesthetist may be very upset by causing an accidental dural puncture.
  As maternity units are often very busy places and turnover of staff is high, there may not be a suitable opportunity to discuss potential problems with colleagues.

Maternity units are areas where different professional groups (anaesthetists, obstetricians and midwives) work closely together, with sometimes different priorities. Therefore, it is important to ensure good communication within this multidisciplinary group.

Management options

Failure of communication is one of the main reasons for complaint, and it is important that the anaesthetist continually informs the patient and her relatives when there are problems.

Communication between staff is also crucial. Trainees must always feel able to discuss a problem with their senior colleagues, without embarrassment, and must see themselves as part of the team whose aim is a high standard of care to all the women. Recent emphasis on team working (e.g. the World Health Organization's surgical safety checklist) has highlighted the need for proper communication between team members.

It is important that there is regular multidisciplinary discussion, and that staff do not automatically blame each other when outcomes are bad. Senior staff of all disciplines should ensure that each major catastrophe is fully discussed in an open fashion, and that all staff involved with the case have a chance to discuss it. Severe adverse events may lead to the development of strong negative emotional responses in some clinicians, triggering feelings of guilt, loss of confidence and even suicidal thoughts. Counselling and a formal support system should be made available to them.

When any member of staff is worried that there has been a problem, it is often helpful to seek advice from their medical protection organisation. It is also useful to go back to the medical record and, where appropriate, expand the account of the events and keep a full copy for personal use.

Post-crisis management also includes identification of any legal and/or financial threats to the hospital and taking steps to avoid or reduce them.

Key points

- All staff are vulnerable to experiencing a catastrophe in the maternity unit.
- Communication with all levels of staff and a non-judgemental approach are essential.
- All members of staff involved in a catastrophe should be offered support and, if necessary, counselling.

Further reading

Association of Anaesthetists of Great Britain and Ireland. *Catastrophes in Anaesthetic Practice: Dealing with the Aftermath*. London: AAGBI, 2005. www.aagbi.org/sites/default/files/catastrophes05.pdf (accessed December 2018).

McCready S, Russell R. A national survey of support and counselling after maternal death. *Anaesthesia* 2009; **64**: 1211–17.

Pratt SD, Jachna BR. Care of the clinician after an adverse event. *Int J Obstet Anesth* 2015; **24**: 54–63.

Research on the labour ward

Research involving pregnant women has particular ethical and practical issues. Perhaps partly because of this, much of obstetric and anaesthetic practice on the labour ward was traditionally based on little available evidence, or else little attention was paid to what evidence there was. Fortunately, there has been increasing reliance on published studies in guiding management, although in the quest for 'evidence-based' decisions, it is often forgotten that the best evidence there is may be far from perfect, because the ideal randomised controlled trial (RCT) has not been done. For example, the question of whether loss of resistance to air is indeed associated with a greater incidence of accidental dural tap than loss of resistance to saline would require a huge study, which would involve more centres and take more time than is practicable. In this situation one is left with methodologically weak studies (e.g. retrospective reviews), which may suggest a causal link but no more.

In the generally quoted hierarchy of evidence, the best of all is the systematic review, in which all known relevant RCTs are screened for correct methodology and the results pooled to increase power. Next, prospective RCTs themselves are still considered the gold standard for comparing different treatments or courses of management, as long as they are of adequate size. Then, in descending order, come non-randomised, single group, cohort or case–control studies; non-experimental studies; and finally case reports and 'expert' opinions.

Despite the fact that RCTs remain the gold standard, they are increasingly difficult to do, owing to constraints on time and funding. Many centres are now collaborating to produce multicentre databases as a way of collecting evidence pertaining to important clinical issues.

Problems and special considerations

Ethical issues are related to:

- The special vulnerability of pregnant women who are going through an intensely emotional time
- The increasing involvement of mothers in decisions affecting their pregnancy and thus their exposure to many potentially difficult choices
- The fact that many drugs in current obstetric anaesthetic practice are not licensed for use in pregnancy (largely related to the cost to manufacturers of separate trials in this group)
- The often uncertain effects of experimental drugs and procedures on the pregnancy, labour or fetus

The issue of consent may be cause for discussion. It has been argued that a woman in labour is unable to give truly informed consent for inclusion in a study (or even for a procedure such as an epidural) because of the pain and distress she may be suffering, especially if drugs such as pethidine have been given. This makes studies of epidural techniques especially difficult, since it may not be possible to identify in advance women who might go on to request epidural analgesia. An especially controversial area concerns the calls for randomised studies of epidural versus non-epidural analgesia, in order to assess side effects in particular; some would consider it unethical to withhold the only really effective form of analgesia from mothers, whereas others claim it is unethical not to do so if it is the only way of properly evaluating the effects of epidurals.

The care of pregnant women has traditionally been something of a battleground between various medical and non-medical staff, and the risk that a well-intentioned study may be viewed as an intrusion into a normal process should not be taken lightly. Most maternity units have multidisciplinary groups or committees for the approval and oversight of proposed studies, in addition to the usual regulatory structures (research and development departments, research ethics committees, etc.), since even purely 'anaesthetic' studies are likely to have implications for obstetric and midwifery practice.

Practical difficulties of conducting obstetric anaesthetic studies relate to:

- Obtaining consent, discussed above (see also Chapter 169, *Consent*)
- Defining a homogeneous group of subjects (the 'standard primip' was suggested over 30 years ago as suitable for the majority of studies; women in this category are aged 25, healthy, with a full-term normal singleton pregnancy and no malposition or malpresentation)
- The fact that labouring women in particular are demanding in terms of requesting information and determining their own management
- The largely unpredictable nature of the workload

In addition, since all subjects must have the right to withdraw from any study at any time without penalty, randomised studies may suffer from considerable drop-out rates (e.g. those studies of epidural versus non-epidural analgesia). Since a mother's situation may change suddenly during labour, this may further increase the drop-out rate. Finally, the records relating to the research may easily become lost among the voluminous paperwork that passes through the labour ward.

Management options

Apart from the considerations mentioned above, research methods are as for any other clinical situation. The practicalities of labour ward research preclude many topics from being suitable for study, even though they may be of interest and clinical value. Many potential or actual studies suffer from either too few subjects or too rare an outcome, or both; thus, for example, many complications that are relatively uncommon can only be meaningfully studied in multicentre trials (e.g. dural taps, neurological complications). On the other hand, studies comparing different regional anaesthetic techniques are relatively easy to conduct in a single unit, since so many anaesthetic interventions involve regional techniques.

As for any project, an obstetric anaesthetic RCT requires appropriate consideration of:

- The primary hypothesis (what question is the study asking – and is it worth asking?)
- The subjects to be studied (inclusion and exclusion criteria)
- The type of data collected (what is being measured and how)

- The methods of analysis (which statistical tests to use)
- The overall power of the study (related to the number of subjects per group, the size of the difference between the groups, and the statistical test used)

Finally, it should be remembered that a statistically significant result may not be clinically significant (e.g. a 30-second difference in onset of epidural block), and also that a statistically significant result found in a single study may still be a chance finding (albeit with a likelihood of less than 5% if a probability of 0.05 was taken to denote 'statistical significance'). In addition, just because the evidence supporting a particular course of action or management may be overwhelming, it does not necessarily follow that clinicians will adhere to it.

Key points

- For research on the labour ward, basic ethical considerations apply.
- Subjects are especially vulnerable but may be especially demanding.
- Practical difficulties include obtaining consent and the unpredictability of labour.

Further reading

American College of Obstetricians and Gynecologists. Committee Opinion no. 646. Ethical considerations for including women as research participants. *Obstet Gynecol* 2015; **126**: e100–7.

George RT, Butcher M, Yentis SM. Pregnant women's views on informed consent for research in labour. *Int J Obstet Anesth* 2014; **23**: 233–7.

Lupton MG, Williams DJ. The ethics of research on pregnant women: maternal consent sufficient? *BJOG* 2004; **111**: 1307–12.

Obstetric anaesthesia organisations

Several organisations and societies relevant to obstetric analgesia and anaesthesia exist. The Obstetric Anaesthetists' Association is the body that represents obstetric anaesthesia in the UK. There are, in addition, several UK-based regional societies and groups, some involving non-anaesthetists as well as anaesthetists.

Obstetric Anaesthetists' Association (OAA)

The OAA was formed in 1969 to promote the highest standards of anaesthetic practice in the care of the mother and baby, and has an international membership in the order of 2500, ~20% of whom are based outside the UK. It provides a focus for all anaesthetists who want to improve the care and safety of women in childbirth. The OAA has charitable status, supports a research fellowship and offers annual research grants and bursaries. It also offers prizes for trainees for research presented at the annual scientific meeting.

The OAA holds three main meetings a year: in March, a one-day meeting in London on cases and clinical challenges in obstetric anaesthesia; in the spring, a two-day meeting at different venues in the UK (and more recently in continental Europe) on current research and practice; and in late autumn, a three-day course in London presenting the latest academic and clinical views on modern obstetric anaesthesia and analgesia. Further smaller refresher courses and meetings on various topics are also held.

The *International Journal of Obstetric Anesthesia* (IJOA) is the official journal of the OAA, carries OAA notices, and is included in the annual subscription. The OAA also supplies educational videos and publications.

Society for Obstetric Anesthesia and Perinatology (SOAP)

Outside Britain, SOAP is the biggest and most active group for obstetric anaesthetists. It was founded in the USA in 1968 to provide a forum for discussion of problems unique to the peripartum period. SOAP comprises anaesthetists, obstetricians, paediatricians and basic scientists who share an interest in the care of the pregnant patient and the neonate; membership currently numbers approximately 900.

The mission of the society is to promote excellence in research and in the practice of obstetric anaesthesia and perinatology. Through its newsletter, website and annual meetings, SOAP allows practitioners of several specialties to meet and discuss clinical practice, basic and clinical research and practical professional concerns. SOAP has a travelling scholarship programme, allowing overseas anaesthetists from developing countries to travel to the annual meeting and to spend a week at a centre of excellence in the USA. The society awards an annual research fellowship, and a smaller research starter grant is also offered.

European societies

There are several national obstetric anaesthetic societies, for example in France (CARO: Club Anesthésie-Réanimation en Obstetrique), Ireland (ISOA: Irish Society of Obstetric Anaesthesia) and Switzerland (SAOA: Swiss Association of Obstetric Anaesthesia). There are also obstetric anaesthetic sections of other regional or national societies, including the Danish, Scandinavian and Spanish societies, and the European Society of Anaesthesiology (ESA) has an Obstetric Anaesthesiology Subcommittee.

Other societies

In Asia, there is the Association of Obstetric Anaesthesiologists – India. In Australasia, the Australian and New Zealand College of Anaesthetists (ANZCA) has a number of subspecialty interest groups, one of these being the Obstetric Anaesthesia Special Interest Group.

Key points

- There are several organisations, national and international, with an interest in obstetric anaesthesia.
- Some are independent, while others are subgroups of anaesthesia societies.

Further reading

Obstetric Anaesthetists' Association. www.oaa-anaes.ac.uk (accessed December 2018).
Society for Obstetric Anesthesia and Perinatology. www.soap.org (accessed December 2018).

Vital statistics

In the UK, figures are collected by three main mechanisms:

- Statutory reporting schemes (e.g. registration of births to the Office of National Statistics (ONS) by the parents; birth notification to the Director of Public Health by midwives or medical staff; reporting of congenital abnormalities to ONS)
- Non-statutory but obligatory schemes (e.g. those organised for accreditation and training by the Royal Colleges; the Confidential Enquiries into Maternal Deaths)
- Specific projects, which may or may not be supported by national or professional bodies (e.g. surveys carried out by the Audit Commission or National Birthday Trust; hospital- or department-based projects; Obstetric Anaesthetists' Association (OAA) or Association of Anaesthetists projects)

Anaesthetists may be involved in some of the above schemes, and the information gained may be of interest to obstetric anaesthetists in particular. There may be considerable overlap between the information gained for public health or political purposes and that gained for research or audit purposes. The bodies that collect the information and support the schemes may also have conflicting interests.

Some of the national figures from recent years are provided in Table 177.1. See also Chapter 89, *Maternal mortality*, and Chapter 161, *Perinatal mortality*.

Problems and special considerations

As with all large information-gathering schemes, there may be inaccuracies in the figures collected, which in turn can be interpreted in different ways. It is also generally easier to collect information about outcome events than about denominators – for example, the total number of births is known but the total number of pregnancies is not (it is estimated from the number of births, the number of ectopic pregnancies and the number of legal and spontaneous abortions from hospital data systems and morbidity reports). There may also be discrepancies between data collected for the UK as a whole and its composite parts. There are also considerable differences between the ability to collect information, and thus contribute to the various reporting schemes, of the approximately 320 National Health Service and independent units in the UK in which babies are born. Finally, centrally collected and administered schemes may report several years after the period of interest.

Table 177.1 UK maternity statistics (per year) for 2017, unless otherwise stated

Total number of live births and stillbirths	~680,000 (680,000–790,000 over past 20 years)
General fertility rate	~60–62 live births per 1000 women aged 15–44 (~90 in 1950s–1960s)
Total number of pregnancies	860,000–875,000
Legal abortions	~190,000
Mothers < 20 years old	3.0%
Mothers > 35 years old	21.3%
Gestation < 37 weeks or > 41 weeks	5–7% each
Caesarean section rate (England)	24–28% since 2006 (emergency rate 12–15% and elective rate 16%)
General anaesthesia for caesarean section	8–10% (> 50% in 1989–90)
Forceps or ventouse delivery (England)	12.4%
Induction rates (England)	29%
Epidural rate in labour	Uncertain; thought to be ~20–30%

Figures from Office for National Statistics and NHS Maternity Statistics.

Key points

- Collection of maternity and related data may be a statutory requirement, an obligatory professional requirement or a non-obligatory but desirable practice.
- A number of national data collection schemes produce reports of interest to anaesthetists.

Further reading

Office for National Statistics. Births, deaths and marriages. www.ons.gov.uk/peoplepopulationand community/birthsdeathsandmarriages (accessed December 2018).

NHS Digital. NHS maternity statistics, England 2017–18. https://files.digital.nhs.uk/ pdf/l/1/hosp-epis-stat-mat-repo-2016–17.pdf (accessed December 2018).

Historical developments in obstetric analgesia and anaesthesia

Knowledge of the major developments in obstetric anaesthesia and analgesia helps to put modern obstetric practice into context. The following brief summary outlines some of these developments, and also those in general anaesthetic practice that have had profound effects on the subspecialty.

General

- Ancient methods of pain relief included various plant-derived sedatives, acupuncture and physical methods such as binding.
- 1881: Matrons' Aid Society founded (becoming the Midwives' Institute and later the College of Midwives).
- 1929: British College of Obstetricians and Gynaecologists founded (granted a Royal Charter in 1947).
- 1932: Association of Anaesthetists of Great Britain and Ireland founded.
- 1933: Grantly Dick-Read, English obstetrician, published his book *Natural Childbirth*, followed in 1944 by *Childbirth Without Fear*. He proposed a link between fear, tension and pain, suggesting that the cycle could be broken by abolishing fear.
- 1941: College of Midwives founded (granted a Royal Charter in 1947).
- 1948: Faculty of Anaesthetists of the Royal College of Surgeons of England founded.
- 1952–54: the period covered by the first report of the Confidential Enquiries into Maternal Deaths, published by the Department of Health.
- 1953: Virginia Apgar, anaesthesiologist at Columbia University, described her scoring system for assessing neonates.
- 1956: Fernand Lamaze, French obstetrician, published his book *Painless Childbirth*, in which he suggested that pain was a conditioned reflex triggered by uterine contractions, and that a period of unconditioning followed by reconditioning (psychoprophylaxis) could reduce pain.
- 1969: Obstetric Anaesthetists' Association founded.
- 1975: Frédérick Leboyer, French obstetrician, published *Birth Without Violence*, in which he advocated delivery in a quiet, darkened room, with minimal stimulation.
- 1988: College of Anaesthetists founded (granted a Royal Charter in 1992).
- 1993: the Department of Health's Expert Maternity Group published its report *Changing Childbirth* (the Cumberlege Report), which placed the expectant mother at the centre of care, emphasising her right to choose and signalling a formal move away from the traditional paternalistic 'medical' approach.

Systemic analgesia

- 1902: morphine and hyoscine first used in labour.
- 1940: pethidine first used in labour.
- 1950: pethidine approved by the Central Midwives Board.
- 1970: pethidine patient-controlled analgesia (PCA) described.
- 1999: remifentanil PCA described.

Inhalational analgesia

- 1847: James Young Simpson, Professor of Midwifery at Edinburgh University, administered the first obstetric general anaesthetic using ether. Considerable opposition came from religious leaders for going against the Bible, and from medical authorities for compromising safety. Simpson went on to advocate chloroform in preference to ether, having used it the same year. He was a major influence in British obstetrics and also designed obstetric forceps, which bear his name.
- 1853: John Snow, London physician, generally considered the father of British anaesthesia, delivered Queen Victoria's eighth child (Prince Leopold) under chloroform, putting an end to the above objections. Snow is also famous for his part in ending the London cholera epidemic of 1854.
- 1881: Stanislav Klikovitch, Russian physician working in St Petersburg, described the use of nitrous oxide (80% with 20% oxygen) for labour, noting its lack of effect on the uterus and the requirement for inhalation before each contraction started.
- 1936: Robert James Minnitt's nitrous oxide/air apparatus approved by the Central Midwives Board.
- 1961: Michael Tunstall, Aberdeen anaesthetist, described the use of premixed nitrous oxide and oxygen in labour. The mixture was marketed 2 years later in the UK as Entonox. Tunstall also described the isolated forearm technique for detecting awareness, developed the Entonox demand valve (from diving equipment) and advocated the 'failed intubation drill' in obstetrics.

Regional analgesia

- 1884: Carl Koller, German ophthalmologist, used cocaine for eye surgery.
- 1885: James Leonard Corning, New York neurologist, produced spinal and epidural blockade in dogs.
- 1899: August Bier, German surgeon, used spinal anaesthesia for surgery. Bier described postdural puncture headache for the first time.
- 1901: Jean-Athanase Sicard and Fernand Cathelin, French neurologist and urologist respectively, introduced caudal analgesia.
- 1921: Fidel Pages, Spanish surgeon, used lumbar epidural blockade for surgery.
- 1931: Eugen Bogdan Aburel, Romanian obstetrician, described continuous caudal plus lumboaortic plexus blocks in labour.
- 1933: John Cleland, American obstetrician, described paravertebral block in labour.
- 1942: Robert Hingson, American obstetrician, described continuous caudals in labour.
- 1949: Cleland described continuous lumbar epidural block in labour.

- 1960s to 1990s: British pioneers included Andrew Doughty (Kingston, 1960s–70s); J. Selwyn Crawford (Birmingham, 1960s–80s); Donald Moir (Glasgow, 1960s–80s); Barbara Morgan (Queen Charlotte's, London, 1980s–90s).
- 1980s: pencil-point spinal needles were first described in 1920s, but advances in their manufacture resulted in their wide availability in the late 1980s/early 1990s.
- 1981–82: combined spinal–epidural technique first described in the UK; popularised in obstetrics in the 1990s; 'mobile epidural' combined spinal–epidural technique popularised at Queen Charlotte's Hospital by Barbara Morgan.
- Late 1980s: microfine spinal catheters used in the late 1980s/early 1990s; withdrawn in the USA by the Food and Drug Administration in 1992.
- 1990s: patient-controlled epidural analgesia (PCEA) introduced.
- 2000s: more sophisticated methods of epidural analgesia (e.g. programmed intermittent bolus, computer-integrated PCEA) described in the mid- to late 2000s.

General anaesthesia for caesarean section

- 1945: Curtis Mendelson, American obstetrician, described the syndrome of acid aspiration both clinically and experimentally, distinguishing it from upper airway obstruction caused by inhalation of large pieces of food.
- 1961: Brian Sellick, London anaesthetist, described cricoid pressure as a means of preventing aspiration of gastric contents.
- 1960s: the problem of intraoperative awareness became topical, with up to 9% of mothers who received thiopental, nitrous oxide and neuromuscular blockade remembering intraoperative events. Donald Moir, Glasgow anaesthetist, described a technique of halothane 0.5% with 50:50 nitrous oxide:oxygen in 1970, with no recall. Tunstall described the isolated forearm technique as a means of monitoring consciousness during general anaesthesia in 1979.
- 2014: the 5th National Audit Project (Royal College of Anaesthetists and Association of Anaesthetists of Great Britain and Ireland) implicated obstetric anaesthesia as a risk factor in accidental awareness under general anaesthesia.

Index

Printed in the United States
by Baker & Taylor Publisher Services